P9-CRN-551

FROM THE LIBRARY OF

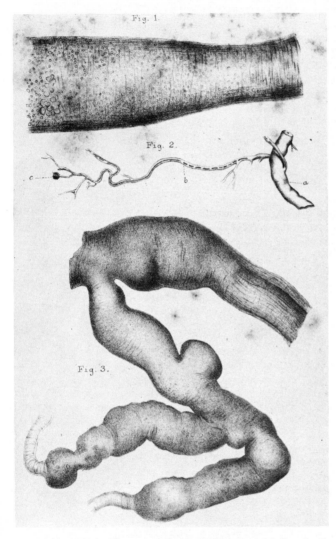

Frontispiece. The miliary aneurysms of Charcot and Bouchard. From New Sydenham Society (1881): *Clinical Lectures on Senile and Chronic Diseases*, J. M. Charcot.

Volume 4 in the Series

Major Problems in Neurology
JOHN N. WALTON, TD, MD, DSc, FRCP
Consulting Editor

OTHER MONOGRAPHS IN THE SERIES

PUBLISHED

Barnett, Foster and Hudgson: **Syringomyelia,** *1973*
Dubowitz and Brooke: **Muscle Biopsy: A Modern Approach,** *1973*
Pallis and Lewis: **The Neurology of Gastrointestinal Disease,** *1974*

FORTHCOMING

Currie: **Immunological Aspects of Neurology**
Cartlidge and Shaw: **Medical Aspects of Head Injury**
Lewis and Pallis: **The Neurology of Renal Disease**

Strokes
Natural History, Pathology and Surgical Treatment

E. C. HUTCHINSON, MD, FRCP

Consultant Neurologist, North Staffordshire Hospital Centre, Stoke-on-Trent, Staffs.

E. J. ACHESON, MD

Lately Research Fellow, Neurology Department, North Staffordshire Hospital Centre, Stoke-on-Trent, Staffs; presently Research Fellow, Department of Medicine, The Royal Infirmary, Manchester.

With contributions by

P. J. H. FLETCHER, MB, MRCPath
Consultant Pathologist, North Staffordshire Hospital Centre, Stoke-on-Trent, Staffs.

L. J. LAWSON, BSc, MB, FRCS
Consultant Surgeon, North Staffordshire Hospital Centre, Stoke-on-Trent, Staffs.

A. J. McCALL, MD, FRCP, FRCPath
Consultant Pathologist, North Staffordshire Hospital Centre, Stoke-on-Trent, Staffs.

1975

W. B. Saunders Company Ltd   London · Philadelphia · Toronto

W. B. Saunders Company Ltd: 12 Dyott Street
London WC1A 1DB

West Washington Square
Philadelphia, Pa. 19105

833 Oxford Street
Toronto, Ontario M8Z 5T9

Library of Congress Cataloging in Publication Data
Hutchinson, Edward C
    Strokes

    (Major problems in neurology)
    1. Cerebral ischemia. I. Acheson, Enid Joan, joint
author. II. Title. III. Series. [DNLM: 1. Cerebral
ischemia, Transient. W1MA492U v. 4 / WL355 H976n]
RC388.5.H87   616.8'1   74-28100
ISBN 0-7216-4870-3

ⓒ 1975 by W. B. Saunders Company Ltd. All rights reserved. This book is protected by
copyright. No part of it may be reproduced, stored in a retrieval system, or transmitted in
any form or by any means, electronic, mechanical, photocopying, recording, or otherwise,
without written permission from the publisher.

Printed at The Lavenham Press Ltd, Lavenham, Suffolk, England.

Print Number: 9 8 7 6 5 4 3 2 1

Foreword

So much has been written in the last few years about cerebral vascular disease that the publication of yet another monograph upon this topic may seem to require special justification. In my opinion, however, readers of this book will find that any doubts they may have felt about its topicality and relevance to modern neurology will be quickly dispelled. Dr Hutchinson and his colleagues were among the first to stress the importance of disease in the great vessels of the neck as a potent cause of cerebrovascular insufficiency, and now with Dr Acheson he has provided a masterly commentary upon the natural history of cerebral ischaemia, based upon their own experience and upon a thorough review of the relevant literature. At a time when the vascular surgeons are turning their attention increasingly to methods of alleviating or preventing minor and major strokes, their results must plainly be assessed against a background of detailed information relating to the prognosis of these disorders in patients not subjected to this form of treatment; it is this information which the authors provide. Wisely they have decided in addition to review the applied anatomy of the cerebral circulation in order to clarify their subsequent discussion, and for similar reasons they have invited their colleagues Drs McCall and Fletcher to contribute a chapter summarising current pathogenetic concepts. They also consider in detail problems of terminology and differential diagnosis and end with a balanced discussion of modern methods of treatment, including a chapter on surgical treatment contributed by Mr L. J. Lawson.

Strokes continue to be a major cause of death and disability, and their management places an increasing burden upon medical and supportive facilities in developed and under-developed countries alike. All neurologists are conscious of their relative therapeutic impotence in many such cases and valid information against which they can judge the effects of their preventive and therapeutic endeavours continues to be needed. This volume represents an important contribution towards the fulfilment of this need and I am sure that it will be widely welcomed.

Newcastle upon Tyne, 1974   John N. Walton

Preface

Cerebral vascular disease embraces a large number of conditions but only subarachnoid haemorrhage, intracerebral haemorrhage and cerebral infarction occur with any frequency.

Subarachnoid haemorrhage is a familiar picture in hospital practice since the majority of short-term survivors are admitted. Since the condition has a mortality of 50 per cent and definitive treatment is in the hands of the neurosurgeon it presents its own well-defined problems. Massive cerebral haemorrhage of the classical type causes death in over 80 per cent of patients and, apart from the exceedingly rare opportunity of surgical treatment in infratentorial haemorrhage, it offers little scope for treatment by the physician.

The last of the three, cerebral infarction, has a much lower mortality and it is with the survivors of initial episodes that the physician and vascular surgeon have been concerned in efforts to prevent further disasters. Progress in knowledge has been slow but, gradually, pathological and clinical studies have led progressively to a better understanding of the mechanisms behind cerebral infarction. This, of course, is an essential prerequisite to rational treatment.

The monograph is concerned almost exclusively with the subsequent clinical behaviour of patients presenting with signs and symptoms leading to a diagnosis of transient cerebral ischaemia or cerebral infarction. Because the precise mechanism of cerebral infarction may be uncertain clinically, these patients will be referred to as 'stroke' patients. It will emerge later in the monograph that the assumption that a clear distinction could be made on traditional clinical grounds between infarction and other forms of cerebral vascular disease directly related to hypertension (i.e. cerebral haemorrhage) has proved fallacious.

The monograph falls naturally into three sections. The first concerns the applied anatomy of the cerebral blood supply as it relates to occlusive cerebral vascular disease. Also discussed are the recent advances that have been made in recognising the various responses of the cerebral circulation and its control mechanisms to cerebral ischaemia.

An account of the pathology of cerebral infarction and cerebral haemorrhage, an essential part of any study of the common types of cerebral vascular disease, has been written by Dr A. J. McCall and Dr P. J. H. Fletcher and we are grateful to them both for this contribution. The first section is completed by an examination of the contribution of epidemiological studies to the knowledge of the natural history of cerebral ischaemia.

The second section is concerned with the natural history of transient cerebral ischaemia and of patients with a stroke. Thereafter, the role of hypertension and the significance of abnormal electrocardiograms and heart size, as determined by x-ray, are considered. Other more indirect factors such as the anatomical site of ischaemia, mode of onset of the stroke, and the significance of the elevated serum cholesterol are also considered. Finally, in this section the causes of death in published series are examined, and here the role of hypertension becomes very much more clear.

The third and last section concerns medical and surgical management. The chapter on surgical treatment is written by Mr L. J. Lawson and we are most grateful to him for agreeing to write this chapter.

We would like to record our gratitude to the Research Sub-Committee of the Birmingham Regional Hospital Board and to the British Heart Foundation for their generous financial support to one of us (J.A.); also to Dr M. C. Hickey for the angiograms of a persisting trigeminal artery (Figures 1.5a and b) and to Dr Leonard Langton of the Midland Centre for Neurosurgery for allowing us to use the angiograms illustrating Moya-Moya disease (Figures 1.7a and b). Dr J. R. Heron kindly allowed us to photograph his patient shown in Figures 1.3a and b. We would also thank Dr Jack P. Whisnant, Professor and Chairman of the Department of Neurology, the Mayo Clinic, for permission to use Figures 5.3, 5.4a, b and c, and for Figures 12.1 and 12.2. Our gratitude goes to Dr C. R. Knappett for permission to use Figure 3.4 and to Dr T. R. Marshall for Figure 3.5. Dr R. W. Ross Russell was kind enough to supply Figure 3.24. We are also indebted to Dr Leslie Bowcock, Director of the Department of Medical Illustration, for his generous help with all of the reproductions, and to Mrs Woosnam and Mrs Bell, librarians of the Medical Institute.

We are indebted to the Editor and Publishers of *Brain* for permission to reproduce the drawing of the vertebral artery in Chapter 1, Figure 1; to the Editor and Publishers of the *Quarterly Journal of Medicine* for permission to reproduce the Tables in Chapters 5.7, 6.6, 7.2, 9.8; and finally to the Editor and Publishers of *Stroke* for permission to reproduce the Figures in Chapters 5.3, 5.4a,b,c, and Figures 12.1, 12.2.

Mr D. C. Manley, BSc, MSc, SSS, gave continuing help and advice on the statistical handling of the data. We are also grateful to the Director of the Pharmaceutical Division, I.C.I. Limited, for the assistance given by Mr F. Grady and other members of the Data Services Section, Research Department, Alderley Park.

We also acknowledge gratefully the contribution of the late Dr J. P. P. Stock who reported upon all the electrocardiograms.

The problems of the follow up study and the management of patients were considerably eased by the supervision and management of the patients by Sister K. Thompson. Finally we would like to express our gratitude to the secretarial staff of the Neurology Department for the preparation of the manuscript.

North Staffordshire Hospital Centre,   Edward C. Hutchinson
May, 1974   Joan Acheson

Contents

CHAPTER ONE

Applied Anatomy

Knowledge of the traditional anatomy of the cerebral blood supply is a necessary framework for an appreciation of the various forms of cerebral vascular disease. However, it is not proposed to consider the basic anatomical facts, as they are adequately described in the standard textbooks. Attention is mainly devoted to congenital anomalies and collateral vascular channels. The congenital anomalies range from interesting rarities such as agenesis of the carotid arteries to common anomalies such as variations in the relative size of the paired vertebral arteries. The collateral vascular channels, both real (e.g. the Circle of Willis) and potential (e.g. the external/internal carotid artery connections), may be vital to survival in occlusive vascular disease.

Gillilan (1959) studied the cerebral blood supply in 300 human and fetal brains and, from her observations on the leptomeningeal anastomoses, suggested that the intracranial part of the cerebral blood supply should be regarded as a single functioning unit. The point she was making was that there had been undue emphasis on the value of the Circle of Willis as a collateral channel when occlusions of the major vessels of supply had occurred. The over-emphasis had tended, in her view, to obscure the clinically important anastomoses between the distal branches of the major cerebral and cerebellar arteries lying in the sulci and fissures of the cortex. Physicians and surgeons concerned with the management of occlusive vascular disease, particularly disease of the major cervical vessels, would certainly extend Gillilan's concept much further.

Radiology has made a major contribution to anatomical and pathological knowledge of disease of the cervical vessels, not only by defining primary sites of atheromatous disease but also by demonstrating in a dynamic way the wealth of potential collateral channels that may develop in response to vascular occlusion. Such channels are frequently a major factor in survival and therefore the modern approach to the anatomy of the cerebral blood supply, particularly for those interested in cerebral vascular disease, is to regard the left atrium and the left ventricle, the great vessels of the thorax and neck and the terminal intracerebral circulation as interdependent units.

Congenital anomalies of the cerebral blood supply and the potential collateral channels are properly considered together for two reasons. The first is that agenesis of the vessels may require the persistence of the embryological collateral circulation. The second is that hypoplasia or agenesis may significantly alter the effectiveness of the normal collateral channels, and this can be well seen in the Circle of Willis.

CAROTID ARTERIES

Anomalies of origin

The right common carotid artery may arise at a higher level than normal at the upper border of the sternoclavicular joint or it may arise as a separate branch from the arch of the aorta or in conjunction with the left common carotid artery.

The left common carotid artery shows anomalous variations more frequently than the right. A common variation is for it to arise in conjunction with the innominate artery or if, as rarely happens, this artery is absent, the two common carotid arteries arise as a single trunk.

The level in the neck of the division of the common carotid artery into the internal and external branches may also vary. The division may be higher than usual, up to a point just below the base of the skull, or it may occasionally divide lower than usual and begin at the lower border of the cricoid cartilage.

Agenesis and hypoplasia

Agenesis of the carotid arteries is a considerable rarity. Boyd (1934) was only able to find a description of absence of the right common carotid artery in only nine instances in the literature up to that date. Later, Turnbull (1962) found only 20 cases of unilateral agenesis of the carotid artery and in two cases the agenesis was bilateral.

In the patient described by Turnbull (1962) the middle and anterior cerebral vessels were supplied to the Circle of Willis by the basilar artery and by the contralateral internal carotid artery. If agenesis is present the internal carotid artery may communicate with the foramen ovale and foramen rotundum, and via this route the ophthalmic artery on the affected side may take origin from the internal carotid circulation. More often, when agenesis of the internal carotid artery is present, the ophthalmic vessel is a branch of the middle cerebral artery. Unless in later years main vessel occlusions develop, Turnbull concluded that these anomalies were probably harmless and represented interesting anatomical variants.

Tharp et al (1965) described two patients who presented with the symptoms of cerebral vascular disease and were shown to have hypoplasia of the carotid artery. In both cases the common and the external carotid artery were normal but the internal carotid artery above the bifurcation was reduced to a thread without evidence of arterial disease. They were able to find only three other examples in the literature. No doubt the not uncommon appearance of hypoplasia of the internal carotid artery seen at angiography is a minor variation of this anomaly.

VERTEBRAL ARTERIES

Anomalies of course, size and origin

The vertebral artery, having ascended the posterior triangle of the neck, enters the vertebral canal in over 80 per cent of the cases at the level of the 6th cervical vertebra (Bell, Swiggart and Anson, 1950). The artery then passes through the vertebral canal and in its course has a close medial relationship to the neurocentral joint. The development of osteophytic spurs at this site is capable of displacing the artery in a lateral or anterio-posterior direction (Figure 1.1).

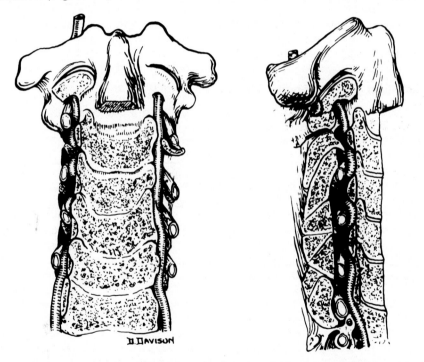

Figure 1.1. Drawing of dissected specimen to show vertebral artery within the vertebral canal and degree of distortion caused by cervical spondylosis. (Reproduced from *Brain* (1956) **79**, 319).

Variations in relative size of the vertebral artery are commonplace. Stopford (1916), Meyer and Loeb (1965) have all emphasised that the two vertebral arteries almost always have a different diameter. In 73 per cent of cases the side-to-side difference is considerable and in one in five the ratio of the diameter between the right and left sides was 1:2.

The vertebral artery usually takes its origin from the subclavian, but it may occasionally arise from the aorta, the subclavian, or the carotid arteries. Very rarely, it arises from the carotid bulb as a hypoglossal vertebral artery (Herndon, Meyer and Johnson, 1960). Awareness of the frequency of variations of origin of the vertebral artery is important before significant conclusions are drawn about occlusion of the vessel.

COLLATERAL CIRCULATION

The contribution of neuroradiology to the study of actual or potential sites of collateral circulation in the presence of occlusive vascular disease has already been emphasised. The development of collateral circulation may be considered at three levels. The first level is in the neck following major vessel occlusion there. The second level is at the Circle of Willis where adjustments may be made to counter major vessel occlusion in one of the supplying vessels. The third level is in the leptomeningeal circulation when the major intracerebral vessels such as the anterior, middle and posterior cerebral vessels are occluded.

Collateral circulation proximal to the Circle of Willis

Fields, Bruetman and Weibel (1965) published a comprehensive study of the collateral circulation of the brain based mainly on a radiological survey of patients with symptoms and signs of cerebral vascular disease. They gave a useful synopsis of the principal anastomoses that are available in the event of occlusion of the major vessels. Weiss (1938) also examined the anatomical connections between the internal and external carotid artery, and the details of the connection are shown in Table 1.1. Meyer and Loeb (1965) have, in a similar manner, detailed the connections between the vertebrobasilar system and carotid circulation which are potential sources of collateral circulation. In clinical practice we are mainly concerned with occlusions of the internal carotid artery at its origin and under these circumstances an adequate intercerebral circulation can be maintained in two ways.

The first is to utilise a naturally available collateral channel provided by the Circle of Willis. This assumes, of course, normal configuration of this structure; this assumption is not infrequently incorrect, a point that will be discussed later. The second is for retrograde flow to develop through the ophthalmic artery by anastomoses with the supraorbital, palpebral and dorsal nasal branches and through the superficial temporal and internal maxillary artery of the internal carotid system. Through this anastomosis retrograde flow down the ophthalmic artery may provide an adequate internal carotid blood supply.

The radiological appearances of this collateral channel are now well known and are shown here (Figure 1.2). Perhaps less well known is the fact that the development of this valuable collateral channel may be associated with enlargement of the ipsilateral temporal artery. Yates and Hutchinson (1961, case 98) demonstrated at post-mortem in a patient with internal carotid

Table 1.1. Potential collateral communications between internal and external carotid arteries according to Weiss (1938).

		Branches of internal carotid artery	Branches of external carotid artery
1		Tympanic	⎧ Anterior tympanic branch of internal maxillary ⎨ ⎩ Stylomastoid branch of posterior auricular
2		Pterygoid	Pterygoid of internal maxillary
3		Cavernous	Cavernous of middle meningeal
4		⎧ Zygomatic branch of lachrymal	⎧ Deep temporal ⎨ Transverse facial
5		Recurrent branch of lachrymal	Middle meningeal
6	Branches of	Supraorbital	Frontal branch of superficial temporal
7	ophthalmic	Posterior ethmoid	Sphenopalatine
8	artery	Superior palpebral	Zygomatic orbital branch of superficial temporal
9		Inferior palpebral	⎧ Transverse facial ⎨ Angular branch of external maxillary
10		Dorsal nasal	⎧ Angular branch of external maxillary ⎨ Lateral nasal branch of external maxillary

artery occlusion that the ipsilateral temporal artery was twice the size of the right and the ophthalmic artery had an internal diameter of 1.5 mm.

This enlargement of the external carotid vessels, and particularly the temporal vessel, may be a useful physical sign in occlusion of the internal carotid artery and is illustrated in Figure 1.3. The angiograms of this patient are shown in Figure 1.2.

The development of alternative channels in response to occlusion of the major arterial blood supply is normally an advantage. But this is not always so, and the point is nicely demonstrated by the 'subclavian steal' syndrome. Contorni (1960) was the first to draw attention to retrograde flow from the vertebral artery to the subclavian vessel distal to an occlusion of the subclavian. This was followed by the demonstration by Reivich et al (1961) that this particular collateral pathway may have clinical significance. They described two patients who presented with symptoms of vertebrobasilar ischaemia developing with the use of an upper limb. At angiography, in both patients there was a marked stenosis of the left subclavian artery proximal to the origin of the vertebral, and to compensate for this there was a reversal of the blood flow in the left vertebral artery which then formed the main blood supply to the upper limb. Clearly, the extra oxygen requirements of the exercising limb caused reversal of flow from the intracerebral circulation and thus could cause temporary embarrassment with symptoms of hind brain ischaemia.

They followed up these clinical observations by a study in experimental animals and observed that after occluding the left subclavian artery proximal to the origin of the vertebral a reversal of flow immediately occurred and the amount of blood taking part in the reverse flow almost equalled the normal forward flow in the vertebral artery. They did find, however, there was an over-all reduction in total cerebral blood flow after the occlusion.

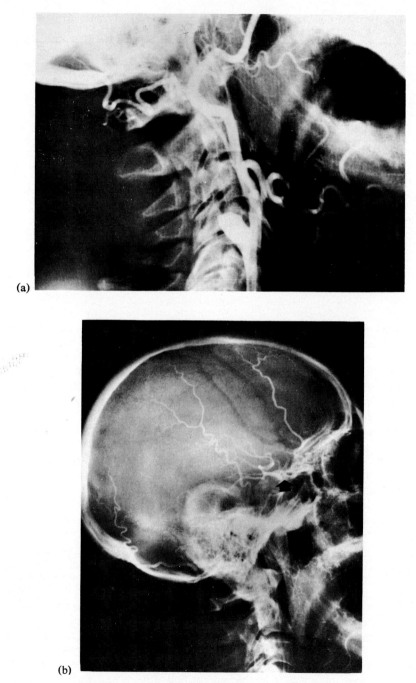

(a)

(b)

Figure 1.2. a. Carotid angiogram showing carotid artery occlusion at origin. b. Later film showing early middle cerebral filling via the ophthalmic artery.

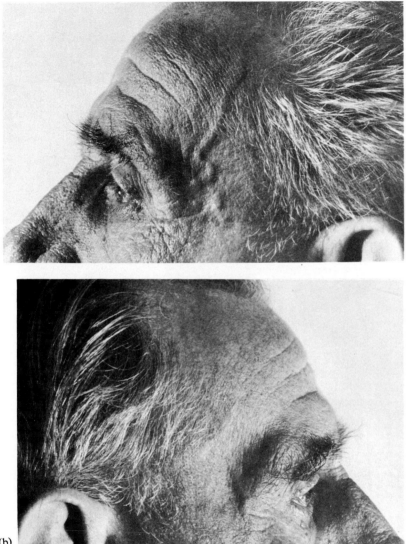

(a)

(b)

Figure 1.3. a. Dilation of temporal artery on side of carotid occlusion shown in Figure 1.2a. b. Normal contralateral side for comparison (courtesy of Dr J. R. Heron).

Not every patient in whom subclavian steal is demonstrated at angiographic examination develops symptoms of hind brain ischaemia. North et al (1962) reported 1500 patients with cerebral vascular disease and selected 59 who showed obstruction to the subclavian artery proximal to the origin of the vertebral artery. Only 33 of these had any neurological symptoms and only in 6 were there recurring symptoms with exercise of the upper extremity on the affected side.

Sample radiographs demonstrating evidence of subclavian steal are shown in Figure 1.4. On this occasion the occlusion of the subclavian artery was bilateral and resulted in deviation of blood from the hind brain circulation.

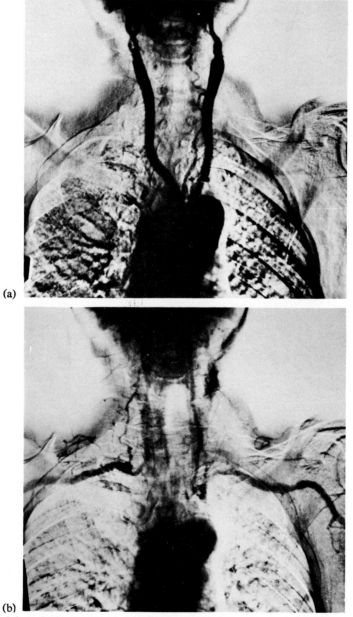

(a)

(b)

Figure 1.4. a. Arch aortogram showing bilateral subclavian artery occlusion (subtraction film). b. Later film demonstrating bilateral filling of both subclavian arteries via both vertebrals.

An extension of the subclavian steal syndrome is the 'triple-steal' syndrome described by Cala and Armstrong (1972). The patient, a 53-year-old female, was admitted with a dense left hemiplegia, and at angiography the left subclavian artery was occluded with retrograde filling of the distal subclavian from the left vertebral artery. The innominate artery was occluded with refilling of the distal right subclavian artery via the right vertebral artery and there was refilling of the right internal and external carotid artery and part of the common carotid artery via the Circle of Willis. Finally, they noticed stenosis of the origin of the left common carotid artery. Surgery successfully restored the patency in all vessels involved.

CIRCLE OF WILLIS AS A COLLATERAL CHANNEL

Although collateral channels of the type discussed and illustrated may occasionally make a vital contribution to maintaining the intracerebral circulation, a major responsibility falls on the Circle of Willis in the event of occlusion of the cervical vessels.

There is a natural tendency to consider only the function of the Circle of Willis as it relates to occlusion of the carotid and vertebral circulation. But Brain (1957) observed that the Circle of Willis is unlikely to have evolved merely to protect the human brain from the later adverse effects of occlusive vascular disease. He indicated that he believed that the real biological function of the Circle of Willis was to protect the brain from ischaemia whatever the position of the head relative to the trunk may be. Kramer (1912) had already pointed out that Willis himself regarded the structure as a means of equalising the blood supply to all parts of the brain and regarded it as a kind of reservoir from which the various arteries of the brain would draw their blood supply. Modern experimental work supports Brain's view, for there is now evidence that variations in blood flow in the carotid and vertebral arteries do occur with change in position of the head relative to the cervical spine (Toole and Tucker, 1960; Hardesty et al, 1962).

But it still remains true that whatever its biological function the Circle of Willis may have a vital role to play in the vascular adjustments necessary for survival after occlusion of the major vessels in the neck.

Kramer's (1912) classical experiments succeeded first of all in demonstrating that injections into both carotid arteries and into the vertebral arteries on different occasions gave a constant area of staining, which indicated that under normal circumstances each vessel contributed blood to its own particular territory. However, immediately the various arteries were ligated, such clear definition of vascular territories disappeared and the stain was carried forward or backward according to the vessel ligated. He concluded that: 'the Circle of Willis is an antero-posterior anastomosis between the carotid and vertebral arteries which, under physiological conditions, does not permit the mingling of blood streams but when, however, either the anterior or posterior arteries are completely blocked then the anastomosis will supply blood to the areas of the central nervous system which were supplied by the blocked vessel.'

McDonald and Potter (1951) repeated Kramer's work with more sophisticated techniques and showed that in the experimental animal there is a point midway along the posterior communicating artery where the anterior and posterior circulations met and where no movement of blood occurred. If, however, the pressure of balance was upset the posterior communicating artery immediately functioned as an anastomosis.

The importance of the posterior communicating vessels in the development of anastomoses was shown by the work of Meyer, Fang and Denny-Brown (1954) which demonstrated that ischaemic change in the cerebral hemisphere of experimental animals following occlusion of the extracranial blood supply was related in its extent to the accuracy of the collateral channels as judged by the size of the posterior communicating arteries.

The normal shape of the Circle of Willis has been described by Alpers, Berry and Paddison (1959) as a 'polygon or closed circuit in which by means of component vessels fluid may circulate from any entrance point to return to that point of entrance; with the components of the mature brain being more than 1 mm in outside diameter with no excess vessels and with the usual paired anterior cerebral arteries'.

Variations in the anatomical structure of the Circle of Willis that may impair its function as a collateral channel can be considered under two headings. The first is the presence of anomalous vessels; the second is an anomalous origin and size of the component vessels of the Circle.

Anomalous vessels

The early dependence of the developing hind brain on the carotid circulation has been demonstrated by embryological studies (Padget, 1945). The embryonic vascular pattern may occasionally be observed continuing into adult life. In two examples, namely, the persisting hypoglossal artery and acoustic artery, the incidence is excessively rare. By contrast, a persisting trigeminal artery is not infrequently recognised at angiography.

In the 4 mm embryo the internal carotid artery can be defined and at this stage its terminal branches are the ophthalmic and trigeminal arteries. The latter is for a short time important as it supplies blood both to the fore brain and to the hind brain. It is soon superseded in this role in relation to the hind brain by the posterior communicating artery which develops anterior to it in the 5 to 6 mm embryo, and thereafter, its function terminated, the trigeminal artery regresses rapidly. When it does persist and is demonstrated at angiography it is approximately the same size as the carotid artery.

The vessel rises in the cavernous portion of the carotid artery and runs either laterally to the posterior clinoid process or else it pierces the dorsum sellae and then joins the basilar artery at the junction of the upper and middle third of that vessel. There is usually an associated hypoplasia or even absence of the vertebral artery and posterior communicating vessels on the same side. Sutton (1950) was the first to describe the angiographic appearances of the artery during life and observed the direction of flow to be from the carotid to the basilar circulation.

In the example illustrated here (Figure 1.5), the anomalous vessel is shown

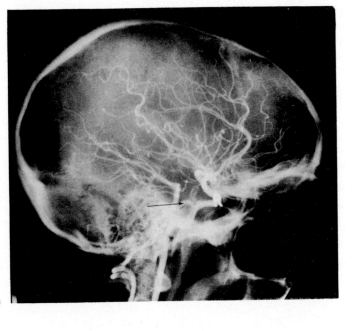

(a)

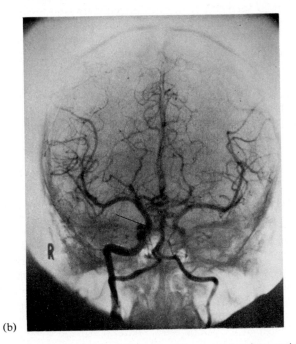

(b)

Figure 1.5. a, and b. A.P. and lateral carotid angiograms, showing persisting trigeminal artery (arrow) (courtesy of Dr M. C. Hickey).

under the conditions of angiography to be capable of filling the whole cerebral circulation.

Attempts to relate the presence of a persisting trigeminal artery to clinical neurological abnormalities (Campbell and Dyken, 1961) are not convincing, and this probably represents in the majority of cases an interesting angiographic finding only. It may, however, as they pointed out, rarely cause significant differences in retinal artery pressure, the pressure being lower on the side of the persisting trigeminal artery; potentially, therefore, this anomaly could cause false positive results on ophthalmodynamometry.

Anomalies in size and origin

Although entities such as a persisting trigeminal artery have an intrinsic interest, the most important anomalies are those that relate to the size of the communicating vessels and, less importantly, to the site of origin of the posterior cerebral vessels.

It is customary in the literature, when component vessels of the Circle of Willis are considered to be so small as to be incapable of acting as a collateral channel, to refer to them as 'string-like' and this practice will be followed here.

Alpers, Berry and Paddison (1959) found the anterior communicating arteries to be string-like in 3 per cent of cases and the proximal portion of the anterior cerebral artery to be similarly defective in 2 per cent. This relatively low incidence of inadequacy in the anterior communicating vessels is fortunate in view of their importance in providing a side-to-side anastomosis in carotid artery occlusions of whatever cause. Much more frequently, however, the posterior communicating vessels were found to be string-like either unilaterally or bilaterally in 22 per cent of the specimens. The appearance of the anomaly is illustrated from dissections (Figure 1.6).

In order to assess the relevance of the anomaly to the development of cerebral infarction Bhattacharji, Hutchinson and McCall (1967) reported an autopsy study of the Circle of Willis in 49 patients with cerebral infarction and compared their findings with those observed in 88 control subjects. The incidence of anomalies was higher in the infarct group than in the controls but statistical significance was only reached when unilateral string-like posterior communicating arteries were associated with stenosis or occlusion of one or more major neck vessels.

No satisfactory explanation could be offered for this apparently anomalous finding since one would reasonably have anticipated that bilateral string-like vessels would be a more effective block to the development of an adequate collateral channel than a similar state of affairs occurring unilaterally.

It would perhaps be unwise to attribute over-riding importance to the Circle of Willis in terms of survival as this may tend to put too much emphasis on the availability of collateral channels and thus obscure the real importance of thrombo-embolic phenomena. There are, however, in the literature some striking examples of the role collateral channels may play. Doniger (1963), for example, described a patient with bilateral carotid artery occlusion in whom there was retrograde filling of both ophthalmic arteries to fill the anterior and middle cerebral circulations; there was also a basilar artery

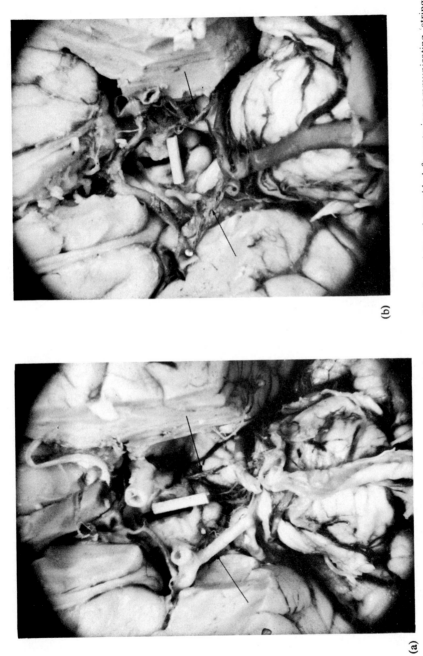

Figure 1.6. a. Circle of Willis displayed. Right posterior cerebral artery arising from internal carotid; left posterior communicating 'string-like'. (Wooden Marker 2 mm approx. in diameter). b. Both posterior communicating vessels represented by a 'leash' of small vessels.

occlusion which was compensated for by blood from the posterior inferior cerebellar artery that supplied the rest of the basilar circulation. A restricted field defect was the only residual neurological lesion.

Fields, Edwards and Crawford (1961) described six patients with bilateral carotid artery occlusion and in three adequate circulation was maintained by retrograde ophthalmic artery flow while in three other patients flow was to the cross-circulation at the level of the Circle of Willis.

The clinical importance of an anomalous origin of the posterior cerebral artery is easy to appreciate since there is no need to take into account the subtleties of pressure gradients and flow. In the study already referred to (Bhattacharji, Hutchinson and McCall, 1967) the posterior cerebral artery arose from the internal carotid artery in 27 per cent of cases in the infarct group and in only 17 per cent of the controls, but the difference was not statistically significant. In one specimen, however, the occipital poles were infarcted as a result of emboli from the carotid artery traversing the posterior cerebrals which themselves arose from the carotid artery. In another specimen with an identical anomaly the occipital poles were spared infarction in the presence of basilar artery occlusion.

Moya-Moya disease

A recently described form of cerebral vascular disease demonstrates yet another form of potential collateral circulation at the level of the Circle of Willis, and the disease entity is that called Moya-Moya. The credit for the first description of this condition is given to Takeuchi (1961) by Suzuki and Takaku (1969). The name Moya-Moya translates a Japanese expression for a haze drifting through the air, a condition that was originally described in young Japanese females. The diagnosis can be made only at angiography where stenosis or occlusion of the terminal portion of the carotid artery is demonstrated, and this is associated with a faint blush of abnormal vessels adjacent to the occlusion. The mechanism by which it arises is first of all an occlusion of a major vessel supply proximal to the Circle of Willis coupled with an inadequacy of the collateral circulation at this level. As a result of the inadequacy at the Circle of Willis the collateral circulation develops from other basal central collaterals which are normally not concerned with the main supply and are not usually prominent (Langton—personal communication). Two examples are illustrated (Figure 1.7).

Somewhat similar collateral channels have been observed at angiography by Handa, Waga and Handa (1971). They described four Japanese children, all over ten years of age, presenting with focal neurological signs indicating a hemisphere lesion. In each child occlusion or stenosis of the internal carotid artery distal to the origin of the ophthalmic was demonstrated. The recurrent meningeal branch of the ophthalmic artery provided collateral channels which directly supplied the cortical leptomeningeal arteries and seemed to be capable of supplying a useful collateral circulation to the hemispheres.

In other cases of carotid artery occlusion the middle meningeals may anastomose with the lachrymal artery and in a retrograde manner supply the ophthalmic and, thus, the internal carotid artery (Tolosa, 1968).

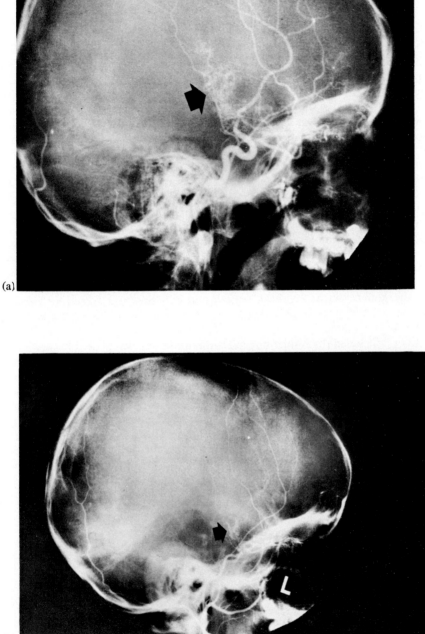

Figure 1.7. a. Right carotid angiogram showing very small internal carotid artery occluded at its termination with basal telangiectatic collaterals. b. Bilateral carotid occlusion with basal telangiectasia—Moya-Moya disease (courtesy of Dr Leonard Langton).

16

Leptomeningeal anastomoses

Reference has already been made to Gillilan's observations that led her to stress the importance of the leptomeningeal anastomoses. Vander Eecken and Adams (1953) in a paper entitled 'The anatomy and functional significance of meningeal arterial anastomoses of the brain' also studied the significance of the anatomical communication between the known meningeal anastomoses between the anterior middle and posterior cerebral vessels in the fore brain and in the major cerebellar arteries in the hind-brain circulation. As they said, there were at that time two extremes of opinion with regard to the cerebral blood vessels; one regarded them as inert pipes which, if occluded by foreign material caused ischaemic necrosis in the tissues supplied by that vessel; the other ignored the morbid anatomical findings altogether and proposed that blood vessels underwent continuous changes in calibre even to the point of partial or complete occlusion by local segmental spasm. They found neither view a satisfactory explanation for certain phenomena associated with apoplexy. By injection and dissection techniques they demonstrated the main leptomeningeal connections between the anterior and middle and posterior cerebral arteries and between the anterior and posterior cerebral arteries. The average width of the loops, which varied in number from four to eight between the anterior, middle cerebral, and three to five between the middle and posterior cerebral, was 311 µm. Subsequent injections of the infarcted brain provided further evidence of their value in restricting the areas of infarction.

They concluded that under normal conditions there was probably very little flow of arterial blood between these anastomoses because there would be an equalisation of pressure in the two arterial beds, but they felt that they were capable (provided arteriosclerotic disease had not supervened) of providing an anatomical pathway for useful collateral circulation through the leptomeninges. As they pointed out, however, since the most devastating effects of vascular occlusion are nearly always in the basal ganglia and brain stem, it is unfortunate that these areas are supplied almost solely by non-anastomosing penetrating vessels derived from the major intracerebral blood vessels.

CONCLUSION

1. Congenital anomalies of the cerebral arterial tree are of theoretical interest only, *provided* occlusive vascular disease does not develop.
2. The Circle of Willis, if not inadequate due to the small size of the posterior communicating arteries, may play a vital role in the survival following occlusion of major neck vessels.
3. The development of potential collateral circulations in the neck between the internal and external carotid arteries may be responsible for survival in occlusive vascular disease.
4. Leptomeningeal anastomoses may be valuable in restricting the damage due to ischaemia in occlusions distal to the Circle of Willis.

REFERENCES

Alpers, B. J., Berry, R. G. & Paddison, R. M. (1959) Anatomical studies of the circle of Willis in normal brains. *Archives of Neurology and Psychiatry*, **81**, 409–418.

Bell, R. H., Swigart, L. L. & Anson, B. J. (1950) The relation of the vertebral artery to the cervical vertebrae. *Quarterly Bulletin of North West University Medical School*, Chicago, **241**, 184–185,

Bhattacharji, S. K., Hutchinson, E. C. & McCall, A. J. (1967) The circle of Willis—The incidence of developmental abnormalities in normal and infarcted brains. *Brain*, **90**, 747–758.

Boyd, J. D. (1934) Absence of the right common carotid. *Journal of Anatomy*, **68**, 551–577.

Brain, R. (1957) Order and disorder in the cerebral circulation. *Lancet*, **ii**, 857.

Cala, L. A. & Armstrong, B. K. (1972) A 'Triple-Steal Syndrome' resulting from innominate and left subclavian arterial occlusion. *Australian and New Zealand Medical Journal*, **3**, 275–277.

Campbell, R. L. & Dyken, M. L. (1961) Four cases of carotid-basilar anastimosis associated with central nervous system dyfsunction. *Journal of Neurology and Psychiatry*, **24**, 250–253.

Contorni, L. (1960) Il circolo collaterale vertebro-vertebrale nella obliterazone dell'arteria succlavia alla sua origine. *Minerva Chirurgica*, **15**, 268–271.

Doniger, D. E. (1963) Bilateral complete carotid and basilar artery occlusion in a patient with minimal deficit. *Neurology*, **13**, 673–678.

Fields, W. S., Bruetman, M. E. & Wiebel, J. (1965) Collateral circulation of the brain. *Surgical Sciences*, **2**, 183–259.

Fields, W. S., Edwards, W. H. & Crawford, E. S. (1961) Bilateral carotid artery thrombosis. *Archives of Neurology*, **4**, 369–383.

Gillilan, L. A. (1959) Significant superficial anastomosis in the arterial blood supply to the human brain. *Journal of Comparative Neurology*, **112**, 55–73.

Handa, J., Waga, S. & Handa, H. (1971) Dural-cortical arterial anastomosis as a collateral channel in carotid occlusive disease. *Clinical Radiology*, **22**, 302–307.

Hardesty, W. H., Roberts, B., Toole, J. F. & Royster, H. P. (1962) Studies of carotid-artery blood flow in man. *New England Journal of Medicine*, **263**, 944.

Herndon, R. M., Meyer, J. S. & Johnson, J. F. (1960) Fibrinolysin therapy in thrombotic disease of the nervous system. *Journal of the Michigan Medical Society*, **59**, 1684–1692.

Kramer, S. P. (1912) Function of the circle of Willis. *Journal of Experimental Medicine*, **15**, 348.

Langton, L. (1974) Personal communication.

McDonald, D. A. & Potter, J. M. (1951) The distribution of blood to the brain. *Journal of Physiology*, **114**, 356.

Meyer, J. S., Fang, H. C. & Denny-Brown, D. (1954) Polarographic study of cerebral collateral circulation. *Archives of Neurology and Psychiatry*, **72**, 296–312.

Meyer, J. S. & Loeb, C. (1965) *Strokes due to Vertebro-basilar Disease*. Springfield, Illinois: Charles C. Thomas.

North, R. R., Fields, W. S., Debakey, M. E. & Crawford, E. S. (1962) Brachial-basilar insufficiency syndrome. *Neurology*, **12**, 810–820.

Padget, D. H. (1945) *The Circle of Willis. Its Embryology and Anatomy, in Intracranial Arterial Aneurysm*, (Ed.) Dandy, W. E. Ch. III. New York: Comstock.

Reivich, M., Holling, H. E., Roberts, B. & Toole, J. F. (1961) Reversal of blood flow through the vertebral artery and its effect on cerebral circulation. *New England Journal of Medicine*, **265**, 878–885.

Stopford, J. S. B. (1916) The arteries of the pons and medulla oblongata. *Journal of Anatomy*, London, **50**, 131.

Sutton, D. (1950) Anomalous carotid-basilar anastomosis. *British Journal of Radiology*, **23**, 617–619.

Suzuki, J. & Takaku, A. (1969) Cerebro-vascular 'Moya-Moya' disease. *Neurology*, **20**, 288–299.

Takeuchi, K. (1961) Occlusive diseases of the carotid artery. *Recent Advances in Research of the Nervous System*, Tokyo, **5**, 511–543.

Tharp, B., Heyman, A., Pfeiffer, J. B. & Young, W. G. (1965) Cerebral ischaemia. *Archives of Neurology*, **12**, 160–164.

Tolosa, E. (1968) Collateral circulation in occlusive vascular lesions of the brain in cerebral circulation. In *Progress in Brain Research*, Vol. **30**, pp. 247–253. (Ed.) Luyendyk, W. Amsterdam: Elsevier.

Toole, J. F. & Tucker, S. H. (1960) Influence of head position upon cerebral circulation. *Archives of Neurology*, **2**, 616–623.

Turnbull, I. (1962) Agenesis of the internal carotid artery, *Neurology*, **12**, 588–590.

Vander Eecken, H. M. & Adams, R. D. (1953) The anatomy and functional significance of the meningeal arterial anastomosis of the human brain. *Journal of Neuropathology and Experimental Neurology*, **12**, 132.

Weiss, S. (1938) The regulation and disturbance of the cerebral circulation through extra-cerebral mechanisms. *Research Publication, Association of Research in Nervous and Mental Diseases.*

Yates, P. O. & Hutchinson, E. C. (1961) Cerebral infarction: The role of stenosis of the extracranial cerebral arteries. *Medical Research Council Special Report Series*, No. 300.

CHAPTER TWO

Cerebral Blood Flow in Cerebral *prevention !* Ischaemia

The vascular lesion responsible for persisting focal signs in the central nervous system will, in the majority of patients, be (due to the late effects of) atheroma, hypertension, or a combination of these two disease processes. In occlusive cerebral vascular disease due to atheroma, whether the occlusion affects the major cervical vessels or the intracerebral blood supply, the end-result will be cerebral infarction, and the extent of the infarction will determine both the immediate short-term survival and the long-term morbidity. The factors that determine the extent of the infarction are many, but an important one is the inherent ability of the cerebral blood vessels to compensate rapidly for sudden changes in the blood supply. This ability, in its turn, depends upon the physiological control of blood flow and the available compensatory or collateral channels. It is appropriate, therefore, to examine the relevant information that has become available due to advances in techniques for determining cerebral blood flow (CBF).

METHODS

The primates, unlike other mammals, demonstrate an almost complete isolation of the intracranial and extracranial blood supply. In health, the intracranial supply is totally dependent upon the internal carotid and vertebral circulations. An equally happy evolutionary chance dictated that venous blood obtained at the level of the internal jugular bulb is almost exclusively that from the intracranial cavity. Kety (1970) has summarised the evidence demonstrating that sampling from one or other internal jugular bulb gives results that are representative of the brain as a whole and there is little side-to-side variation. It is for these two reasons that studies on the cerebral circulation have usually been performed on the higher apes and man.

Kety and Schmidt (1945) published their classic paper entitled 'Determination of cerebral blood flow in man by the use of nitrous oxide in low concentrations'. Their method, utilising the Fick principle, is based on the fact that

19

'the rate at which the cerebral venous content of inert gas approaches the arterial blood content depends upon the volume of blood flowing through the brain'. The method, which commits the patient to minimal discomfort, involves the inhalation of small quantities of nitrous oxide, and specimens for analysis are obtained from puncture of the internal jugular bulb and from a peripheral artery. The original communication described 16 determinations of CBF carried out on 11 human volunteers. Later results showed that the work had a reproducible degree of accuracy and the method was widely applied. Within 15 years, Lassen (1959), in a review of the publications up to that date, was able to consider nearly 200 contributions. Modifications of the nitrous oxide technique were introduced by Scheinberg and Stead (1949) and some years later McHenry (1964) and Lassen and Munck (1955) introduced a radioactive inert gas technique following the same principles as those of Kety and Schmidt.

The method introduced by Kety and Schmidt and subsequent modifications express a quantity that represents the total blood flow through the entire brain. Immediately, investigations yielded valuable information on the basic physiology of the cerebral circulation and also on the factors that control it. At the same time, neuroradiology was emerging as a growing discipline and with it the ability to demonstrate with precision the site of vascular pathology. It was natural therefore that methods of comparing blood flow through individual hemispheres should be sought.

The next important milestone was the description by Ingvar and Lassen (1962) of a technique that permitted the study of regional blood flow in the brain. The method calls for techniques more complicated than the original method of Kety and Schmidt and have not yet reached a point where they can fairly be regarded as a clinical investigation applicable for general use.

The method involves catheterising the internal carotid artery in order to avoid contamination of blood from the external carotid circulation and then the rapid injection, over 1 to 1.5 seconds, of 1 milli-curie of 133 Xenon dissolved in 5 ml of sterile saline. The clearance of the isotope is then followed by 16 scintillation crystals placed laterally over the head. The technique can be further combined with serial angiography which can be done almost simultaneously, and Shah et al (1972) in fact believe that the combination of the two examinations gives a better understanding of the dynamics of flow disturbance in cerebral vascular disease than using either method alone.

Although these procedures are admittedly complex, experts in this field are generally agreed that the method gives an accurate assessment of regional hemisphere flow with an ability to differentiate between flow rates in white and grey matter and of recognising, with precision, variations in regional flow.

There have, of course, been many other methods described measuring CBF. The electromagnetic flow-meter to measure carotid artery flow was used in man by Hardesty et al (1960) but this has the significant disadvantage that it requires exposure of the carotid artery in the neck. Nylin et al (1960) used radioactive erythrocytes and studied the dilution curve in the jugular bulb. Gotoh, Meyer and Tomita (1966) described a method using hydrogen gas and recorded the partial pressure of the gas in the arterial and venous blood by means of hydrogen electrodes. However, in clinical studies, the method of Ingvar and Lassen (1962) and modifications of this method are the most extensively used.

NORMAL VALUES

Normal values for total CBF by the method of Kety and Schmidt (1945) are expressed as ml of blood per 100 g of brain per minute. If the arterial and venous oxygen is estimated at the same time, the cerebral oxygen utilisation (CMRO$_2$) can be calculated, and by further monitoring the mean arterial pressure, a value for the cerebral vascular resistance (CVR), can also be expressed. There is general accord among investigators as to normal results, as the following sample figures show:

	Age (years)	CBF	CVR	CMRO$_2$
Kety and Schmidt (1948)	28	54	1.7	3.5
Lassen and Munck (1955)	38	51	1.8	3.4
McHenry (1964)	27	57.5	1.52	3.37

$$CVR = \frac{\text{Mean arterial B.P.}}{\text{CBF}}$$

$$CMRO_2 = \frac{\text{A-V (0}_2\text{)}}{\text{CBF}}$$

CONTROL OF CEREBRAL BLOOD FLOW

Before considering the relevant information available in cerebral vascular disease it is necessary to examine briefly the factors regulating CBF. The CBF is controlled by two factors, namely, the perfusing pressure and the cerebral vascular resistance, and associated with these two factors is the phenomenon of autoregulation of the cerebral blood supply. Autoregulation, a term used by Fog (Lassen, 1966) is defined as the ability of the brain to maintain a normal blood supply in spite of variation of these factors.

Perfusing pressure

Since the pressure in the jugular bulb is virtually zero in the resting subject under normal conditions the perfusing pressure is represented by the arterial blood pressure.

The original concept was that the CBF responded passively to changes in the arterial pressure. Therefore, by definition, it was indirectly controlled by the recognised homeostatic mechanism based on pressure sensors in the aorta and the carotid arteries that control the systemic blood pressure. This concept of passive response was abandoned as soon as direct measurements of blood flow were possible.

Lassen (1959), in his review of the literature, plotted the CBF against blood pressure using the mean values observed in 11 groups of subjects reported by different observers. These 11 groups provided a total of 376 determinations of CBF, all of which gave figures for blood flow in association with hypotension, hypertension, and in normal subjects.

Severe and moderate hypotension was usually induced by drugs. Normal values were obtained from pregnant women and physically normal men. The hypertension of toxaemia, hypertension induced by drugs, and essential hypertension were also studied.

In summary, Lassen demonstrated that these studies showed that it required marked hypotension, that is, a pressure fall to half the initial values, to produce a reduction in the CBF to 60 per cent of the control value and thus to induce physical signs of cerebral hypoxia. In hypertension, whatever the cause, the cerebral vasculature showed a similar ability to maintain a normal flow.

The striking ability of the brain to maintain an adequate flow in spite of wide variations in the mean systemic pressure clearly demonstrates that the brain possesses the quality of autoregulation of a very high order, which is not surprising in terms of biological survival.

Cerebral vascular resistance

The second factor controlling CBF is the CVR which is, in the main, the state of 'tone' of the intracerebral arterial vascular tree. It is true that the viscosity of the blood is a factor in CVR because in polycythaemia resistance is increased and in anaemia the reverse is the case. But the most important factor in determining CVR is the variation in the diameter or tone of the muscle wall of the vessels comprising the intracerebral blood supply. But the heart of the problem was the nature of the regulating mechanism or mechanisms that control the vascular tone.

It is an anatomical fact that fibres from the stellate and superior cervical ganglion accompany the internal carotid and vertebral arteries, but Schmidt (1950), reviewing the evidence, came to the conclusion that cerebral vasomotor innervation is probably without physiological importance in controlling the CBF flow or in playing a part in the process of autoregulation.

Modern views on the mechanisms underlying autoregulation had, of course, been presaged by the experiments described by Fog (1939a) in his studies of reaction of the pial arteries to variations in blood pressure and to epinephrine. He showed that a local application of epinephrine in cats caused the local arteries of the pia to constrict slightly but the arterioles showed no change in calibre; intravenous epinephrine gave similar results. He concluded that sympathetic vasoconstrictive mechanisms were not only feeble but were confined to the larger vessels. He also showed (Fog, 1939b) that changes in the intravascular pressure produced changes in the physiological state of 'tonus' of the wall. A fall in pressure caused relaxation and a rise in pressure contraction of the arterial muscle fibres. Bilateral section of the cervical sympathetic and vasosensory nerves of the aorta and the carotid sinus had no effect on this response. He concluded that 'the mechanism by which tonus of these vessels is regulated is not yet established'.

Thirty-five years later this is no longer true, and the importance of the blood gases, and particularly of carbon dioxide and oxygen as controlling mechanisms is now recognised. Of the two gases, carbon dioxide is the more important and a considerable amount of work both in man and in experimental animals over the last two decades has been directed towards elucidating the site and mode of its action.

Role and mode of action of carbon dioxide

The major controlling factor in CVR is the CO_2 tension of the arterial blood. Kety and Schmidt (1948) demonstrated that 7 per cent CO_2 could double the CBF whereas hypocapnia induced by hyperventilation caused a marked fall in such flow (Kety and Schmidt, 1946). The mode of action of the varying CO_2 tension was a matter for debate for a long time. Patterson et al (1955) studied both patients and volunteers, using the nitrous oxide technique to measure the total blood flow and combined with the nitrous oxide concentrations of 2.5 per cent and 3.5 per cent CO_2 in inspired gas. They observed little or no change in the total blood flow, oxygen utilisation, or CVR with 2.5 per cent CO_2. In contrast with 3.5 per cent CO_2 there was a significant increase (10 per cent) of the total flow together with a comparable fall in the CVR but no change in oxygen utilisation. It is clear therefore that the threshold for a cerebral vasodilator effect lies just beyond the level of 2.5 per cent inspired CO_2 which induces a mean increase in the arterial tension of the gas of 4.1 mm Hg.

Later work indicated that it was the level of CO_2 tension itself and not a change in pH that was important. This point has been well made by Harper and Bell (1963). They measured the cortical blood flow in the dog and, keeping the arterial CO_2 pressure constant, they varied the pH by infusions of lactic acid and sodium bicarbonate. They demonstrated that neither metabolic acidosis nor alkalosis produced any significant change in the cortical blood flow.

Reivich (1964) studied the full range of responsiveness of the cerebral vasculature in the rhesus monkey. In the experiments the cerebral perfusion pressure and the arterial oxygen saturation were kept constant and sources of error, such as temperature, the effects of anaesthesia and metabolic acidosis, were carefully controlled. Varying the CO_2 tension from 5 mm to 148 mm Hg, he observed minimal and maximal values for the CBF of 18 and 40 ml per 100 g of brain per minute. These values of CBF were obtained when the arterial PCO_2 was in the range of 10 to 15 mm Hg and 100 mm Hg respectively.

It is important to recognise the interplay between perfusing pressure and CO_2 tension in view of suggestions in the literature that varying the CO_2 tension may have some relevance in the treatment of the acute stroke. Harper (1966) measured the CBF using Krypton 85 and varied the blood pressure in dogs by bleeding. In normocapnic dogs with a $PACO_2$ of 30 to 40 mm Hg autoregulation of the blood flow to the brain continued unimpaired in spite of variations in the arterial pressure of 90 to 100 mm Hg, showing that of the two factors a level of $PACO_2$ was the more important. In hypercapnic animals with a $PACO_2$ of 70 to 90 mm Hg, which would cause a pre-existing cerebral vasodilatation, a passive pressure flow relationship was observed, indicating that autoregulation had been lost. He suggested that lack of awareness of the fact of the effect of hypercapnia on autoregulation might explain the failure of some workers to demonstrate the autoregulation of the CBF in response to changes in the arterial blood pressure.

Site of action of CO_2

It only remained to attempt to define the precise site and mode of action of CO_2. Gotoh, Tazaki and Meyer (1961) reported a crucial series of experiments where the rate of transport of oxygen and nitrogen through the living cat's brain was compared to that through the dead brain. In the same experiment they examined the effect of extravascular gases on cerebral vasomotor activity.

The results indicated that extravascular CO_2 was a potent vasodilator and was more effective than a varying hydrogen ion concentration. Other studies (Caldwell, 1958; Gotoh, Tazaki and, Meyer, 1961) had already demonstrated that CO_2 passes more readily through the cell membrane of smooth muscle than the hydrogen ion and lowered the intracellular pH more rapidly. They concluded that the final factor responsible for the control of cerebral vasomotor activity is a change in the intracellular hydrogen ion concentration in the smooth muscle fibres of cerebral arterioles.

Lassen (1968) indicated in a review of the problem that the evidence that had accumulated from various sources supported Gotoh et al (1961) in the view that the local extravascular pH is probably the main factor regulating CVR. This would mean that the intracerebral arteriole acts like a PCO_2 electrode. In the latter, CO_2 diffuses freely through the endothelial membrane, whereas hydrogen ion and bicarbonate cannot do so freely. Hence, it is the intravascular CO_2 and the extravascular bicarbonate that determines the pH around and, presumably, inside the vessel wall.

Oxygen

Kety and Schmidt (1946) demonstrated that in the normal young male at physical and mental rest at sea level about 20 per cent of cardiac output and about 24 per cent of the total oxygen consumption of the body catered for the requirements of the brain.

Variations in the partial pressure of oxygen in the blood had the reverse effect of those demonstrated with CO_2. Whereas moderate variations in value for oxygen tension above and below the normal range did not affect the CBF Heyman, Patterson and Whatley Duke (1952), demonstrated that inhalation of mixtures of high oxygen tension caused a moderate vasoconstriction whereas inhalation of low oxygen tension caused dilatation of the pial vessels. This latter response may have a vital role in the face of severe anoxic states as it may help appreciably to combat the degree of arterial oxygen unsaturation.

CEREBRAL VASCULAR DISEASE

When an acceptable technique for measuring CBF in a living patient became available it was natural that focal cerebral vascular disease would be studied in its many aspects. The literature can be categorised under two headings.

The first concerns information obtained using the inert gas technique which expresses total CBF. This information, in retrospect, is particularly valuable in patients with extracranial occlusions as it demonstrates a ready ability to compensate for these lesions in the absence of small vessel disease. These initial studies used the techniques of inhalation of either nitrous oxide or radioactive inert gas (Kety and Schmidt, 1948; Scheinberg and Stead, 1949; McHenry, 1964; Lassen and Munck, 1959).

The second is the valuable information obtained over the last few years following the introduction by Ingvar and Lassen (1962) of techniques for studying regional blood flow following cerebral infarction. These techniques have allowed focal areas of the brain to be examined over the presumed site of infarction and have thus monitored dynamic changes taking place there.

Unspecified cerebral vascular disease

Many of the early communications calculating total CBF in the presence of cerebral vascular disease lack sufficient clinical detail to correlate sensibly with the results. This is not to be unduly critical of the work but rather to emphasise that modern angiographic techniques were not readily available at that time.

Scheinberg (1950) studied a group of middle-aged patients and all, with one exception, had hypertension complicated by cerebral vascular disease. He sub-divided the patients into two groups on the basis of their mental state, the sub-division being based on the normality or otherwise of their mental function. The results showed a clear difference between the two groups since the patients with abnormal mental states had lower blood flow values. He suggested that assessment of the CBF might offer a means of monitoring the progress of cerebral vascular disease.

However, other investigators found considerable disparity in the values for the total blood flow and the clinical signs of cerebral ischaemia. Alman and Fazekas (1957), reviewing 700 observations of their own, stated that previously a critical flow was considered to be about 30 to 35 ml per 100 g of brain per minute. That this view should be modified was shown by their own series where they observed patients with values that fell well below this. Indeed, in one group with a mean age of 62 years and a mean CBF of 28.1 ml/100 g/min the patients were quite alert and possessed adequate cerebral function. They further found that it was possible to vary the flow to a remarkably low degree without any interference with cerebral function. Again, however, the results were not constant. In one patient they reduced the flow from 36.4 to 19.7 ml/100 g/min without any obvious disturbance of cerebral function but in another a similar reduction resulted in loss of consciousness.

In acute cerebral vascular accidents with focal signs investigations have shown that the mean CBF tends to fall. Heyman et al (1953) found that in such circumstances the mean CBF was reduced to 40 ml per 100 g of brain per minute together with a reduction in the cerebral metabolic rate and an increase in CVR. In a contrasting group of seven patients who were believed on clinical grounds to have chronic progressive vascular disease with a history of multiple strokes the mean CBF was 35 ml per 100 g of brain per min together with a fall in the cerebral metabolic rate and an increase in CVR. In a group of patients who were examined in an acute phase and then re-examined five weeks after the initial episode the mean CBF increased significantly although it did not return to normal values. In general, however, flow studies showed that patients with a greater neurological deficit had a greater fall in cerebral blood flow and in cerebral metabolic rate.

Kempinsky et al (1961) obtained similar results and in their studies they compared the results of bilateral CBF. They could not detect any significant difference in the flow values obtained from the side of the cerebral infarct as compared with the unaffected hemisphere.

Correlation of vascular occlusion and cerebral blood flow

With the development of the widespread use of angiography it was possible to study CBF against a background of more precise knowledge of the site of vascular occlusion and thus to examine the potentially different effects of extracranial and intracranial vascular occlusion.

Fazekas et al (1962) described three patients with extracranial vascular occlusion who were studied in considerable detail. The first patient had bilateral occlusion of the internal carotid artery with a collateral circulation supplied through the external carotid arteries, and also marked narrowing of the right vertebral artery. The second patient had a complete occlusion of both internal carotid arteries and stenosis of the left vertebral artery. Both patients had adequate cerebral function and a normal or near normal CBF. In the second patient described, it was demonstrated by compression studies that 80 per cent of the CBF was maintained through the vertebral channels. In the third patient there was complete occlusion of the right internal carotid artery and 60 per cent occlusion of the left, together with a small right vertebral artery. In contrast to the first two patients studied the CBF was much reduced.

The speed with which the circulation may adjust to occlusion using alternative available channels is remarkable. Shenkin et al (1951) observed the immediate changes that followed acute carotid occlusion. It was acute because the occlusion was produced by carotid ligation in the treatment of intracranial aneurysms. They observed an immediate increase after ligation in the CVR by 47 per cent and a mean increase in the mean arterial pressure by an average of 20 per cent. No change occurred in either the CBF or the cerebral oxygen uptake, clearly indicating an immediate compensatory increase in blood flow through the remaining patent carotid artery and the vertebral circulation.

Symon et al (1963) examined the immediate haemodynamic adjustment in monkeys in response to major vessel occlusions in a degree of detail not permissible in man. They used electromagnetic flow meters to record the blood flow. The extent to which readjustments can be effected was shown by two cases of bilateral occlusion of the internal carotid artery where one showed a normal total blood flow and the other achieved 70 per cent of normal flow. Eklof and Schwartz (1969) also confirmed this remarkable adaptive facility. In acute experiments in baboons, where progressive stenosis of the major neck vessels was carried out, they found that with bilateral occlusion of vertebral arteries a 15 per cent increase in carotid flow was noted. When occlusion of one carotid artery was carried out the flow in the companion vessel increased by 88 per cent of normal values.

Stenosis or known occlusions of the middle cerebral artery (McHenry, 1966) were in line with the previous observations, namely, that in cerebral vascular disease there was a reduction in total CBF. Fieschi et al (1966) reported a study of 50 patients with acute cerebral lesions and they found, again, that there was a total reduction of blood flow in most cases affecting the entire brain, but in some it was found that reduction was greater in the infarcted hemisphere in cases of middle cerebral occlusion.

O'Brien and Veall (1970) from their own data summed up the effects of occlusion or stenosis of the major neck vessels. They believed that neither marked stenosis nor complete occlusion had any constant effect on blood flow in the cerebral cortical territory of the affected vessel and this they attributed to the development of a collateral supply. They felt that asymmetries of blood flow in the hemispheres was a good indication of disease at or above the level of the Circle of Willis and since their technique involved examining cortical perfusion they felt it was the state of the small blood vessels that was the ultimate determinant of the CBF.

It seems reasonable to assume therefore that in major cervical arterial occlusion the integrity of the total CBF can be maintained by increasing the flow through the remaining patent vessels or by utilising collateral channels. That variations in total flow from one patient to another with apparently similar angiographic findings are an expression of small vessel disease appears likely in the absence of an alternative explanation but is difficult to prove.

CO_2 levels and total cerebral blood flow

As soon as it was apparent that increasing the concentration of CO_2 in inspired air rapidly increased the CBF, it was not surprising that the potential therapeutic effect of such treatment in cerebral vascular disease came to be assessed.

In unilateral carotid obstruction Hegedus and Shackleford (1965) reported a 40 per cent increase in total CBF and recommended CO_2 inhalation as an adjunct to vascular surgery in the treatment of unilateral carotid obstruction, but it had already been demonstrated by Fazekas et al (1962) that the response was not always consistent.

In the three patients, already referred to, with multiple extracranial vascular occlusions demonstrated at angiography, two responded well to CO_2 whereas the third showed no response whatsoever. Again, in the experiments of Eklof and Schwartz (1969) in baboons with experimental occlusions the total blood flow responded briskly to CO_2 and here, of course, the question of small vessel disease did not arise.

Fazekas and Alman (1964), in a further communication, described 22 patients who had had four-vessel angiography carried out and were shown to have a demonstrable lesion in at least three of the four major vessels of the neck. Of the 22 patients, nine were observed to lack any appreciable response in the total CBF to inhalations of 5 per cent CO_2 whereas the remaining patients responded normally. It was not possible on clinical or radiological grounds to differentiate between the two groups of patients. Certainly, the mean CBF was reduced in the unresponsive group when compared with the group that responded in a normal manner. The CVR was also higher in the unresponsive group and the cerebral oxygen consumption reduced.

They concluded that the failure of an adequate cerebral vascular response to 5 per cent CO_2 was due to an existing maximal dilatation of the cerebral arterioles and that this dilatation, in its turn, was due to reduced perfusion pressure due to disease of the small cerebral vessels. They felt that this reaction represented an exhaustion of the haemostatic reserve which, they felt, was implicit in maximal arteriolar dilatation and indicated that the use of CO_2 may very well be harmful under certain conditions. The percipience of this cautionary note became apparent very rapidly when estimations of the CBF studied in a regional manner were reported.

REGIONAL BLOOD FLOW IN CEREBRAL VASCULAR DISEASE

Luxury perfusion syndrome

Lassen (1966) introduced into medical terminology a syndrome which he attractively labelled the luxury perfusion syndrome. He defined it as an acute derangement of the cerebral circulation associated with brain damage and claimed that it was characterised by an over-abundant CBF relative to the metabolic needs of the brain. In discussing the subject, Lassen pointed out that Meyer, Fang and Denny-Brown (1954) who examined the ischaemic hemisphere in the experimental animal with polographic platinum electrodes, had already demonstrated an increase in oxygen tension in many areas surrounding the hypoxic zones.

The phenomenon of over-abundant blood supply can be directly observed since bright red blood is seen in the venous drainage of the area of brain damage. According to Feindel, Yamomoto and Hodge (1968) it was first observed by Penfield in 1937 after electrical stimulation of the cortex. Feindel, Yamomoto and Hodge (1968), during neurosurgical procedures, had seen the phenomenon not only in arterial venous shunts but also in what they referred to as a 'metabolic shunt.' They indicated, as did Lassen, that the cause lay with the inability of the damaged cell tissue to utilise oxygen adequately. They instanced necrotic tumour, cortical cyst, brain scars and cerebral infarction as conditions under which red venous blood can be observed. Waltz (1969) also discussed the phenomenon of red venous blood and found it to occur following increased arterial CO_2 tension, following the relief of general hemisphere anoxia and after local trauma. He also observed it in association with neoplasms, with cystic scars and with acute and chronic ischaemia.

Lassen (1966) indicated that in all the conditions in which the phenomenon of red venous blood had been observed there was one factor they all had in common, namely, hypoxia. Hypoxia will induce acid metabolites and this acute metabolic acidosis, which may be focal or general in the brain, depending upon the nature of the disease process, will produce vasodilatation. He deduced that in clinical practice an early phlebogram in patients with cerebral vascular accidents may well be helpful and Cronquist and Laroche (1967) did in fact describe transitory hyperaemia indicated by early venous filling at angiography and emphasised that these could be differentiated from tumour circulations by the normal anatomy of the veins.

Regional cerebral blood flow in cerebral vascular disease

Høedt-Rasmussen et al (1967) examined how the concept of the luxury perfusion syndrome could contribute to the understanding of the haemodynamic changes associated with the acute stage of apoplexy. Using the 133 Xenon technique they examined 16 regions of the hemisphere following the acute vascular episode. In seven control patients without evidence of focal cerebral disease no systematic difference was found between the regional CBF in different regions. Six patients were studied and all were in the acute phase of a stroke; each had a clear-cut clinical history of hemiparesis of sudden onset; none was unconscious and the cerebrospinal fluid was free of blood. The longest time the examination was carried out after the acute vascular lesion was four days and the shortest half a day.

Their most important observation was that hypertension induced by drugs increased blood flow locally in the area of the presumed site of the vascular lesion. In four of the six patients local hyperaemia in relation to other regions of the hemisphere was present and the area did not show the normal anticipated response to increased concentrations of CO_2 in the inspired air. In view of what is known of the control of the cerebral blood supply these two findings indicated that in the area of the infarct there was an impairment of the inherent quality of autoregulation of the cerebral blood supply and a loss of the normal response to hypercapnia. These findings were in accord with those of Fieschi, Bozzao and Agnoli (1965).

They interpreted this focal vasomotor paralysis as the basic abnormality of the local circulation surrounding an area of vascular damage and because of its presence a normal perfusion pressure would cause excessive perfusion whereas if perfusion pressure was reduced ischaemia would result.

They felt that their observations supported the view put forward by Lassen (1966), namely, that hypoxia initiated a local tissue acidosis which, in its turn, induced vasodilatation and loss of autoregulation.

They discussed the possibility that ischaemic areas, which lie adjacent to the areas that are hyperaemic, produce acid metabolites, principally lactic acid, which may spread locally and thus cause vasodilatation in areas with normal perfusion pressure.

One significant point the authors made was that, in the four cases showing the luxury perfusion syndrome in the area of the infarct the investigation had been carried out within 36 hours of the onset of symptoms whereas in the two patients not showing this abnormality the time interval was between three and four days.

They believe that their findings indicate that therapy designed to cause vasodilatation, either by using carbon dioxide or by pharmacological agents, would not only be ineffective—since the vessels concerned were incapable of responding to the stimulus—but, they argued, might actually be harmful in the acute stroke. They reasoned that since vasodilatation may occur only in non-affected areas and not in the territory where vasomotor control was paralysed this would deviate blood from an ischaemic focus. This they referred to as 'a sort of intracerebral steal syndrome'.

Paulson, Lassen and Skinhøj (1970) reported on a more extensive study in a group of 31 patients. All patients had cerebral angiography carried out and in none was there an occlusion of major intracerebral vessels. There was a history of hemiparesis in all patients and in 20 of them the investigation was carried out within 14 days of the stroke.

They indicated that the abnormalities that could occur in the regional cerebral circulation in association with cerebral infarction were as follows:

1. HYPERAEMIC FOCI

In the areas of hyperaemic foci, flow values of 30 to 40 per cent above the hemisphere average could be found in the very acute phase of the disease and were combined with a loss of responsiveness in the vasomotor apparatus. Four of the five patients studied in the first one-and-a-half days after the onset of the symptoms showed a hyperaemic focus but they were not present in any of the patients studied later than this, and in one patient studied on two succeeding days the hyperaemic focus disappeared. Thus, it was a transitory phenomenon with a close temporal relationship to the onset of symptoms.

2. VASOMOTOR PARALYSIS

Vasomotor paralysis, like the hyperaemic foci, was a phenomenon observed in the acute phase of the disease, although it was not confined strictly to the first few days. In one patient it was observed as long as 14 days after the onset of symptoms.

In areas where the vasomotor paralysis was well marked paradoxical flow could be observed, that is, regional blood flow in the affected area decreased during vasodilatation and increased during vasoconstriction. They emphasised, however, that in many patients, the changes observed were only small and not far removed from the normal variations observed in the non-diseased parts of the brain.

3. ISCHAEMIC FOCI

Ischaemic foci showed a reduction of flow of the order of 10 to 20 per cent of the normal values but their presence bore no particular temporal relationship to the onset of symptoms.

4. PARADOXICAL FOCAL FLOW DECREASE

When hypertension was induced they observed the phenomenon which they described as paradoxical focal flow decrease. These patients showed in the unaffected areas of the hemisphere the anticipated response to hypercapnia and hypocapnia in contrast to the focal areas of abnormality of regional blood flow where no such response was observed.

During drug-induced hypertension they demonstrated a global loss of autoregulation since the total hemisphere flow followed the changes in the perfusion pressure passively. In the focal areas of abnormality, however, blood flow was decreased. They pointed out that this paradoxical reaction, which they referred to again as the steal syndrome, had been commonly observed in cerebral tumours. The five patients in their study all showed a loss of autoregulation throughout the hemisphere.

5. ISOLATED LOSS OF VASODILATATION WITH HYPERCAPNIA

In one patient they found a loss of vasodilatation during hypercapnia but preserved vasoconstriction following hypocapnia and hypertension. They demonstrated this in an area between the territories of the anterior and middle cerebral arteries and, they felt, this was an area with marginal blood supply and that the cerebral vessels in this region were probably already maximally dilated even at rest.

Very similar findings to these were reported by Paulson (1970) in a series of patients with occlusion of the middle cerebral artery demonstrated at angiography.

In transient ischaemic attacks Skinhøj et al (1970) demonstrated focal disturbance of CO_2 responsiveness at time intervals of up to four days after the attack but they found no persisting abnormality. However, Rees et al (1970) found persisting areas of disturbed flow in patients with a history of transient cerebral ischaemia which could be observed persisting for as long as 90 days.

Potential danger of altering inspired CO_2

This new information on the phenomenon of focal or general loss of autoregulation with impaired response to hypercapnia has not unnaturally provoked further consideration on the advisability of administering CO_2 in inspired air to patients with known infarcts. Lassen (1966), when putting forward the luxury perfusion syndrome as an appropriate title, suggested that perhaps giving CO_2 to patients may in fact be actively harmful by decreasing the blood flow in ischaemic areas.

If hypercapnia is harmful, then it is natural to consider whether hypocapnia would have the reverse effect. There is certain experimental evidence that hyperventilation with its associated hypocapnia may influence the extent of infarction. Soloway et al (1968) occluded the middle cerebral artery in the dog at its origin and the internal carotid artery at a point between the posterior communicating and the anterior cerebral artery. Following occlusion the arterial CO_2 was maintained at 38 mm Hg for two hours in a control group of four animals, whereas in the experimental group the CO_2 was kept at 25 mm for two hours.

At postmortem all control animals were shown to have extensive cortical damage as well as infarcts in the lenticular nucleus, the internal capsule and the thalamus. In contrast, in the experimental group with a maintained reduction of arterial CO_2 tension, only two-thirds of them showed infarction and this only at a cortical level and with no evidence of infarction of the deeper structures.

They felt that their results supported the view that hyperventilation does not produce cerebral ischaemic hypoxia. They also felt that a significant increase in arterial CO_2 may well divert blood from an ischaemia area by the 'steal mechanism' in association with vasodilatation and an increased total CBF. In contrast, hypocapnia may in fact increase collateral flow by producing vasoconstriction in the normal collateral channels and thus increase the perfusing pressure to the ischaemic area.

More recently, Paulson, Oleson and Christensen (1972) reported a study on six patients, four of whom were suffering from cerebral tumour and two from apoplexy. The purpose of the study was to examine the effect of hypocapnia on the phenomenon of global loss of autoregulation which may be observed in the non-diseased parts of the brain but which are associated with a retained responsiveness or sensitivity in the cerebral vasculature to the level of the arterial CO_2 (Paulson, 1970; Paulson, Lassen and Skinhøj, 1970; Palvolgyi, 1969).

In the six patients they demonstrated a loss of autoregulation in the non-diseased hemisphere in the resting state. Hypocapnia was then induced by hyperventilation to a level of about 25 mm Hg and maintained at this level for nearly an hour. Autoregulation was completely restored in four of the patients, in one of the remainder a partial restoration was observed, and in the last patient no effect was noted.

Meyer et al (1973) published a detailed study on 32 patients who were variously categorised as cases of TCI, rapidly recovering strokes, presumed cerebral infarction with moderate residual disability and, finally, a group of patients with presumed cerebral infarction but with severe disability which persisted for more than three weeks and with little evidence of recovery. Hemisphere blood flow was calculated from the hydrogen clearance curve measured in blood from the transverse sinus following the injection of a bolus of hydrogen through the carotid arteries.

Their results indicated an inverse relationship between impaired cerebral autoregulation and the time following an acute episode. An important aspect of their results was that while severe hemisphere lesions showed a more prominent loss of autoregulation than minor hemisphere lesions there was evidence that subcortical lesions were associated with a greater impairment of autoregulation than cortical lesions. The most important observation, however, was that brain stem lesions, including transient cerebral ischaemia, had a greater effect on impairment of cerebral autoregulation than lesions at any other site. Not only were they more marked but they also persisted for a longer time.

These observations led them to conclude that control of autoregulation was mediated by structures situated in the brain stem and in the deep cerebral structures.

If these observations are confirmed then a major step forward will have been taken in the problem of cerebral vascular control both in normal subjects and in survivors from a stroke.

CONCLUSION

1. The normal value for total cerebral blood flow in a healthy adult brain is of the order of 55 ml of blood per 100 g of brain tissue/min.
2. Autoregulation (the ability of the brain to adapt to variations in perfusing pressure and cerebrovascular resistance) is developed to a high degree in normal subjects.
3. The arterial CO_2 concentration plays a vital role in varying cerebrovascular resistance and, therefore, influencing the total cerebral blood flow.
4. Experimental evidence now seems to indicate that it is the local extra-vascular pH at arteriolar level which is the operative factor in determining cerebrovascular resistance.
5. The mean total cerebral blood flow falls in cerebrovascular disease but the adjustment after occlusion of main vessels occurs rapidly.
6. There is no constant effect on total blood flow with neck vessel occlusion. There is evidence that small vessel disease dictates the level of blood flow.
7. Inhaled CO_2 may cause a normal response (i.e. doubling of the flow) in presence of neck vessel occlusion. Failure to respond probably indicates exhaustion of the haemostatic reserve.
8. Regional blood flow studies have shown that ischaemia may affect autoregulation either locally in the area of ischaemia or generally over a hemisphere.
9. Following local ischaemia there may be hyperaemic foci, vasomotor paralysis and ischaemic foci. Paradoxical focal flow increase in response to hyper- and hypocapnia may be observed.
10. There is some evidence that hypocapnia may transiently restore loss of autoregulation.
11. Recent work indicates that control of autoregulation may be mediated by structures in the brain-stem and by deep cortical structures.

REFERENCES

Alman, R. W. & Fazekas, J. F. (1957) Disparity between low cerebral blood flow and clinical signs of cerebral ischaemia. *Neurology*, **7**, 555–558.

Caldwell, P. C. (1958) Studies of the internal pH of large muscle and nerve fibres. *Journal of Physiology*, London, **142**, 22–62.

Cronquist, S. & Laroche, F. (1967) Transitory hyperaemia in focal cerebral vascular lesions studied by angiography and regional cerebral blood flow measurements. *British Journal of Radiology*, **40**, 270–274.

Eklof, B. & Schwartz, S. I. (1969) Effects of critical stenosis of the carotid artery and compromised cephalic blood flow. *Archives of Surgery*, **99**, 695–701.

Fazekas, J. F., Yvan, R. H., Callow, A. D., Paul, R. E. & Alman, R. W. (1962) Studies of cerebral hemodynamics in aortocranial disease. *New England Journal of Medicine*, **266**, 224–228.

Fazekas, J.' F. & Alman, W. R. (1964) Maximal dilatation of cerebral vessels. *Archives of Neurology*, **11**, 303–309.

Feindel, W., Yamomoto, Y. L. & Hodge, C. P. (1968) Red cerebral veins as an index of cerebral steal. *Scandinavian Journal of Laboratory and Clinical Investigations, Supplement*, **102** X:C.

Fieschi, C., Bozzao, L. & Agnoli, A. (1965) Regional clearance of hydrogen as a measure of cerebral blood flow. *Acta Neurologica Supplementum*, **14**, 46–52.

Fieschi, C., Agnoli, A., Battistini, N. & Bozzao, L. (1966) Regional cerebral blood flow in patients with brain infarct. *Archives of Neurology*, **15**, 6, 653–663.

Fog, M. (1939a) Reaction of pial arteries to epinephrine by direct application and by intravenous injection. *Archives of Neurology and Psychiatry*, **41**, 109–118.

Fog, M. (1939b) Reaction of pial arteries to increase in blood pressure. *Archives of Neurology and Psychiatry*, **4**, 260–267.

Gotoh, F., Tazaki, Y. & Meyer, J. S. (1961) Transport of gases through brain and their extravascular vasomotor action. *Experimental Neurology*, **4**, 48.

Gotoh, F., Meyer, J. S. & Tomita, M. (1966) Hydrogen method for determining cerebral blood flow in man. *Archives of Neurology*, **15**, 549–559.

Hardesty, W. H., Brook, R., Toole, J. F. & Royster, H. P. (1960) Studies of carotid artery blood flow in man. *New England Journal of Medicine*, **263**, 944–946.

Harper, A. M. & Bell, R. A. (1963) The effect of metabolic acidosis and alkaloses on the blood flow through the cerebral cortex. *Journal of Neurology, Neurosurgery and Psychiatry*, **26**, 341–344.

Harper, A. M. (1966) Auto-regulation of cerebral blood flow. Influence of the arterial blood pressure on the blood flow through the cerebral cortex. *Journal of Neurology, Neurosurgery and Psychiatry*, **29**, 398–403.

Hegedus, S. A. & Shackleford, R. T. (1965) Carbon dioxide and obstructed cerebral blood flow-correlation between cerebral blood flow crossfilling and neurological findings. *Journal of the American Medical Association*, **191**, 279–282.

Heyman, A., Patterson, J. L. jr. & Whatley Duke, T. (1952) Cerebral circulation and metabolism in sickle cell and other chronic anaemias with observations on the effects of oxygen inhalation. *Journal of Clinical Investigation*, **31**, 824–828.

Heyman, A., Patterson, J. L. Whatley Duke, T. ,& Battey, L. L. (1953) The cerebral circulation and metabolism in arteriosclerotic and hypertensive cerebrovascular disease. *New England Journal of Medicine*, **249**, 223–229.

Høedt-Rasmussen, K., Skinhøj, E., Paulson, O., Ewald, J., Bjerrum, J. K., Fahrenkrug, A. & Lassen, N. A. (1967) Regional cerebral blood flow in acute apoplexy. The 'luxury perfusion syndrome' of brain tissue. *Archives of Neurology*, **17**, 271–281.

Ingvar, D. & Lassen, N. A. (1962) Regional blood flow of the cerebral cortex determined by Krypton[85]. *Acta Physiologica Scandinavica*, **54**, 325–338.

Kempinsky, W. H., Boniface, W. R., Keating, Jose B. A. & Morgan, P. P. (1961) Serial hemodynamic study of cerebral infarction in Man. *Circulation Research*, **9**, 1051–1058.

Kety, S. S. & Schmidt, C. F. (1945) The determination of cerebral blood flow in man by use of nitrous oxide in low concentrations. *American Journal of Physiology*, **143**, 53–66.

Kety, S. S. & Schmidt, C. F. (1946) The effects of active and passive hyperventilation on cerebral blood flow. Cerebral oxygen consumption, cardiac output and blood pressuer of normal young men. *Journal of Clinical Investigation*, **25**, 107–119.

Kety, S. S. & Schmidt, C. F. (1948) Oxide method for the quantitative determination of cerebral blood flow in man. Theory, procedure and normal values. *Journal of Clinical Investigation*, **27**, 476–484.

Kety, S. S. (1970) The cerebral circulation. *Handbook of Physiology—Neurophysiology*, **II**, 1751–1760.

Lassen, N. A. & Munck, O. (1955) The cerebral blood flow in man determined by the use of radio-active Krypton. *Acta Physiologica Scandinavia*, **33**, 30–49.

Lassen, N. A. (1959) Cerebral blood flow and oxygen consumption in man. *Physiological Reviews*, **39**, 183–238.

Lassen, N. A. (1966) The luxury perfusion syndrome. *Lancet*, **ii**, 1113–1115.

Lassen, N. A. & Palvolgyi, R. (1968) Cerebral steal during hypercapnia and reverse reaction during hypocapnia observed by the 133 Xenon technique in man. *Scandinavia Journal of Clinical Laboratory Investigations*, Supplement **102** X III D.

McHenry, L. C. jr. (1964) Quantitative cerebral blood flow determination application of Krypton[85] desaturation technique in man. *Neurology*, **14**, 785–793.

McHenry, L. C. (1966) Cerebral blood flow in middle cerebral and internal carotid artery occlusion. *Neurology*, **16**, 1145–1151.

Meyer, J. S., Fang, H. C. & Denny-Brown, D. (1954) Polargraphic study of cerebral collateral circulation. *Archives of Neurology and Psychiatry*, Chicago, **72**, 296–312.

Meyer, J. S., Shimazu, K., Fukuuchi, Y., Ohuchi, T., Okamoto, S., Koto, A. & Ericsson, A. D. (1973) Impaired neurogenic cerebrovascular control and dysautoregulation after stroke. *Stroke*, **4**, 169–186.

Nylin, G., Silfverskiold, B. P., Lofstedt, S., Regnstione, O. & Hedlund, S. (1960) Studies of cerebral blood flow in man using radioactive-labelled erythrocytes. *Brain*, **83**, 293–335.

O'Brien, M. D. & Veall, N. (1970) The influence of carotid stenosis on cortex perfusion. *Research in Cerebral Circulation, 3rd International Salzburg Conference*, 165–167.

Palvolgyi, R. (1969) Regional cerebral blood flow in patients with intracranial tumors. *Journal of Neurosurgery*, **31**, 149–163.

Patterson, J. L., Heyman, A., Battey, L. L. & Ferguson, R. W. (1955) Threshold of response of the cerebral vessels of man to increase in blood carbon dioxide. *Journal of Clinical Investigation*, **34**, 1857–1864.

Paulson, O. B. (1970) Regional cerebral blood flow in apoplexy due to occlusion of the middle cerebral artery. *Neurology*, **20**, 66–77.

Paulson, O. B., Lassen, N. A. & Skinhøj, E. (1970) Regional cerebral blood flow in apoplexy without arterial occlusion. *Neurology*, **20**, 125–138.

Paulson, O. B., Olesen, J. & Christensen, M. S. (1972) Restoration of autoregulation of cerebral blood flow by hypocapnia. *Neurology*, **22**, 286–293.

Rees, J. E., Bull, J. W. D., Ross-Russell, R. W., Marshall, J. & Symon, L. (1970) Regional cerebral blood flow in transient ischaemic attacks. *Lancet*, **ii**, 1210–1213.

Reivich, M. (1964) Arterial PCO_2 and cerebral hemodynamics. *American Journal of Physiology*, **206**, 25–35.

Scheinberg, P. (1950) Cerebral blood flow in vascular disease of the brain with observations on the effects of stellate ganglion block. *American Journal of Medicine*, **8**, 139–147.

Scheinberg, P. & Stead, E. A. (1949) Cerebral blood flow in various physiological states. *Journal of Clinical Investigation*, **28**, 1163–1171.

Schmidt, C. F. (1950) *The Cerebral Circulation in Health and Disease*. Springfield, Ill.: Charles C. Thomas.

Shah, S., Bull, J. W. D., DuBoulay, G. H., Marshall, J., Ross-Russell, R. W. & Symon, L. (1972) A comparison of rapid serial angiography and isotope clearance measurements in cerebrovascular disease. *British Journal of Radiology*, **45**, 294–298.

Shenkin, H. A., Cabieses, F., Van-Den Noordt, G., Sayers, P. & Copperman, R. (1951) The hemodynamic effect of unilateral carotid ligation of the cerebral circulation of man. *Journal of Neurosurgery*, **8**, 38–45.

Skinhøj, J., Høedt—Rasmussen J., Paulson, O.B. & Lassen, N. A. (1970) Regional cerebral blood flow and its autoregulation in patients with transient focal cerebral ischaemic attacks. *Neurology*, **22**, 485–493.

Soloway, M., Nadel, W., Albin, M. S. & White, R. J. (1968) The effect of hyperventilation on subsequent cerebral infarction. *Anesthesiology*, **29**, 975–980.

Symon, L., Ishikawa, S., Lavy, S. & Meyer, J. S. (1963) Quantitative measurement of cephalic blood flow in the monkey. *Journal of Neurosurgery*, **20**, 199–218.

Waltz, A. G. (1969) Red venous blood. Occurrence and significance in ischaemic and non-ischaemic cerebral cortex. *Journal of Neurosurgery*, **31**, 141–148.

CHAPTER THREE

Pathology

A. J. McCALL
P. J. H. FLETCHER

CEREBRAL INFARCTION

We adopt Adam's (1967) definition of a cerebral infarct as an area of brain in which the blood flow has fallen below the critical level necessary to maintain the viability of the tissue. Infarction is, of course, the cause of nearly all completed strokes except those due to haemorrhage.

Morbid anatomy of infarcts

A recent infarct due to ablation of a sizeable vascular territory presents as a swollen softened area of brain involving both cortex and white matter, and often the deep grey matter as well. When well established its limits are usually evident. Some small infarcts will escape detection if the brain is cut before fixation and very early infarcts may be undetectable with certainty without microscopy.

SPECIAL FEATURES OF EMBOLIC INFARCTS—HAEMORRHAGIC INFARCTS

Embolic infarcts are often multiple and bilateral, and the finding of multiple contemporary infarcts is strongly suggestive of embolism. Emboli of cardiac origin may enter both carotids very closely in time and emboli entering either vertebral artery may finish in either or both posterior cerebral arteries. The infarcts may be minute or may involve a very large area, as when the middle cerebral artery is blocked proximal to its perforating branches. Embolic infarcts may be pale but are very frequently haemorrhagic, and the finding of haemorrhagic infarcts suggests embolism. Punctate haemorrhages within or at the periphery of otherwise pale infarcts are commonplace but many embolic infarcts are haemorrhagic throughout. They are seen most often in the cortical grey matter and may involve only the cortex in the depth of the sulci.

Fisher and Adams (1951) found that only 3 out of 66 haemorrhagic infarcts they examined were not clearly embolic. We subscribe to the explanation offered by Fisher and Adams that they result from disintegration of the embolus or from its movement distally beyond the site of initial arrest. In either case blood under normal pressure flows through previously unperfused vessels into brain softened by ischaemia and in which the small arteries are themselves partly necrotic. In 8 out of 30 embolic infarcts examined by Fisher and Adams they found fragments of embolic material within the infarcted area, indicating disintegration of the embolus. Old haemorrhagic infarcts show heavy orange or brown pigmentation resulting from deposition of haemosiderin.

CELLULAR CHANGES IN INFARCTS

Microscopically, early brain infarcts show acute ischaemic changes in neurons, followed by disintegration, destruction of glial cells, necrosis of the small blood vessels, accumulation of interstitial fluid, and destruction of axons and myelin. In pale infarcts there is minimal extravasation of erythrocytes but in haemorrhagic infarcts the larger perivascular haemorrhages are virtually confluent. The early acute swelling of pale infarcts is due mainly to the accumulation of interstitial fluid; this is followed by cellular infiltration. Experimentally, it has been found that irreversible changes can occur within five minutes of induced ischaemia. Chiang et al (1968) produced cerebral ischaemia in rabbits by clamping the aorta, and found that after five minutes some areas remained ischaemic when the blood supply was restored. They showed that many capillaries were obstructed by swelling of the feet of perivascular astrocytes and by bleb formation in the capillary endothelium. When ischaemia was prolonged for 15 minutes, half the brain failed to reperfuse (Digiacinto, Cantu and Cantu, 1970).

The cerebral infarct ceases to increase in size after four or five days. Microscopically it is seen to be infiltrated by numerous compound granular corpuscles. These cells are swollen microglia stuffed with products of degenerating myelin. Newly formed capillaries are prominent (Figure 3.1). Ultimately shrinkage, cavitation, and scarring in the surrounding tissue occur; glial fibres and collagen both contribute to the scar tissue. Most infarcts of any size show some central cavitation after three weeks and the cavity may be traversed by septa. Shrinkage of the lesion may distort either the surface convolutional pattern, the ventricles, or both.

SECONDARY EFFECTS OF INFARCTION

All recent cerebral infarcts are rapidly expanding lesions and haemorrhagic infarcts must occupy more space than would a pale infarct in the same territory. Most of the acute deaths and many of the clinical features of cerebral infarction are attributable to the rapid expansion of these lesions. When a

38   STROKES

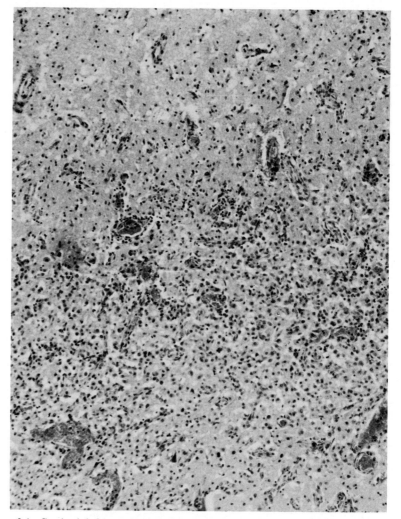

Figure 3.1. Cerebral infarct, sixth day. Infiltration by microglia and prominent small vessels. (Haematoxylin and Eosin × 100.)

sizeable infarct is examined at autopsy the affected hemisphere usually shows obvious swelling and flattening of the convolutions. Herniation of the ipsilateral cingulate gyrus across the midline beneath the free edge of the falx may result in a groove on the herniated gyrus. Pressure of the falx on this gyrus results in loss of neurons and, eventually, glial scarring occurs if survival is sufficiently prolonged. Downward displacement of the brain through the tentorial incisura results in herniation of the hippocampus which may show a well-marked groove or even obvious necrosis; again, loss of neurons or scarring may indicate previous herniation.

Another important effect of transtentorial herniation is compression of the posterior cerebral vessels with resulting infarction of a medial part of the ipsilateral occipital lobe. The infarct is usually haemorrhagic and a possible explanation of this is that, initially, the veins are obstructed and arterial occlusion occurs later. Adams (1967) states that patency of the posterior cerebral artery has been demonstrated angiographically just before death in patients showing these occipital lesions at autopsy (Figure 3.2).

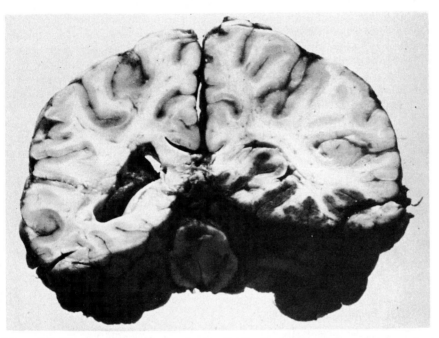

Figure 3.2. Haemorrhagic infarction in the distribution of the right posterior cerebral artery; the result of ipsilateral transtentorial herniation from supratentorial haemorrhage.

These changes are accompanied by distortion of the ventricular system and rotation of the corpus callosum; occasionally, compression of the contra-lateral cerebral peduncle results in haemorrhagic necrosis of this structure, thus giving rise to one of the false localising signs of expanding supratentorial lesions. Haemorrhage into the midbrain and pons are well recognised consequences of a rapidly expanding supratentorial lesion. These haemor-rhages may be multiple and small or large and confluent, and it is now widely accepted that they are a consequence of rupture of small arteries which become stretched by caudal displacement of the brain stem (Johnson and Yates, 1956).

Haemorrhage may also occur into the oculomotor nerve where it crosses the posterior cerebral artery. These and other phenomena can result from any rapidly expanding supratentorial lesion and are seen in primary cerebral haemorrhage, tumour, trauma, and in many cases of ruptured berry aneurysm. Detailed consideration of the secondary effects of brain swelling and of the structural changes and physiological consequences of raised intracranial pressure will be found in Miller and Adams's (1972) review.

Varieties of cerebral infarcts and their pathogenesis

When perfusion of an area of brain is reduced by local obstruction of a cerebral artery, the inflow of blood from an adjacent arterial territory through anastomotic vessels will often reduce the size of the area infarcted or may occasionally prevent infarction from occurring. If, however, there is an overall perfusion failure, the area of brain at the periphery of the two adjacent underperfused territories suffers most and may become the site of infarction.

Two groups of brain infarcts can, therefore, be recognised: those lying within the area of supply of one of the cerebral arteries, and the so-called watershed or boundary zone infarcts (see later section) situated at or near to the junction of two major arterial territories.

We shall apply the term *single territory infarcts* to lesions lying *within* the area of supply of a cerebral artery. We include, of course, cases where more than one 'single territory' is involved; for example, simultaneous infarction in the middle and anterior cerebral artery territories.

Single territory infarcts will be subdivided into (1) *occlusive single territory infarcts*, where occlusion of the territorial artery is considered responsible though it may no longer be demonstrable at autopsy, and (2) *non-occlusive single territory infarcts*, in which there is no evidence to suggest that occlusion of the territorial artery has occurred.

We exclude from the present discussion very small randomly distributed infarcts resulting from various forms of angiitis or microemboli; e.g. fat embolism.

Occlusive single territory infarcts

When autopsy reveals a cerebral artery occluded by embolus or thrombus the mechanism of infarction is clear but a central problem has been the brain infarct where occlusion of the relevant artery is not demonstrated. Thus, Foix, Hillemand and Ley (1927) examined 63 infarcted brains and found an occluded cerebral artery in only 2, and in 100 infarcted brains studied by Hicks and Warren (1951) no occluded vessel was found in 60 of them.

Confusion is caused, and understanding of the pathogenesis of infarction has been delayed, by the continuing use of the term cerebral thrombosis as a virtual synonym for cerebral infarction. It is, of course, now well established that many infarcts that would formerly have been considered examples of cerebral artery thrombosis are a result of propagation thrombosis from the internal carotid or vertebral arteries. Again, many cases of infarction without demonstrable cerebral arterial occlusion result from embolisation.

CEREBRAL EMBOLISM

The frequency of cerebral embolism was for long underestimated for two reasons. In the first place it was not sufficiently appreciated how rapidly emboli could disintegrate, and the angiographic techniques capable of demonstrating their impaction and dissolution have been applied only in recent years. In the second place the importance of the neck vessels, aorta, and heart as embolic sources was not fully realised. Two groups of cases have presented problems to pathologists. Firstly, there were cases of recognisable embolism of a cerebral artery and resulting brain infarction in which they found no embolic source, and, secondly, there were cases with one or more embolic sources and brain infarcts with features associated with embolism but no embolus could be found.

Recognition of emboli or thrombi at autopsy. When recent, local thrombotic occlusion presents as a red laminated intravascular plug broadly attached to the arterial wall, and if more than a few days old, invasion by capillaries and fibroblasts occurs over a wide segment of the vessel.

A recent embolus is usually softer than a locally formed thrombus and may consist of a detached fragment of propagation thrombus only. It is usually free from the vessel wall, or, at most, attached over a small segment only. Microscopically it may show platelets and leucocytes entrapped in strands of fibrin. Fibroblasts and endothelial cells may be present, but they must not derive from the arterial walls. There must be no local angiitis, but we would not insist on the absence of local atheroma provided the atheromatous plaque was clearly not involved in the occlusion.

Castaigne et al (1973) classified as old emboli thrombi occluding the artery and surrounded by a normal elastica and a normal outer vessel wall, when found in association with haemorrhagic infarction and an embolic source. Old organised emboli and organised local thrombi are indistinguishable on microscopy and both thrombi and emboli may become incorporated in the arterial wall, where they may form an atherosclerotic plaque (Duguid, 1949; Peters and Chandler, 1971).

The increasing recognition of embolic cerebral infarction. Chiari (1905) had encountered the problem of middle cerebral artery embolism in which no source for the embolus could be discovered and after examining the internal carotid arteries in 400 unselected autopsies found thrombosis in 7, and 4 of these had produced cerebral emboli. Hultquist (1942) found 38 cases of carotid occlusion in 1300 unselected autopsies. Examination of the carotids, however, remained largely neglected for some time. Thus, in the 100 cases with cerebral infarcts reported by Hicks and Warren (1951), in which they failed to find an occluded cerebral vessel, no mention is made of the carotid arteries, although the autopsies were described as complete.

We owe the beginning of renewed interest in the neck vessels largely to Fisher (1951). He remarked that in case after case of cerebral infarction coming to autopsy he failed to confirm the clinical impression of disease of the middle cerebral artery, and in 200 of these cases he found no thrombosis of this vessel. He described 8 cases of atheromatous carotid artery occlusion, and emphasised the occurrence of associated thrombosis. Later, Fisher (1954) described 4 cases of cerebral embolism arising from thrombus in the carotid sinus.

Further support for the role of embolism in brain infarction was provided by Symonds and MacKenzie (1957) whose paper on cortical blindness is a model of clinical and pathological correlation. The bilateral calcarine infarcts found at autopsy in these cases are sometimes of different ages and the visual field loss from the first infarct may have passed unnoticed. Often, however, the infarcts have obviously occurred simultaneously, when immediate cortical blindness results. The mechanism remained a mystery until Symonds and MacKenzie pointed out that embolism through the basilar artery or originating in it provided the explanation. In 8 out of the 9 cases they described the source of embolism was found at autopsy. Symonds (1927) had previously recorded 2 patients with subclavian artery thrombosis who developed contralateral hemiplegia of sudden onset which he attributed to embolism.

A paper by Gunning et al (1964a) drew attention to the importance of mural internal carotid thrombus in cerebral embolism and indicated the role of platelet emboli in causing recurrent and often transient symptoms.

The autopsy diagnosis of cerebral embolism in the absence of an occluded vessel must be based on circumstantial evidence; e.g. multiplicity and haemorrhagic character of the brain infarcts, healthy cerebral arteries, demonstrable embolic source, and evidence of embolism in other organs. The disintegration and disappearance of the occluding embolus appeared plausible and the demonstration of embolic fragments within the infarct supported this assumption. Experimental brain emboli had been shown to disappear (Hill et al, 1955), but the final proof that these events actually occurred awaited their demonstration by angiography.

Bladin (1964), Dalal et al (1965), and Dalal, Shah and Aiyar (1965) showed that angiographically demonstrable emboli could disintegrate or disappear, often quite rapidly. Dalal, Shah and Aiyar (1965) demonstrated an embolus angiographically nine hours after the ictus, which, in a second angiogram taken 10 minutes later, had disappeared. An embolus shown angiographically three days after the ictus was not demonstrable at autopsy seven days later although haemorrhagic infarction was present in the territory of the previously occluded vessel. Zatz et al (1965) found a middle cerebral artery occlusion angiographically which could not be demonstrated at autopsy three days later although there was infarction in the middle cerebral artery territory.

Frequency of embolic infarction.   Although there has been increasing recognition of the importance of embolism, estimates of the proportion of infarcts resulting from it have differed greatly. There must clearly be a difference of opinion and interpretation between pathologists who are prepared to diagnose embolism on strong circumstantial evidence and those who insist on the demonstration of the embolus. It is clear, if only from the angiographic evidence, that the last group will underestimate the frequency of embolism.

Adams and vander Eecken (1953) thought about 50 per cent of brain infarcts were embolic, and Lhermitte, Gautier and Derouesné (1970) found 68 per cent of 41 middle cerebral artery occlusions that were embolic.

Bhattacharjii (1965) who made a detailed examination of the heart, aorta, neck vessels, and cerebral arteries in 57 infarcted brains thought embolism might be the cause in 68 per cent.

The sources of cerebral emboli

One of us (McCall, 1967) reviewed 11 500 autopsies performed at the North Staffordshire Royal Infirmary from 1946 to 1966; there were brain infarcts in 581 cases (N.S.R.I. series). The mean age of cases with infarcts was 65.3 years. The autopsy material examined by Bhattacharji (1965) was included. The cervical internal carotid arteries were inspected in all cases, and in 90 the entire lengths of the carotid and vertebral arteries were examined. In 338 (58 per cent) a possible source of brain embolism was recorded.

Table 3.1 shows the distribution of the potential embolic sources; often more than one was found. When thrombus was found in the neck vessels it was given precedence over the aorta or heart. Cardiac lesions were given precedence over aortic lesions.

Table 3.1. Potential sources of embolism in 581 autopsies on patients with brain infarcts.

Embolic source	Infarcted brains (%)
No source of embolism found	42
Heart disease	34
Thrombi in carotid, vertebral, innominate, or subclavian arteries	12
Aortic thrombi	8
Paradoxical embolism	4

It is not claimed that when an embolic source was found the infarct was necessarily embolic. In fact, some with neck vessel thrombi were demonstrably due to propagation thrombosis, and many infarcts were too old for critical assessment. It is felt, however, that a retrospective review of this kind will have underestimated the role of embolism. In the earlier years, the observers were not searching for embolic sources with special diligence, and examination of the neck vessels was incomplete in all but 90 cases.

CARDIAC EMBOLI

In all published series the heart has provided more emboli than any other source. Blackwood et al (1969) found that cardiac emboli accounted for 46 per cent of all their carotid strokes and the observations of Vost, Wolochow, and Howell (1964) suggest that the incidence of embolism in all varieties of heart disease may be higher than is suspected. These authors studied the incidence of cerebral infarcts in patients dying from various heart diseases. The infarcts were sought in thin slices of fixed brain, if necessary using a hand lens. There is no doubt that these workers discovered infarcts that would not have been found in a routine autopsy. They examined the brains of 340 patients dying with heart disease and found that 53.8 per cent had brain infarcts compared with 12 per cent of 100 patients who were free from heart disease. As the average age of the controls was seven years less than that of the heart disease group they compared 99 patients in each group matched for age and sex. The incidence of brain infarcts in the heart disease group was more than three times than that in the controls—39 per cent against 12 per cent. The incidence of infarcts within the different varieties of heart disease is shown in Table 3.2, which is taken from their paper. Apart from the very high incidence of infarcts in bacterial endocarditis the incidence of brain infarcts in the other varieties of heart disease is surprisingly similar. They found that mural thrombi in the left heart chambers had only the same incidence of brain infarcts as the whole series, though cases with atrial thrombi only did have a higher incidence. Congestive cardiac failure did not increase the

Table 3.2. Incidence of cerebral infarction in patients with various forms of heart disease.

Disorder	No. of patients	No. with cerebral infarction	Percentage with cerebral infarction
Old myocardial infarction	133	80	60.2
Fresh myocardial infarction (without evidence of old myocardial infarction)	39	19	48.7
Pure hypertensive heart disease	55	28	50.9
Pure chronic cor pulmonale	18	6	33.3
Cardiomyopathy	32	16	50
Myocarditis	10	5	50
Thrombotic non-bacterial endocarditis	10	5	50
Bacterial endocarditis	10	9	90
Rheumatic heart disease	22	8	36.4
Other forms of heart disease	11	7	62.7
All forms of heart disease	340	183	53.8
Heart disease with hypertension	123	65	52

From Vost, A., Wolochow, D. A. & Howell, D. A. (1964), *Journal of Pathology and Bacteriology*, **88**, 465, with kind permission of the authors.

incidence of brain infarcts in the whole series or in the largest sub-group, i.e. cases with old cardiac infarcts. The severity of the cardiac lesion did not, therefore, appear to be a determining factor. None of their cases gave a history suggesting a hypotensive episode and only 24 arterial occlusions were found in association with 340 infarcts. They thought that embolisation from the heart must be the explanation for most of the brain infarcts in their material. This implies that hearts diseased from any cause are liable to develop mural thrombi which will often have disappeared or become un-recognisable at autopsy. We think the explanation of their findings offered by Vost and his colleagues is reasonable.

In the N.S.R.I. series half the potential embolic sources lay in the heart. A breakdown of the cardiac lesions in this series is given in Table 3.3.

Table 3.3. Varieties of lesions found in 198 hearts with potential sources of embolism, in 581 autopsies on patients with brain infarcts.

Nature of heart lesion	Total cardiac embolic sources (%)
Myocardial infarcts, old and recent	50
Rheumatic heart disease	26
Congestive cardiomyopathy, myocarditis, and unexplained cardiac thrombi	15
Infective endocarditis	7
Thrombotic endocarditis	2
Atrial myxoma	1 case

Ischaemic heart disease. In the N.S.R.I. series, 50 per cent of the embolic cardiac sources were associated with ischaemic heart disease, and we have already noted the high incidence of brain infarcts found by Vost et al in this group, i.e. 60 per cent of old myocardial infarcts and 49 per cent in recent cases.

The persistent menace of cardiac thrombi following myocardial infarction deserves emphasis. It is not uncommon for cardiac lesions to have been forgotten when a stroke occurs some years later. Hymen and Parsonnet (1932) noted the long interval that might elapse and described basilar embolism from cardiac thrombus five years after the myocardial infarction.

Rheumatic heart disease. In the N.S.R.I. series rheumatic heart disease provided potential embolic sources in 26 per cent of the abnormal hearts with brain infarcts. Vost and his colleagues found brain infarcts in 36 per cent of patients with rheumatic heart disease.

Mitral stenotics may produce emboli indefinitely. Figure 3.3 shows a thrombus in an atrial appendage amputated during mitral valvotomy. The collagenous base indicates that it is of longstanding but there is a freshly formed friable platelet leucocyte thrombus on the surface providing a ready source of emboli.

Wood (1968) stated that up to 14 per cent of mitral stenotics developed embolism and 60 per cent of the emboli were cerebral, while Fleming and Bailey (1971) have drawn attention to the high incidence in patients with sinus rhythm and in those with rheumatic mitral incompetence. It is not always possible to demonstrate an atrial thrombus at autopsy when there is unequivocal evidence of cerebral embolism from mitral stenosis. Wood (1968) stated that in 36 per cent of cases with a history of embolism no atrial thrombus could be found.

Congestive cardiomyopathy, myocarditis, and unexplained cardiac thrombi. No attempt was made in the N.S.R.I. series to distinguish between these conditions, and together they accounted for 15 per cent of potential emboli originating in the heart. In the paper by Vost and his colleagues, cardiomyopathy and myocarditis are listed separately and in each group 50 per cent were associated with brain infarcts. Batsakie (1968) estimates that 50 per cent of patients with congestive cardiomyopathy are found at autopsy to have systemic emboli.

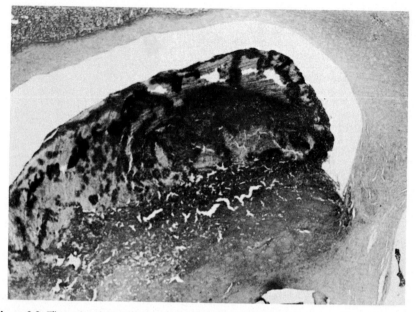

Figure 3.3. Thrombus in left atrial appendage excised during mitral valvotomy. (Carstair's trichrome stain × 14.5). It is an old thrombus with a collagenised base but there is a substantial cap of recently formed leucocyte-platelet thrombus that is a ready source of embolism.

Infective endocarditis. The incidence of systemic embolism is high in this disease (Spain, 1968) and brain emboli outnumber all others. Vost and his colleagues found the highest incidence of brain infarcts (90 per cent) in this group. It accounted for 7 per cent of cardiac emboli in the N.S.R.I. series (from 1946 to 1966); all cerebral infarcts in this group were considered embolic. Although its incidence has been greatly reduced in the last two decades the diagnosis is not infrequently delayed or, occasionally, even overlooked in the elderly, in whom it may present as an unexplained cerebral infarction.

Thrombotic endocarditis. Sterile thrombotic vegetations are encountered almost exclusively in the left heart, where they are found on the line of closure of the mitral or aortic valve; they are occasionally attached to the atrial endocardium. They do not deform the valve and their clinical manifestations are exclusively embolic. The emboli are usually quite small and are unlikely to cause trouble except when they obstruct cerebral or coronary arteries.

Thrombotic vegetations may be found in cachectic individuals and in patients dying slowly from a variety of diseases and have a well-recognised association with carcinoma. MacDonald and Robbins (1957) reviewed 18 486 autopsies and found 78 cases with thrombotic endocarditis, 8 of whom had brain emboli. The highest incidence was in the seventh and eighth decades. Cancer of the stomach, lung, and pancreas, were the tumours most frequently responsible.

Although most commonly encountered in advanced malignant disease, thrombotic vegetations sometimes develop while the growth is small and localised. In this respect thrombotic endocarditis resembles the unexplained venous thrombi and thrombophlebitis migrans that sometimes herald malignant disease.

Barron, Siqueira and Hirano (1960) found that thrombotic endocarditis accounted for 10 per cent of the cerebral infarcts in their autopsy material. This high figure is attributable to the high incidence of terminal malignant disease in the Montefiori Hospital.

Vost and his colleagues found that 50 per cent of their cases with this condition had cerebral emboli. The predilection for the old-age group and the association with malignancy will determine the incidence of thrombotic endocarditis in any autopsy series; in the N.S.R.I. series it provided only 2 per cent of the total probable cerebral emboli. It is, however, the commonest cause of stroke attributable to extracranial malignancy.

Cardiac myxoma. This is an uncommon cause of brain embolism; we have observed three cases. The first (which is included in the N.S.R.I. series) occurred in the early days of valvotomy when an unsuspected left atrial myxoma was explored and vertebral embolism followed. The second case was a child, aged 8 years at death, who died from middle cerebral embolism and had suffered a previous embolic episode. Atrial myxoma was again responsible.

The third case was an example of the rare ventricular myxoma. This case had multiple emboli and was recorded by Danta and Williams (1969).

Paradoxical embolism

Paradoxical embolism is only occasionally mentioned in discussing cerebral embolism. In the N.S.R.I. series it was thought to be the cause of cerebral infarction in 24 cases (4 per cent). This high incidence reflects the special interest in the condition within the department; in each case the diagnosis was made at the time by the pathologist conducting the autopsy.

Thompson and Evans (1930) pointed out that nearly all paradoxical emboli traverse the atrial septum and transit usually occurs through a patent foramen ovale guarded by a left atrial flap-valve that is normally closed because the pressure in the left atrium is higher than in the right. This is so. Embolism through atrial defects with two-way patency makes a much smaller contribution and the contribution from other forms of congenital heart defects is negligible.

Thompson and Evans adopted the earlier suggestion of Beattie (1925) that right to left passage of an embolus might occur when a pulmonary embolism transiently raised the pressure in the right atrium and so opened the valve. They thought about 30 per cent occlusion of the pulmonary arterial tree was necessary to open the valve.

In one of our cases with a valvular foramen ovale there was chronic pulmonary hypertension, a right atrial appendage thrombus, but no pulmonary embolism. Huber (1965) has drawn attention to the importance of chronic pulmonary hypertension in facilitating the passage of emboli through the atrial septum. Our remaining cases all complied with Thompson and Evans's criterion of 30 per cent embolic occlusion of the pulmonary arteries in cases with a valvular foramen, although we now think that paradoxical passage may occur without the assistance of this valve-springing mechanism. Thompson and Evans found probe patency of the foramen in 29 per cent and pencil patency in 6 per cent of adults.

At autopsy the presence of venous thrombus, pulmonary embolism and infarction of several organs provide suggestive evidence of paradoxical embolism. It is, of course, necessary to exclude other possible sources of systemic emboli. Cases with atrial fibrillation or chronic lung sepsis are excluded and the pulmonary veins must be inspected for thrombi.

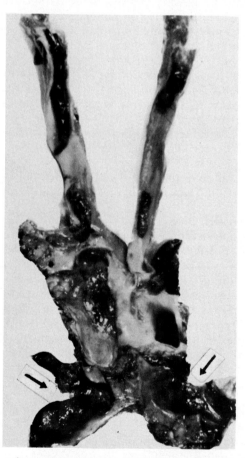

Figure 3.4. Massive pulmonary and paradoxical embolism. Arrows show left and right pulmonary arteries completely occupied by embolus. Two paradoxical emboli are seen in each carotid and one in the left subclavian artery. Valvular foramen ovale admitted a 1.5 cm 'probe'. (Dr C. R. Knappett's case.)

It should be emphasised that it is not necessary to find thrombus in the foramen to make the diagnosis. The massive paradoxical emboli shown in Figure 3.4 make the point; the heart was free from thrombus in this case. We have found emboli astride the foramen nine times in an extended series of cases (Figures 3.5, 3.6, 3.7), and free in the left ventricle once. It is astonishing how tightly an embolus may be gripped by the slit-like passage through the atrial septum (Figure 3.5). Trapped emboli may give rise to recurrent episodes of systemic embolism (Le Mar, 1962), but in several of our examples, and in others in the literature, entrapment was clearly a premortal event and systemic embolism had apparently not occurred.

Huber (1965) estimated that about 8 per cent of systemic emboli might be paradoxical, and the brain is certainly the commonest site for paradoxical systemic embolism. In 34 cases that we observed in an extended series, 25 had brain emboli. Thompson and Evans suggested that paradoxical embolism accounted for about 4 per cent of cerebral emboli.

Pulmonary embolism is the commonest cause of death in patients with paradoxical embolism and the cerebral lesion easily escapes clinical recognition in patients dying in this way. In other cases, however, the cerebral catastrophe overshadows the pulmonary embolism, but any evidence suggesting this combination of lesions should suggest the diagnosis. Recurrent paradoxical cerebral embolism may occur after an interval. In one of our cases a woman developed hemiplegia four days after injection of varicose veins. She died four years later, and at autopsy had a pulmonary embolism from varicose veins, a fresh middle cerebral embolism, and a valvular foramen ovale. We believed that both strokes were due to paradoxical embolism.

CAROTID ARTERY EMBOLISM AND THROMBOSIS

Some 22 per cent of carotid strokes result from cardiac emboli as compared with 9 per cent of strokes involving the vertebrobasilar territory (Castaigne et al, 1970).

Large cardiac emboli may block the internal carotid artery at its origin where they straddle the common carotid bifurcation. Smaller emboli may block the entrance of the petrous canal or the bifurcation of the internal carotid, which is the commonest site of arrest. Smaller emboli still often arrest in the middle cerebral artery trifurcation. Embolism in any of these situations is likely to be followed by a thrombosis and occlusion, if this was not already complete. Occlusion of the internal carotids by thrombus, whatever its pathogenesis, may cause infarction of the brain by its haemodynamic consequences, by release of emboli, or by propagation of thrombus beyond the Circle of Willis. We are at present concerned only with the last two mechanisms. The first is considered elsewhere (p. 65ff.).

Atherosclerosis of the internal carotid arteries. Atherosclerosis accounts for the great majority of thromboses in the internal carotid arteries. Severe atherosclerosis is seen in the carotid sinus more frequently than in any other site, and ulceration, calcification, and haemorrhage into atheromatous plaques are common in this situation. As with comparable arteries, raised

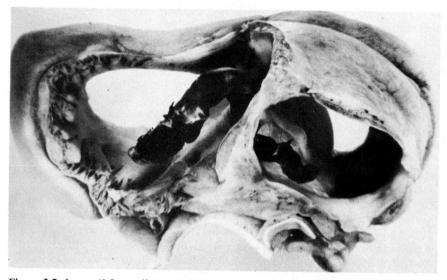

Figure 3.5. Large (1.0 cm diameter) embolus in transit through valvular foramen ovale which grips it tightly. Death from pulmonary embolism. (Dr T. L. Marshall's case.)

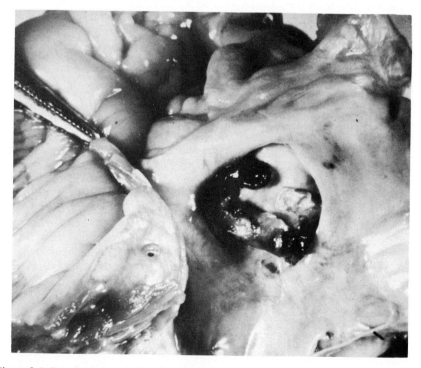

Figure 3.6. Paradoxical embolism in transit through valvular foramen ovale. View from right atrium.

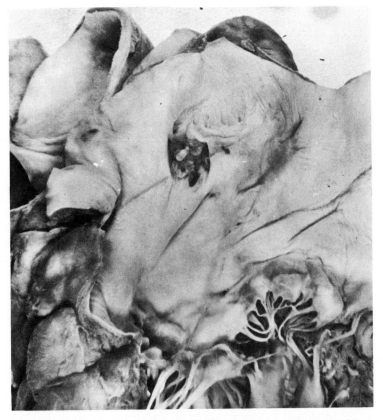

Figure 3.7. View from left atrium of paradoxical embolus shown in Figure 3.6, emerging from foramen ovale.

atheromatous plaques are very frequently associated with an inflammatory reaction extending to the adventitia and its surrounding connective tissues. Fibrosis, increased vascularity, and lymphocytic infiltration were seen by Mitchell and Schwartz (1965) in some 70 per cent of the blocks they examined from vessels affected by atherosclerosis. This lesion is particularly common in relation to the carotid sinus and accounts for the frequent observation by surgeons of the adhesion of this vessel to the surrounding structures. The tortuous terminal portion of the vessel is the next most severely affected, and calcification is commoner here than in any other part of the artery. Thrombosis starts most frequently in these two sites and there is agreement between all observers that pre-existing stenosis is a most important predisposing cause of thrombotic occlusion.

In our experience, the sinus is the commonest site for thrombosis and in this we are in agreement with Yates and Hutchinson (1961) and with Lhermitte, Gautier and Derouesné (1966). Torvik and Jörgensen (1966) found that the incidence of brain infarction was the same whether the intracranial or extracranial part of the vessel was occluded.

Emboli either originating in, or passing through, the carotid most commonly enter the middle cerebral artery, and isolated anterior cerebral emboli are much less frequent. Infarction of the posterior cerebral artery territory may occasionally occur when the vessel arises from the internal carotid (p. 14). Small emboli usually reach the cortical branches; large emboli may impact proximal to the ganglionic branches and infarction of deep grey matter and most of the middle cerebral artery territory follows.

Propagation thrombosis and embolism from thrombotic carotid occlusions. Anterograde propagation thrombosis beyond the Circle of Willis is a common mechanism of cerebral infarction. The extent of the infarct depends on whether or not the thrombus extends to block the anterior and posterior communicating vessels as well as the middle cerebral artery. Hultquist (1942) remarked on the large size of infarcts when thrombus extended beyond the origin of the anterior cerebral vessels. It might be supposed that reduction in the diameter of the communicating vessels from atherosclerosis would influence the size of the infarcts observed, but Torvik and Jörgensen (1966) found no evidence to support this from their autopsy studies. They found that brain infarction was about equally common whether the carotid was occluded within the skull or in the neck, but that the intracranial thrombotic occlusions produced the larger infarct. They attributed this to the greater tendency of the intracranial thrombi to block the Circle of Willis. In 21 cases in which the circle was blocked, 17 of the thrombotic occlusions were intracranial, but in cases with no blocks in the Circle of Willis only 13 out of 22 had intracranial thromboses.

The relative frequency of embolism and thrombus propagation from carotid thrombi in cases with cerebral infarction has been variously estimated. In the N.S.R.I. series, 54 brain infarcts were found to be associated with thrombotic lesions in the appropriate carotid artery. In 22 of these, propagation thrombosis had occurred beyond the Circle of Willis, in 14 the middle cerebral artery was embolised, and in 18 there was uncertainty about the role of the carotid thrombus as there was an alternative source of cerebral embolism. Lhermitte, Gautier and Derouesne (1966) found that when atherosclerotic occlusive thrombosis of the carotid was the primary event, embolism was finally responsible for about half the middle cerebral artery occlusions.

The most detailed study of the pathology of internal carotid occlusion is that reported by Castaigne et al (1970) who analysed the autopsy data on 50 patients with these lesions. Thirteen of the occlusions were embolic and of these 11 originated in the heart. All the atherosclerotic occlusions resulted from thrombosis in or near the pre-existing stenosis; 73 per cent of the stenoses were tight. The commonest site for thrombosis was the carotid sinus, and here a tight stenosis was found in 90 per cent of the cases. In about 1 in 4 of the whole series, anterograde thrombosis extended from the site of primary thrombotic or embolic occlusion beyond the bifurcation of the internal carotid artery. As was to be expected when thrombus extended beyond the internal carotid bifurcation large infarcts were common. The mean survival in this group with large infarcts was ten days, and the main cause of death was temporal lobe herniation. When propagation thrombosis was arrested before the bifurcation or discrete embolism had occurred into the middle cerebral artery causing the infarction, large infarcts were uncommon and the mean survival was 63 days. These observers found that angiographic evidence of filling of the ophthalmic artery always indicated that the propagation thrombus had been arrested below this vessel. They found that anterograde thrombosis from thrombus starting in the sinus might reach the internal carotid bifurcation in a matter of hours. Torvik and Jörgensen (1964), while agreeing that propagation thrombosis could be very rapid, pointed out that it did not necessarily extend up to the skull even after a considerable time, and in one case it measured only 2 cm after six weeks. In 13 of the cases described by Castaigne et al with anterograde thrombosis, the occlusion in six stopped below the ophthalmic artery, in two it was short of the posterior communicating artery, in three it extended into the middle cerebral artery, and in two into the middle cerebral and anterior cerebral arteries. Eleven of the 25 cases with thrombotic occlusion finally had embolic infarction from detachment of a portion of the thrombus.

Transient ischaemia and prodromal symptoms in carotid strokes. Fisher (1967) drew attention to the fact that the ictus from embolic infarction did not always appear as a bolt from the blue and one or more ischaemic attacks might occur in the preceding 24 hours. There is now ample evidence that recurrent transient ischaemia occurs from release of unstable emboli, most often from the carotid sinus, and it is probable that platelets are the main constituent of these emboli. It is reasonable to suppose, though difficult to establish, that the release of very small unstable emboli from carotid thrombi may be responsible for the premonitory ischaemic symptoms immediately preceding the ictus, whether final cerebral artery occlusion results from embolism or from a propagation thrombosis. It seems very likely that emboli passing through the carotids (for example from the heart) and entering the middle cerebral artery would be associated with an abrupt onset, while emboli arrested in the carotid might be accompanied by prodromata consequent upon the thrombosis that follows the arrest of the embolus. Torvik and Jörgensen (1966) paid special attention to the presence of platelet aggregates in the leptomeningeal vessels in infarcted areas. They found such aggregates in nearly all infarctions with an intermittent, stepwise, or gradual onset, but in only a third of those with a sudden onset.

Injury and manipulation of the carotid artery in relation to infarction. Strokes have been observed following manipulation of the carotid sinus and the evidence points clearly to an embolic mechanism. Most cases are, no doubt, due to detachment of thrombus but atheromatous embolism has also contributed. Askey (1946) collected 7 cases of hemiplegia following stimulation of the sinus. Calverley and Millikan (1961) reviewed the literature. They pointed out that all the infarctions occurred on the manipulated side so that haemodynamic failure from cardiac inhibition was an unlikely explanation.

Thrombosis of the carotid and subsequent cerebral infarction may follow either closed or open neck injuries. The so-called 'pencil' injuries that occur when children fall with a pencil or similar object in the mouth are well recognised. They result from injury to the carotid in the region of the tonsillar fossa.

We have observed two cases of middle cerebral embolism in young men following carotid injury and thrombosis. One attempted to hang himself by leaping through a window with a rope fastened round his neck. He died a week later from middle cerebral embolism. The second patient was wounded in the neck and developed dense hemiplegia within 24 hours. In each case middle cerebral embolism followed thrombosis in the internal carotid artery in relation to an intimal tear (Figure 3.8). Hughes and Brownell (1968) have reviewed the literature on traumatic carotid occlusion.

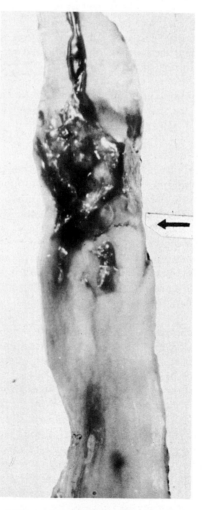

Figure 3.8. Traumatic carotid thrombosis. Left middle cerebral embolism within 24 hours of open injury to the neck. Arrow points to intimal tear at origin of internal carotid artery. Small mural thrombus in common carotid.

Crawford (1956) discussed the complications of angiography. In 75 cases coming to autopsy he found occlusive thrombosis in 4 cases in a single carotid and in 1 patient both vessels were occluded. All these cases had advanced atherosclerosis. In the same series he encountered 9 dissecting aneurysms. Bilateral dissecting aneurysms following angiography were observed by us in a patient with a cerebral glioma (Figure 3.9). Middle cerebral artery infarction resulted.

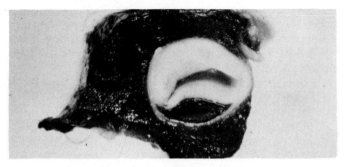

Figure 3.9. Dissecting aneurysm from angiography. The lumen is compressed by the crescentic mural haematoma. There is a large haematoma in the carotid sheath. About 3.2 times natural size.

Vertebral artery embolism and thrombosis

The role of the vertebral arteries in cerebral infarction. The difficulties attendant upon the complete examination of the vertebral arteries at autopsy account for the relatively scanty information about these vessels compared with the carotids. Hutchinson and Yates (1956) were the first to make a systematic examination of the vertebral arteries. They examined these vessels throughout their lengths after decalcifying the spine and skull base in a 100 patients with clinical evidence of cerebrovascular disease. They were followed by Schwartz and Mitchell (1961) who dealt with unselected autopsies.

It was plain from these studies that the vertebral arteries were very frequently the site of severe atherosclerosis, not only in people with cerebrovascular lesions but also in those without. Additional studies were made by Fisher et al (1965a), by Bhattacharji (1965), and by Bhattacharji, Hutchinson and McCall (1967a). Mitchell and Schwartz (1965) found that one patient in four in an unselected autopsy series, aged 35 years and over, had severe stenosis of the vertebral arteries and the other observers quoted are in broad agreement. The first part of the vertebral artery was found by Mitchell and Schwartz to be the most common site for severe stenosis but Fisher et al (1965a) and Bhattacharji, Hutchinson and McCall found the ostium most often severely affected. The terminal portion comprising the tortuous and intracranial parts was found by Bhattacharji, Hutchinson and McCall (1967a) to be a frequent site of severe atheromatous lesions. Mitchell and Schwartz pointed out that there is a higher incidence of severe narrowing in the vertebral arteries than in the carotids because the diameter of these vessels is so much less and small plaques produce relatively severe obstruction. Ulceration is, however, much less common than in the carotids.

Fisher et al (1965a) thought that intracranial vertebral artery occlusions were commonly associated with brain infarcts but occlusions of these vessels in the neck, in marked contrast with cervical carotid occlusions, were not. In a later paper, Fisher (1970) described cases with bilateral occlusion of the first part of the vertebral arteries and recurrent transient symptoms of brainstem ischaemia similar to those found with subclavian steal.

Infarction in the vertebral and basilar territories. Haemodynamic mechanisms are discussed elsewhere (p. 65ff.); we are concerned here with embolism via the vertebral arteries and the basilar artery, and thrombosis in these vessels with subsequent embolism or propagation thrombosis.

The most complete account and discussion of vertebrobasilar occlusion is given in the detailed paper by Castaigne et al (1970) who dealt both with vertebral and basilar occlusions. They studied 44 patients with thrombotic occlusions of one or more of these vessels, half of which had caused infarctions. In 5, the cause of the occlusion remained uncertain, 35 resulted from primary thrombosis associated with atheroma, and in 4, cardiac emboli were responsible. They pointed out that only 9 per cent of vertebral and/or basilar occlusions resulted from cardiac emboli as against 22 per cent in the carotids. They noted the almost invariable location of occlusive thrombi in or very near to severe stenosis and found that 90 per cent of these stenoses were tight, whereas in the carotids only 73 per cent of the stenoses associated with thrombosis were tight.

The terminal portion of the vessel (from the second cervical vertebra to the junction with the contralateral vessel) was the site of primary thrombosis in 12 cases. The proximal portion showed 4 primary thromboses and the intermediate (intraosseous) portion only one.

Propagation thrombosis in the vertebral arteries. Castaigne et al found that anterograde thrombosis might spread to the junction with the contralateral vessel; it might then spread into the basilar artery, or, finally, even extend into a posterior cerebral artery. In agreement with Yates and Hutchinson (1961) they found that thrombus originating in the first (proximal) part of the vertebral artery very rarely extended throughout the entire length of the vessel. Hutchinson and Yates thought this limited propagation might be related to the numerous branches given off in the intravertebral canal. Castaigne and his colleagues gave details of anterograde thrombosis in 6 patients and thought it had determined infarction in 3 of them.

Thrombotic and embolic basilar artery occlusion. Castaigne and his colleagues found 18 occlusions of the basilar artery, one of which was embolic. The remaining 17 occlusions were thrombotic and 14 of them were at the site of atherosclerotic stenoses.

Propagation thrombosis from the basilar artery. Both retrograde and anterograde thrombosis may occur. There was retrograde thrombosis in 28.5 per cent of the 18 cases in Castaigne's series; it is likely to occlude the posterior inferior cerebellar artery and the medullary branches of the vertebrals. Anterograde thrombosis was found in 7 of Castaigne's cases.

Castaigne et al considered, especially, the effect of patency of the opposite vertebral artery and the Circle of Willis in limiting anterograde thrombosis from the basilar artery. They concluded that patency of a vertebral artery had some limiting effect but it could not be relied upon to arrest propagation.

Embolism from basilar artery thrombi. The posterior cerebral artery was embolised in two of the cases described by Castaigne et al. They emphasised that the usual cause of posterior cerebral artery occlusion was embolism from a basilar or vertebral artery thrombus. This is in accord with the observations of Symonds and MacKenzie (1957).

In the case illustrated in Figure 3.10, bilateral occipital lobe infarction followed vertebral artery thrombosis by propagation of thrombus through the basilar into one posterior cerebral artery, and by embolism into its fellow on the opposite side.

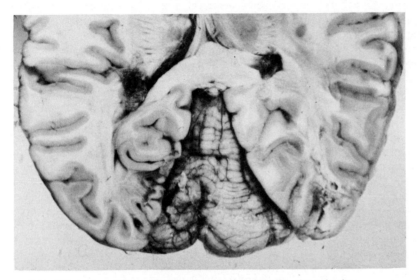

Figure 3.10. Bilateral occipital infarction from vertebral artery thrombosis.

Embolism from subclavian and innominate arteries

There is a high incidence of atherosclerosis in the subclavian and innominate arteries. Bhattercharji, Hutchinson and McCall (1967a) found atheroma in over 90 per cent of these vessels in 145 bodies of average age about 66 years, but severe stenosis was uncommon. Unlike the carotid and vertebral arteries there was no significant difference between the severity and prevalence of atherosclerosis in the subclavians and innominate arteries in patients with and without brain infarction. Indeed, disease of the subclavian arteries makes only a very small contribution to cerebral infarction.

Spontaneous thrombosis may occur in the subclavian vessels but cervical rib and trauma account for most cases. In an angiographic study, Callow et al (1968) found the incidence of thrombosis in the left subclavian to be three times greater than in the right. In spite of this, most brain infarcts attributed to subclavian thrombosis have, because of the differing anatomical arrangements, been associated with thrombosis in the right subclavian artery. Symonds (1927) described two cases of thrombosis of the right subclavian artery with contralateral hemiplegia that he attributed to embolism. In the N.S.R.I. series embolism was seen from spontaneous thrombosis of the innominate artery once and the subclavian once. Most of the recorded cases of cerebral embolism from subclavian thrombosis have been associated with cervical ribs, but it is an uncommon complication. Gunning et al (1964b), who discussed exhaustively the role of embolism in the upper limb in patients with cervical rib, did not encounter brain embolism in their material. Shucksmith (1963) drew attention to the syndrome and de Villiers (1966) reviewed 8 published cases and added one of his own. Clearly the vertebral artery can be embolised from thrombi in either subclavian artery and, of course, emboli traversing either vertebral artery may infarct either or both posterior cerebral vessels. All the cases reviewed by De Villiers (1966) involve the right subclavian, and he accepts Hoobler's (1942) view that carotid embolism could occur only on the right side, and that there must be retrograde spread of thrombus into the innominate artery to provide the source of the carotid embolism.

We have observed left middle cerebral embolism with thrombosis of the left subclavian artery associated with cervical rib. There was thrombosis of the left common carotid from its origin and the thrombus extended through the internal carotid to the skull base (Figure 3.11). We think that reflux embolism may occur from subclavian—derived thrombus carried proximally during diastole to cover the carotid orifice. Thrombi occupying the ostia of the great vessels can be seen, when fresh, to project into the aortic lumen (see Figure 3.18). Reflux of blood through the arch occurs during diastole from leakage through the aortic valve before complete valve closure and from coronary artery filling. A similar mechanism may also explain brain emboli from aortic thrombi distal to the left subclavian orifice (see later section).

Reflux brain embolism from unblocking of Scribener's arteriovenous shunts. Cerebral disturbances have been observed in a considerable number of patients following forcible unblocking of the arterial side of shunts established for haemodialysis and there seems no doubt that embolism has been responsible.

Gaan et al (1969) described two cases where vertebral artery embolism apparently occurred when the arterial side of the shunt was cleared by forcible injection of saline. They calculated that as little as 7 ml rapidly injected into the radial artery would suffice to carry a clot to the vertebral artery. Shunts in the right radial artery may deliver emboli into the carotid artery. Marshall, Epstein and Kincaid Smith (1970) described three cases that occurred after clearing shunts and they considered reflux embolism was

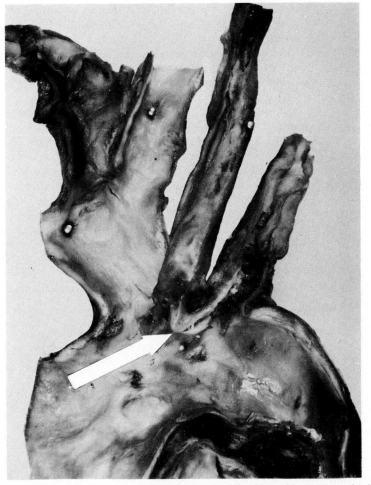

Figure 3.11. Reflux embolism from subclavian to carotid artery. Thrombosis of left sub-clavian artery from cervical rib. Reflux embolism into common carotid with propagation thrombosis to skull base and final left middle cerebral embolism. Cracks in aortic intima (arrowed) are artefacts.

a likely explanation. The same workers were joint authors in a paper by Clyne et al (1970) where the mechanism of reflux flow was investigated. They found that 20 ml of Hippuran labelled with radioactive iodine injected into the radial artery gave a strong signal in the temporal region. Using a dye dilution procedure, 10 ml sufficed to give a signal in the ear. Retrograde angiography, using 25 ml of dye, showed the dye in both the carotid and vertebral systems.

Emboli from the aorta

Brain embolism from aortic lesions was more generally recognised when syphilitic aortitis was a familiar disease (Albutt, 1921). Modern accounts make little mention of aortic syphilis or atheroma as a cause of cerebral infarction, but Carter (1964) and Crawford and Crompton (1968) both refer to it. Emboli from the aorta may consist of detached thrombus or atheromatous material, and atheromatous embolism is well documented (p. 000).

The article by Bruetsch (1971a) may be consulted for an account of the aortic arch syndrome, Takayasu's arteritis, and giant-cell arteritis as it effects the arch and great vessel ostia. Slow occlusion and thrombosis of the great vessels rather than embolism have been considered to be the cause of the cerebral lesions.

In the N.S.R.I. series of 581 infarcted brains an embolic source was present in the aorta, proximal to the left subclavian artery in 18 cases, and the infarcts were thought to be a consequence of embolism from these lesions. Seven of these lesions lay in the ascending aorta and of these 3 were atherosclerotic, 3 syphilitic, and 1 was a case of aortitis of undetermined origin with masses of fibrin covering the aortic intima. In the arch, there were 11 lesions; 9 atherosclerotic and 2 syphilitic with aneurysm formation. The mean age of the 5 patients with syphilitic aortitis was 70 years which was nearly 5 years older than the average for the entire series. All the neck vessels were embolised from one or other of these lesions. Lesch and Engelhardt (1966) described embolism in the left anterior, middle, and posterior cerebral arteries from an aortic thrombus.

Reflux embolism. In the N.S.R.I. series there were eight cerebral infarcts that were thought to be embolic where an ulcerated plaque was found situated at, or close to, the aortic isthmus and, therefore, distal to the left subclavian ostium (Figure 3.12). No other source of embolism was found in these cases after a complete examination of the carotid and vertebral arteries. It is suggested that reflux during diastole, as was discussed in connection with subclavian derived emboli, may carry emboli from this source to the great vessel openings.

Atheromatous cerebral embolism was described by Price and Harris (1970) as a complication of retrograde aortic perfusion during cardiac surgery.

Transient ischaemia from aortic lesions. The cases of atheromatous cerebral embolism described by McDonald (1967) presented fluctuating symptoms; it seems possible that the aorta may also supply unstable platelet emboli and that transient cerebral ischaemia may result. A constantly recurring pattern of symptoms such as occurs with carotid sinus thrombi would not be expected with the greater choice of routes open to aortic-derived emboli.

Embolism from material other than thrombi

Brain embolism by fat globules and air are well recognised; they do not produce macroscopic infarcts. Tumour fragments may occasionally block sizeable cerebral arteries; cardiac myxoma is the most important tumour in this context for it is surgically remediable (see earlier section).

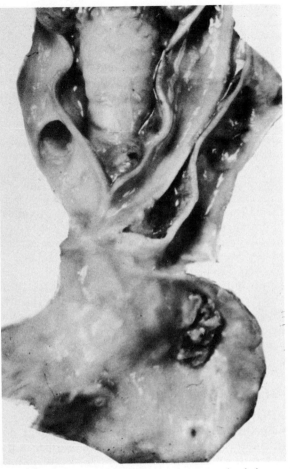

Figure 3.12. Aorta with ulcerating atherosclerotic plaque at the isthmus. Reflux during diastole might carry material from the plaque proximally so that the vertebral or carotid arteries might be embolised.

Following injury, or operation, various translocated tissues have caused embolic infarction. The literature of embolism, in general, is littered with collector's pieces that the authors believe have not been previously observed, and a number of these have been cerebral emboli. We have noted some of these en passant.

A portion of papillary muscle was described by Gerounlanos (1969) occluding the middle cerebral artery following a mitral valve replacement for bacterial endocarditis. Schröter (1967) described an embolus of tuberculo-silicotic material in the middle cerebral artery.

Foreign-body emboli in the middle cerebral artery were reviewed by Piazza and Gaist (1960). The delayed brain embolism described by Sandok and Spiegel (1968) is of clinical interest. Their patient suffered middle cerebral artery embolism from a lead shot 12 years after a shotgun wound to his left arm and chest.

Atheromatous embolism. Since atherosclerosis is seen predominantly in the abdominal aorta, the abdominal viscera and lower limbs must receive atheromatous emboli much oftener than the brain; it seems clear that most of these are asymptomatic.

Atheromatous emboli to the brain were found by Sturgill and Netsky (1963) to occlude vessels from 8 μm to 900 μm in diameter. When impacted they often induce an inflammatory reaction, and the atheromatous material may be extruded into the media or even into the perivascular tissue. These emboli are not susceptable to lysis, but disintegration seems possible, and migration of the smaller refractile bodies that result from atheromatous embolism in the retina has been observed (Russell, 1963a).

The brain infarcts described by Sturgill and Netsky (1963) were frequently multiple, and usually small. In two cases recorded by Meyer (1947) both had multiple small haemorrhagic lesions.

Soloway and Aronson (1964) reported 16 cases of atheromatous brain embolism and reviewed a further 14 published by others. The aorta was apparently considered to be the source of emboli in all these cases, although the state of the carotids was not described. In one of McDonald's (1967) two cases, the internal carotid was the source of the embolism.

Atheromatous embolism was reviewed by Retan and Miller (1966), and a more recent autopsy study was made by Maurizi, Barker and Truehart (1968). These authors described 28 cases of atheromatous visceral embolism in which they had examined the brain in 23 and found emboli in 7.

Occlusive cerebral infarction from disease of the cerebral arteries

We have already discussed occlusive territorial infarcts due to embolism and propagation thrombosis, and we have indicated that most infarctions due to occlusion of a cerebral artery fall into one or other of these categories. There is, indeed, now widespread agreement that, although infarcts are much commoner in the middle cerebral artery territory than elsewhere, primary thrombotic occlusion of this vessel is rarely encountered. Fisher's (1954) series contained no examples; Crawford and Crompton (1968) remarked on the rarity of the condition, as did Lhermitte, Gautier and Derouesné (1970). Bhattercharji (1965) found convincing evidence of middle cerebral artery thrombosis in only 2 out of 57 infarcted brains. Primary thrombosis of the anterior cerebral arteries is of comparable rarity and we have already pointed out that occlusion of the posterior cerebral artery is usually embolic, apart from cases that result from tentorial herniation. This relative immunity of the principal cerebral arteries from thrombosis does not, of course, extend to the intracranial portions of the neck vessels or the basilar artery. It is true that Moossy (1965) has reported a high incidence of thrombotic territorial artery occlusion associated with infarction. He recorded cerebral arterial thrombosis in 55 per cent of 152 infarcted brains, but the neck vessels and the petrous portion of the internal carotids were not examined.

In the coronary arteries, ulceration with extrusion of material into the lumen and haemorrhage into atherosclerotic plaques are recognised causes of sudden arterial occlusion, but these events do not occur in the cerebral arteries. There is good evidence that atherosclerotic stenosis of the cerebral vessels is a determinant of cerebral infarction (p. 000), but thrombosis resulting from atheromatous lesions seems rarely to be the cause.

Winter and Gyari (1960) made a detailed study of *small* cerebral infarcts and the lesions in the arteries supplying them. They excluded cases with occlusions in the main arterial trunks, and the vessels they examined required a hand lens for their inspection. Their main concern was to discount arterial spasm or hypotensive episodes as explanations of the infarcts. In 21 cases they were able to demonstrate 19 occlusive lesions in these small leptomeningeal arteries, and in 6 the occlusion was recognisably embolic. They considered that only recent emboli were recognisable with certainty in this size of vessel, and in older lesions the recognition of embolism must depend on circumstantial evidence.

Occlusion of territorial arteries unassociated with atheroma. Most of the recognised varieties of angiitis have been found responsible for occluding cerebral vessels. Syphilis causes occlusion of cerebral arteries; aneurysms have been described on the vertebral and intracranial carotid vessels. Occlusive arteritis is a well-known consequence of tuberculous meningitis, and occasionally the first clinical manifestation may be a consequence of brain infarction.

Cerebral infarction from mycotic infection is uncommon, at least in Britain, and mucormycosis (phycomycosis) has usually been responsible. These fungi have a propensity for invading blood vessels, usually spread from the paranasal sinuses or pharynx, and attack diabetics and other patients with reduced resistance to opportunistic infections (Stehbens, 1972).

Giant cell arteritis. Common synonyms are cranial or temporal arteritis. This disease is a well-recognised cause of blindness, which is usually due to retinal damage and only occasionally to cortical lesions, though one of the cases described by Heptinstall, Porter and Barkely (1954) had bilateral infarction of the occipital cortex with thrombosis of both vertebral arteries.

Cardell and Hanley (1951) concluded that half the deaths attributable to giant cell arteritis resulted from cerebrovascular accidents, and 2 of the 3 cases autopsied by Heptinstall, Porter and Barkley died from cerebral infarction.

Missen (1966) found that the lesions responsible for cerebral infarction usually lay in the vertebral or carotid arteries. Vertebral obstruction with consequent lesions in the hind brain predominated. He confirmed his findings (Missen, 1974) from a study of 23 cases examined at autopsy. Lesions of the cerebral arteries themselves are certainly uncommon, but Morrison and Abitol (1955) described a case with involvement of the cerebral arteries in the granulomatous process.

Polyarteritis nodosa. The peripheral nerves are very frequently involved in this disease but the brain suffers much less frequently. Stehbens (1972) gives estimates from 8 to 20 per cent quoted in the literature. The vessels involved are usually small and if ischaemic lesions result they are small and multifocal. Occasionally, the cervical or basilar arteries are involved but macroscopic infarction is unusual.

Buerger's disease (thromboangiitis obliterans). It is a controversial question whether Buerger's disease of the cerebral arteries is a recognisable entity. We have not encountered any case of cerebral artery occlusion that could be attributed to this disease and we agree with Fisher (1957) that the evidence for a cerebral form is tenuous. Thread-like silvery leptomeningeal arteries have been considered characteristic but we endorse Fisher's view that these arterial lesions result from organisation following stasis thrombosis distal to an obstruction. In our experience, the obstruction is often an embolus arrested at one of the divisions of the more distal branches of the middle cerebral artery. A lesion of this kind is illustrated in Figures 3.13 and 3.14.

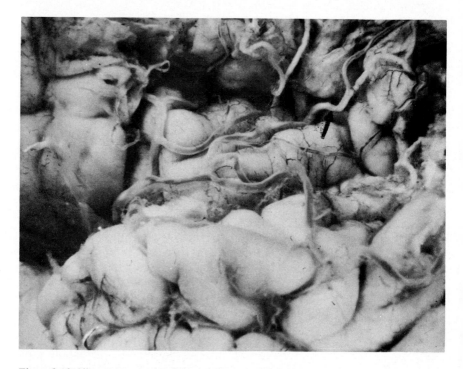

Figure 3.13. Silver-wire arteries (arrow) with middle cerebral embolic infarct. Propagation thrombosis along some middle cerebral artery branches was followed by organisation. These appearances have been incorrectly interpreted as Buerger's disease.

A critical assessment of the problem will be found in the article by Bruetsch (1971b). He takes the view that a variety of obliterative vascular lesions, including rheumatic arteritis, have been mistaken for cerebral thrombo-angiitis obliterans.

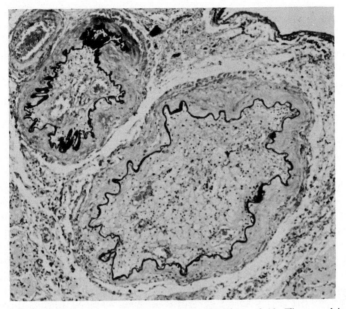

Figure 3.14. Section from silver-wire arteries shown in Figure 3.13. The vessel is occluded by organised thrombus. There is no angiitis (Elastic van Gieson stain, × 45).

Miscellaneous arterial lesions. Systemic lupus erythematosus and Moschowitz's platelet thrombosis syndrome (thrombotic microangiopathy) are essentially small vessel diseases and are considered under this heading (see later). An unusual case of Moschowitz's syndrome was, however, described by Tapp, Geary and Dawson (1969) who found the larger cerebral arteries occluded with consequent macroscopic infarction.

Non-occlusive single territory infarcts

Cerebral infarction within the territory of a vessel depends on the sudden or rapid development of ischaemia within the relevant vascular territory, and the problem is to explain infarction when the territorial artery is not occluded and there is no evidence to suggest that it has been. In general, it has been suggested, in explanation of these lesions, that the blood supply, rendered precarious by one or more stenotic lesions, is suddenly further reduced by some circulatory disturbance the effects of which might be aggravated by inadequacy of the anastomotic channels. There are clearly considerable difficulties in establishing the mechanism in individual cases at autopsy, and angiography may well have more to offer. The observations of Yates and Hutchinson (1961) were summarised in their report on cerebral infarction and the role of stenosis of the extracranial cerebral arteries. After demonstrating the high incidence of severe carotid and vertebral artery stenosis and occlusion in 100 cases with cerebrovascular disease, they sought explanations for the infarctions that they found in 35 of these cases, and they concluded that cerebral infarction had rarely a single cause. It was usually the result, they thought, of a combination of systemic disease and stenosis of the extra-cranial and intracranial arteries, or both. The precipitating haemodynamic factors were attributed to heart disease, which was usually ischaemic, or perhaps to intermittent hypotension resulting from stimulation of the carotid sinus. Vascular spasm and blood sludging were also considered as possibilities. It is clear in retrospect that they underestimated the possible significance of cerebral embolism.

Subsequent observations by Mitchell and Schwartz (1965) cast doubt on the significance of stenosis in the neck arteries. These authors found that severe stenoses occurred as frequently in unselected autopsies as they did in the cases with cerebrovascular disease investigated by Hutchinson and Yates. Mitchell and Schwartz pointed out that reduction in the lumen of the cervical vessels would make a negligible contribution to the total vascular resistance which was largely dependent on the intracranial arteries. Further doubts were thrown on the significance of cervical vessel occlusion by the demonstration by Brice, Dowsett and Lowe (1964) that the internal carotid artery lumen needed to be reduced to about 2 mm² before there was significant reduction in the arterial pressure beyond the constriction. Kameyama and Okinaka (1963) investigated 400 patients at autopsy, all over 60 years of age. In all of these the carotid and vertebral arteries were examined throughout their length. They concluded that cerebral infarction was not closely related to stenosis of neck arteries, but was closely associated with stenosis of the cerebral arteries.

The significance of stenosis of the intracerebral vessels was discussed by Bhattercharji, Hutchinson and McCall (1967a) who made a detailed examina-tion of 57 cases with cerebral infarction and 88 routine autopsies without infarction, all of patients over the age of 40 years. The degree of stenosis was recorded in grades, and the most severe grade was found in the middle cerebral artery in 33 per cent of the cases with infarction, and in only 5 per cent of those without. Smaller but significant differences were found in the anterior and posterior cerebral arteries. Baker, Dahl and Sandler (1963) reported on the vessel changes associated with 290 areas of infarction and found that in half of these there was severe stenosis of the middle cerebral artery supplying the softened area. Atheromatous stenosis of the cerebral vessels, no doubt, operates not only by reducing the supply through the territorial artery; stenosis in the anastomotic channels on the brain surface or in the Circle of Willis must clearly play a part.

There is ample angiographic evidence that the Circle of Willis permits an adequate circulation to areas of brain that would otherwise be hopelessly compromised by vascular occlusion, and it is reasonable to suppose that this compensatory mechanism may prove inadequate in the presence of atherosclerotic or congenital lesions of the circle. The presence of string-like posterior communicating vessels has attracted the attention of many observers, most of whom have found this and other abnormalities occur more fre-quently in the infarcted brains than in normal controls. The most comprehen-sive study was that of Alpers and Berry (1963) who found that the circle was normal in 33 per cent of cases with cerebral infarction, and in 52 per cent of cases without. Bhattercharji, Hutchinson and McCall (1967b) made similar observations but found that the incidence of unilateral string-like posterior communicating vessels was strikingly higher in the group with brain infarcts when this anomaly was associated with severe stenosis of one or more of the neck vessels.

In the discussion of border-zones (watershed) infarcts (in the section following) the crucial importance of hypotensive episodes is emphasised. It seems reasonable to suppose that this mechanism, which can produce infarction in the brain bordering two vascular territories, can also produce a single territorial infarct in the presence of arterial stenosis; but this has proved singularly difficult to establish. A case described by Eastcott, Pickering and Robb (1954) and referred to by Mitchell and Schwartz (1965) illustrated the importance of a combination of vascular stenosis and cardiac insufficiency. Their patient had recurrent attacks lasting 10 minutes to half an hour, which included hemiparesis and aphasia and which were related to attacks of paroxysmal tachycardia. There was angiographic evidence of stenosis of the left internal carotid artery and excision of this segment prevented recurrence of the cerebral attacks, although the paroxysmal tachycardia persisted. The cerebral damage in this case, of course, stopped short of actual infarction.

In general there is agreement between observers that it is quite unusual to be able to produce clear evidence of a hypotensive episode as an explanation for these single territory non-occlusive infarctions. We would only add that when territorial infarcts are associated with thrombotic occlusion of any neck vessel, the possibility of embolus must be carefully considered.

Jörgensen and Torvik (1966) remarked that there is some indication that the great majority of all infarcts are caused by thromboemboli. The combination of multiple atherosclerotic stenoses and episodic circulatory failure is probably responsible for less than 20 per cent of cerebral infarcts.

BOUNDARY ZONE (WATERSHED, BORDER ZONE) INFARCTS

Several mechanisms by which infarcts could be brought about in the boundary zones between the territories of major cerebral arteries have been suggested (see Romanul and Abramowicz, 1964). Factors considered important in the pathogenesis of boundary zone infarction include systemic hypotension and stenosis or occlusion of cerebral and/or cervical arteries (Romanul, 1970).

When the internal carotid artery is occluded, a boundary zone infarct may occur between the anterior and middle cerebral artery territories (Figure 3.15). If the occlusion extends to involve the origin of the ophthalmic artery, the size of the boundary zone infarct is larger because the important anastomosis between the internal and external carotid arteries is obliterated. Occlusion beyond the carotid bifurcation results in single territory infarction (p. 40). The above patterns of infarction occur when the Circle of Willis is of normal adult configuration, but when the fetal configuration persists and the posterior cerebral artery is a branch of the internal carotid artery, the boundary zone between middle and posterior cerebral arteries becomes in-

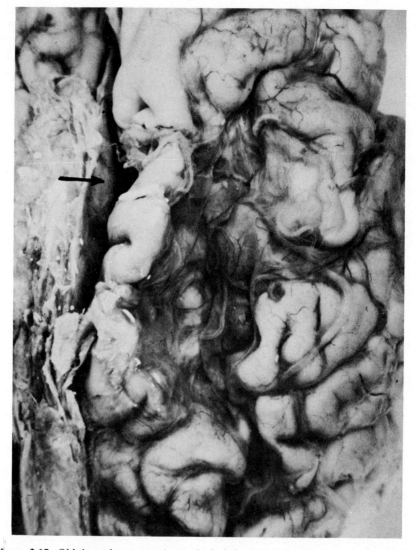

Figure 3.15. Old boundary zone (watershed) infarct. Longitudinal parasagittal infarct along border of right anterior and middle cerebral artery territories. Arrow indicates superior longitudinal fissure.

volved. There is, therefore, an infarct in the temporal region adjacent to the middle temporal gyrus and the most severe lesions occur in the parieto-occipital region in the boundary zone between the anterior, middle and posterior cerebral arteries.

When stenosis without actual occlusion affects two cerebral arteries with adjacent territories, the other factors probably play a more important part in precipitating boundary zone infarction. Patients with disease of the cervical and cerebral arteries often have coexistent heart disease which could give rise to sudden decrease in cardiac output and periods of systemic hypotension. Single or multiple periods of systemic hypotension are important determinants of boundary zone infarcts in patients with and without cerebrovascular disease. Three of Romanul and Abramowicz's 13 cases suffered acute boundary zone infarcts following episodes of profound systemic hypotension. There was no evidence of cerebrovascular disease in these three patients and the boundary zone infarcts were undoubtedly due entirely to the reduction in cerebral blood flow brought about by the systemic hypotension. Zülch and Behrend (1961) believe that ischaemic damage in boundary zones in the brain is due to systemic hypotension.

Adams et al (1966) showed that when a reduction in cerebral blood flow is due to systemic hypotension, the resulting ischaemic brain damage is distributed as follows—

1. Boundary zone ischaemia occurs between the major cerebral and cerebellar arteries (Figures 3.16, 3.17). Maximal lesions, which may amount to haemorrhagic infarcts, occur in the parieto-occipital region at the junction of the anterior, middle and posterior cerebral artery territories. The severity of the lesions decreases towards the frontal poles along the anterior/middle cerebral artery boundary zones and towards the temporal poles along the middle/posterior cerebral artery boundary zones. In Adams et al's (1966) series, cases with this distribution included syncope in pregnancy and syncope occurring during intravenous pyelography. The experimental work of Brierley and others (Brierley and Excell, 1966; Brierley et al, 1969; Meldrum and Brierley, 1969) confirmed the distribution of lesions in profound systemic hypotension.

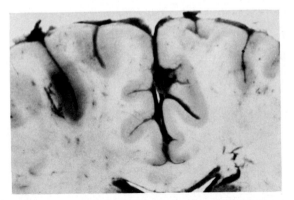

Figure 3.16. Boundary zone infarction in the anterior/middle cerebral artery boundary zone. The patient was severely hypotensive following aortic valve replacement.

2. The cortex of cerebrum and cerebellum showed diffuse ischaemic changes with discrete lesions in the boundary zones. Severe, patchy lesions were also present in the thalamus. Cases showing this distribution of lesions consisted of syncope during pregnancy and labour, and postoperative cardiac arrest or hypotension.

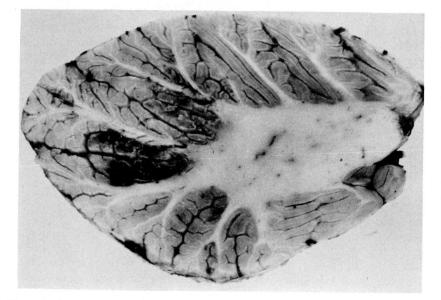

Figure 3.17. Haemorrhagic boundary zone infarct on the dorsal aspect of the cerebellum. Same patient as Figure 3.16.

3. Cases in this group showed generalised ischaemic changes in the cerebral and cerebellar cortex. The cerebellar lesions were constantly severe and the thalamus was involved. Lesions with this distribution in such situations as anaesthetic cardiac arrest with massage, or postoperative hypotension of unknown cause.

As pointed out by Brierley (1970), the modification in the neuropathology of systemic hypotension brought about by the presence of stenosis in major extracranial and/or intracranial arteries needs further investigation.

DIFFUSE ATHEROSCLEROTIC AND HYPERTENSIVE CEREBRAL ARTERIAL LESIONS

Hypertension and ageing are the principal determinants of degenerative lesions in the cerebral arteries of about 500 μm diameter or less. The structural changes in these vessels are discussed by Baker and Iannone (1959) and Arendt and Bachmann (1966) have made a detailed study of the cerebral arteries in known hypertensive patients.

We draw attention elsewhere to the close association of 'lacunes', whatever their pathogenesis, with hypertension. These are often multiple and bilateral and may cause symptoms (p. 88). Degenerative lesions in arteries less than 500μm in diameter play little part in the pathogenesis of gross infarction but their obliteration must reduce the anastamotic flow to areas where the circulation is precarious from other causes.

There is difficulty in assessing the significance of arterial lesions that may accompany cerebral diseases in the aged. The association of Parkinsonism with arterial disease is now thought to be a coincidental finding in cases of idiopathic Parkinsonism occurring in the aged (Kurland and Kurtzke, 1972). The contribution of arterial disease to dementia in the aged has been the subject of detailed and carefully planned studies by Tomlinson and his colleagues (Tomlinson, Blessed and Roth, 1968, 1970). They examined the brains of 50 old demented people (Tomlinson, Blessed and Roth, 1970) and concluded that only 12 per cent could be confidently classified as arteriosclerotic dementia although a further 5 per cent were probably in this category. Their cases of arteriosclerotic dementia included examples of gross infarction but in some the ischaemic lesions were very small and microscopy often revealed multiple minute areas of ischaemic scarring. The age incidence of arteriosclerotic dementia was significantly less than that of senile dementia.

Uncommon varieties of small vessel disease. Under this heading we consider Moschowitz's syndrome, systemic lupus erythematosus and granulomatous and allergic angiitis. Polyarteritis nodosa and giant cell arteritis involve larger arteries (p. 63).

Moschowitz's syndrome. Synonyms are numerous. They include platelet thrombosis syndrome, thrombotic thrombocytopenic purpura, and thrombotic microangiopathy.

Cerebral symptoms are usual in this disease and are characteristically relapsing and varying. Arterioles and capillaries are blocked with acellular material which is 'fibrinoid' in appearance. It stains strongly with the periodic acid Schiff procedure and presents a smudged appearance. It is sometimes referred to as thrombotic material and infiltrates the vessel walls resulting in microaneurysm formation (Orbison, 1952). In a case described by Bornstein et al (1960), there was peri-vascular deposition of the fibrinoid material in quite large amounts. The pathology was reviewed by Adams, Cammermeyer and Fitzgerald (1948) .Microscopic ischaemic damage resulting from these vascular lesions is usual, but macroscopic infarction of the brain is very uncommon (p. 65). We have ourselves, however. observed bilateral infarction of the globus pallidus where the vascular lesions were confined to arterioles and capillaries.

Systemic lupus erythematosus. The neurological manifestations of systemic lupus were reviewed by Johnson and Richardson (1968) and more recently Berry (1971) has reviewed the pathology. Berry remarked that "despite neurologic involvement clinically, there is often a disconcerting lack of gross and even microscopic findings in the nervous system". He found focal softening in 37 per cent of 54 autopsied cases reported in the literature (Berry and Hodges, 1965). Perisulcal softening is a feature.

The vessels affected in subacute lupus erythematosus are usually less than 200 μm in diameter and the characteristic acute lesion is a fibrinoid necrosis of the vessel wall without cellular infiltration, although mononuclear peri-vascular infiltrate may be seen.

Granulomatous and allergic angiitis. The syndrome of polyarteritis nodosa may present as a necrotising small artery disease causing diffuse cerebral lesions (Winkelman and Moore, 1950).

The allergic granulomatous angiitis described by Churg and Strauss (1951) involves both arteries and veins and extravascular granulomas with giant cells are found. The brain and peripheral nerves are commonly involved, together with other viscera. An unusual form of granulomatous angiitis with a strong predilection for the central nervous system has also been recorded. It appears not to be identical with the condition described by Churg and Strauss (Cravioto and Feigin, 1959).

Nurick, Blackwood and Mair (1972) described two apparently similar cases and found an additional 17 cases described. They noted that both arteries and veins were involved.

ORAL CONTRACEPTIVES AND CEREBRAL INFARCTION

Lorentz (1962) seems to have first suggested the possibility that oral contraceptives might be responsible for cerebrovascular lesions. Angiography was not performed and he thought that venous sinus thrombosis was the most likely explanation. There is a review of the English language literature by Masi and Dugdale (1970).

Using data from cases of cerebral artery occlusion in women aged 18 to 45 years seen at the National Hospital, Queen Square, London from 1955 to 1965, Illis et al (1965) found no increase in the incidence following the introduction of oral contraceptives but they were impressed by the fact that in 3 cases infarction occurred within a few weeks of first taking them. Bickerstaff and Holmes (1967) found that 18 out of 25 women under 45 with cerebral arterial insufficiency were taking the 'pill', i.e. 72 per cent compared with an estimated 9 per cent of the female population of reproductive age.

The data referred to in this section derive from the era when contraceptives were mainly of high oestrogen content and it is clear that many clinicians believe this type of contraceptive is sometimes responsible for cerebral infarction. This view is supported by a good deal of evidence but has not been universally accepted. Jennett and Cross (1967) found no evidence from their records that contraceptives precipitated arterial occlusion in young women. They saw 42 non-pregnant women (ages 15 to 45 years) with carotid stroke from 1956 to 1965 and found no increase in the incidence after 1961, when the pill became freely available. Of the 26 women seen after 1961 24 were known not to be taking contraceptives. Masi and Dugdale (1970), however, pointed out that less than 1 per cent of British women were estimated to be taking oral contraceptives in 1961 and thought a comparison of cases before and after 1963 might have produced a different result. Similar considerations apply to the observations of Illis et al (1965) already referred to.

Epidemiological studies have generally supported the association of brain infarction and the 'pill'. Vessey and Doll (1969) estimated that there was a sixfold increased risk of cerebral infarction in 'pill' takers. In a study of 598 women aged 15 to 45 with cerebral vascular lesions (Collaborative Group for the Study of Stroke in Young Women, 1973) it was estimated that there was a ninefold increase in risk and the data suggested that smoking might potentiate the effect of the contraceptive.

We think that the evidence from these studies clearly indicates an associaion between oral contraceptives and cerebrovascular lesions, although Schoenberg et al (1970), working from the comprehensive medical indexing system of the Mayo Clinic, concluded that it would be premature to claim an association.

Mechanism and site of contraceptive-associated infarction. There is now general agreement that infarction in these cases is almost always a result of arterial occlusion. Infarction from venous sinus thrombosis is infrequent and this is perhaps surprising in view of the increased tendency to venous thrombosis with oral contraceptives. Kutas and Bodosi (1971), who described an autopsied case with sagittal sinus thrombosis, found only 4 previously described acceptable cases with intracranial venous thrombosis. Two additional examples were, however, recorded by Mulder, Evenblij and Endtz (1971).

Although most contraceptive associated infarcts are due to occlusion of the carotid or middle cerebral artery, an unexpectedly high incidence of lesions in the vertebrobasilar territory has been recorded. The arterial occlusions responsible for contraceptive-associated infarcts may involve either the cervical or intracranial vessels, and distal embolism or propagation thrombosis may follow.

Bickerstaff and Holmes (1967) drew attention to the fact that in 6 of the 28 contraceptive associated infarcts which they reported, the vertebrobasilar territory was involved. Jennett and Cross (1967) tabulated the cases published up to 1967; in 8 out of 48 the vertebrobasilar territory was affected. Ask-Upmark, Glas and Stenram (1969) also referred to the high incidence of vertebral artery occlusion in these young women. It is of interest that all the cerebral infarctions in the series published by Jennett and Cross (1967), in which contraceptives certainly made no significant contribution, were in the carotid territory.

Bickerstaff (1973) remarked that he had become increasingly convinced, from angiographic and clinical evidence, that embolism accounted for most cases of contraceptive associated infarction, and Enzell and Lidelmalm (1973) found clear evidence in 4 out of 14 cases that the lesion was embolic, while several of the remaining cases were probably embolic also. They failed, however, to demonstrate any source of embolism. Thrombus formation in the pulmonary veins was suggested by Enzell and Lindelmalm as a source of unexplained embolism. It will be very difficult, at autopsy, to exclude a pulmonary venous thrombus as the cause of embolism, but careful search of these vessels is clearly indicated.

We have encountered one case which we attributed to paradoxical middle cerebral embolism. There was a small but unguarded atrial septal defect, thrombi were present in the pelvic veins, and there was a renal infarct with no microscopic evidence of angiitis. In view of the incidence of venous thrombosis, paradoxical embolism might be expected to explain a few contraceptive associated infarctions. One of Enzell and Lidelmalm's cases had a patent ductus arteriosus.

In the case illustrated in Figure 3.18, similar and contemporary thrombi were present in the left common carotid and the innominate arteries. Embolic infarction in the left middle cerebral territory occurred. No angiogram was done but conventional carotid angiography would have failed to demonstrate these two massive sources of emboli.

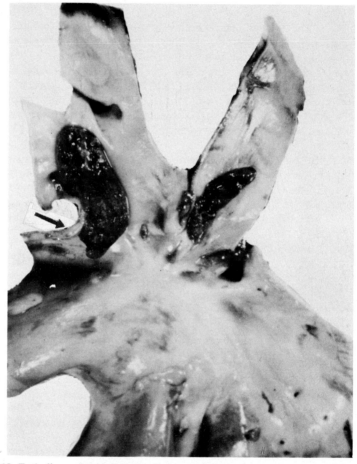

Figure 3.18. Embolic cerebral infarction in woman of 36 years taking oral contraceptives. Large thrombi in the innominate and left common carotid arteries. There is a small plaque of atherosclerosis (arrow) at the innominate ostium where the thrombus is attached. The innominate thrombus projects a little into the aortic lumen (p. 000).

The role of arterial disease in contraceptive associated infarction. In most recorded fatal cases the thrombosed artery has been free from atheroma. In the case illustrated in Figure 3.18 there was a small atherosclerotic plaque at the origin of the innominate, and a flat, scarcely raised plaque in the left common carotid. The possibility that small-vessel disease plays a part has been ventilated but the infarcts seen in women on contraceptives have not differed morphologically from those due to atherosclerosis and it seems unlikely that small-vessel disease is an important determinant of infarction. The case described by Altschuler, McLaughlin and Neuberger (1968) was exceptional. They observed multiple small haemorrhagic necroses in the brain associated with disseminating arteriolar and small artery necroses. The kidneys and myocardium showed similar lesions. It is impossible to know whether the contraceptive was implicated in this solitary case, although it appears that both internal carotid arteries were also thrombosed.

Irey, Manion and Taylor (1970) observed what they thought were distinctive vascular lesions in 22 women taking oral contraceptives. Autopsy details were not given but 21 of the deaths appear to have been due to pulmonary artery embolism or thrombosis and one was attributed to thrombosis of the hepatic veins. All their observations were made on pulmonary vessels, with the exception of one temporal artery. Many of the vascular lesions they saw lay beneath well-established thrombi and could possibly have been a consequence of embolism, since Sayler, Sayler and Hutchins (1974) have shown that destructive mural lesions occur in the arterial wall, in both systemic and pulmonary vessels, following sterile embolism. Irey, Manion and Taylor (1970) found conspicuous endothelial proliferation in pulmonary arteries unassociated with thrombi but no similar lesions were seen in women *not* taking contraceptives who died with thrombo-embolic disease. Further work is clearly required to clarify these observations.

In seeking an explanation for a relatively high incidence of vertebrobasilar strokes we may note the observation of Castaigne et al (1970) that only 9 per cent of occlusions in this territory arise from cardiac emboli as against 22 per cent in the carotids, and we know that ulcerating carotid atheroma is common while ulcerating vertebral atheroma is rare, and lesions of this type make a large contribution to carotid strokes. Contraceptive associated strokes occur in young women who are generally free from heart disease or severe atheroma, and the absence of these two determinants of carotid strokes might explain the smaller proportion of carotid strokes in this group.

If we assume that contraceptives induce strokes by a systemic effect, e.g. hypercoagulability, and that their incidence is not dependent on atherosclerosis, we can postulate that thrombi may form in the subclavian arteries although these vessels only rarely provide embolic sources in atherosclerotic strokes. In other words, the larger area available for thrombus formation under the influence of contraceptives may exert an effect in favour of strokes in the vertebro-basilar region in the absence of cardiac emboli and severe carotid atheroma.

The mortality from contraceptive strokes is low, and autopsy information in this group is scanty. Aortography seems to have been undertaken very rarely and thrombi in these subclavian and innominate vessels are unlikely to be discovered.

Hypercoagulability and oral contraceptives. The occurrence of thrombi in apparently normal arteries has been repeatedly recorded in contraceptive associated infarction. In our case illustrated in Figure 3.18, atherosclerosis was minimal and the thrombi were massive. These observations, together with the association with venous thrombosis, have led many observers to postulate that hypercoagulability plays an important role. The increased incidence of thrombo-embolism associated with the administration of oestrogens to suppress lactation (Daniel, Campbell and Turnbull, 1967), the raised incidence of thrombosis in patients with cancer of the prostate receiving oestrogen (Veterans Administration, 1967), and the incidence of venous thrombosis in women receiving oestrogen-containing contraceptives have all tended to support this conclusion and have focussed attention on the importance of the oestrogen component in the contraceptive preparations.

Increased activity of factors VII and X, increased platelet adhesiveness, enhanced platelet aggregation, and increased fibrinogen have been found (Poller and Thomson, 1966; Poller, 1969; Thomson, 1970). Poller (1969) considers that there is good evidence that a state of hypercoagulability develops with oestrogen-containing contraceptives.

CEREBRAL INFARCTION IN PREGNANCY AND THE PUERPERIUM

Carroll, Leak and Lee (1966) collected 177 cases of pregnancy or puerperal non-haemorrhagic strokes from the literature and added four cases. They considered that the infarctions were due to intracranial venous sinus thrombosis. Indeed, following the publications of Martin (1941), Martin and Sheehan (1941) and Stevens (1954) it had been generally accepted that sagittal sinus thrombosis was the usual explanation of pregnancy infarction. Pruitt and Mole (1967) accepted that venous sinus thrombosis was responsible for most infarctions associated with pregnancy. They reported a case with angiographically confirmed middle cerebral artery occlusion and found only 8 others recorded, with angiographic evidence in 5 and autopsy confirmation in one. The autopsied case (Sauer, 1955) was of a paradoxical embolism from the N.S.R.I. series.

In 1968, Cross, Castro and Jennett challenged the assumption that venous sinus thrombosis was the most important cause of these cerebral infarctions when they analysed their findings in 31 pregnant or puerperal patients. In 70 per cent, carotid angiograms demonstrated occlusions of arteries or ischaemic disease unrelated to venous occlusion. They concluded that the majority of non-haemorrhagic strokes in pregnancy and the puerperium were due to arterial obstruction, and they estimated that cerebral infarction might occur in about 1 in 20 000 pregnancies. They found it very uncommon in the first three months, while the puerperium, up to the sixteenth day, accounted for as many cases as the last six months of pregnancy.

There is no doubt that sagittal sinus thrombosis is an important cause of these strokes; autopsy verification was found in 34 of the 181 cases listed by Carroll, Leak and Lee (1966). It now seems likely, however, that arterial occlusion accounts for a substantial proportion of pregnancy and puerperal strokes. Failure to appreciate that carotid angiograms may be negative in embolic infarction (see earlier section), if they are not undertaken soon after the ictus, may have contributed to under-estimation of the importance of arterial obstruction.

It is perhaps surprising that the relatively high incidence of vertebrobasilar strokes recorded with contraceptives does not appear to have been noted in pregnancy. The blood changes suggesting hypercoagulability associated with contraceptives (see earlier section) have been found also, by the same authors, to occur in pregnancy.

POLYCYTHEMIA AND ERYTHROCYTOSIS

Polycythemia vera. Transient ischaemic attacks, cerebral infarction, and cerebral haemorrhage are all recognised consequences of polycythemia vera. The condition is characterised by an increased blood volume, increased total red cell mass, and an abnormally high peripheral erythrocyte count. There is commonly an increase in leucocytes and platelets, and a few cases develop myeloid leukaemia or myelosclerosis. Brown and Giffin (1926) emphasised the clinical significance of increased blood viscosity which Zadek (1927) found might be some five to eight times greater than normal. Kety (1950) stated that a 50 per cent reduction in cerebral blood flow could be demonstrated in these patients.

In spite of a tendency to thrombosis in both arteries and veins, clotting defects occur, and these, together with the over-distension of vessels, are presumed to contribute to the haemorrhagic episodes.

The condition appears late in life so that atherosclerosis is common in the neck and cerebral vessels in the age group affected. Transient cerebral ischaemia is common and can presumably occur from detachment of unstable emboli from great vessels and from the haemodynamic effects of stenosis aggravated by increased blood viscosity. Millikan (1965) remarked on the almost uniform cessation of attacks that followed successful treatment of the polycythemia or the institution of anticoagulant therapy, and it seems likely that both restoration of normal blood viscosity and the cessation of thrombus formation might be responsible for the therapeutic response. A detailed account of the cerebral manifestations of polycythemia vera was given by Millikan, Siekert and Whisnant (1960).

Cerebral infarction in other erythraemic states. Modan and Modan (1968) discussed a group of patients whom they considered suffered from benign erythrocytosis and characterised by an increased total red cell mass and peripheral erythrocytosis but no abnormality of leucocytes or platelets, and no association with leukaemia or myelosclerosis. The increase in total red cell mass distinguishes this condition from stress erythrocytosis attributable to reduced plasma volume. Fessel (1965) has denied the existence of this form of erythrocytosis, but the interest of Modan and Modan's observations lies in their statement that thrombo-embolic episodes occur with the same frequency as in polycythemia vera. If their findings are confirmed, they support the view that increased viscosity is an important determinant of the thrombo-embolic episodes.

Erythrocytosis resulting from cerebral infarction. The possibility that cerebral infarction may actually cause erythrocytosis has been considered by a number of writers. The association of brain lesions of various types with increased erythrocyte counts has been reviewed by Gilbert and Silverstein (1965). They accepted the well-established association of erythrocytosis with cerebellar haemangioblastoma but thought that anoxia or dehydration could explain the remaining cases in which erythrocytosis had been attributed to brain lesions. They did, however, describe a single case of their own, of cerebral infarction in which a convincing but temporary increase in total red cell mass occurred associated with peripheral erythrocytosis. Anoxia and dehydration could be excluded.

CEREBRAL INFARCTION IN CHILDREN AND YOUNG ADULTS

Aronson and Rabiner (1958) reviewed five hundred consecutive autopsies and found infarcts in 16 per cent of these below the age of 15 years. No details were given but most of them probably resulted from cardiac emboli from rheumatic heart disease. Infective endocarditis superimposed on congenital heart disease accounts for some cerebral emboli in this age group. An uncommon cause of cerebral embolism in the very young and in young adults is congenital atrial aneurysm. Williams (1963) reviewed 10 examples of this lesion and in 3 of them cerebral embolism had occurred. The cardiac abnormality is surgically remediable. We have already mentioned cerebral embolism from atrial myxoma with cerebral emboli.

Bickerstaff (1964) described his findings in 15 children developing sudden hemiplegia, with angiographic features suggesting embolism from thrombosis of the internal carotid artery. He noted a high incidence of antecedent throat infections in his cases and thought the close proximity of the internal carotid artery to the tonsillar fossa might be significant.

Strokes in patients ranging in age from infancy to adolescence have been attributed to most of the varieties of angiitis we have already described and, of course, venous and intracranial venous sinus thrombosis are well-recognised causes of infarction in infants and young children. Occlusive disease of the carotid arteries in children was reviewed by Davie and Coxe (1967) and a bibliography of the literature of strokes in this age group was given by von Deisenhammer, Hammer and Tulzer (1970). The mortality of arterial occlusion in children was estimated by Wishoff and Rothballer (1961) at about 25 per cent. Pathological evidence is scarce. In carotid and basilar artery strokes there has often been no satisfactory explanation for the arterial occlusion; Figure 3.19 illustrates an unexplained basilar thrombosis in a youth of 17 years. Brihaye, Retif and Jeanmart (1971) and Brihaye et al (1971) observed 5 cases of basilar artery occlusion in patients aged 21, 22, 23, 25 and 43 years. Three of these patients had dissecting basilar aneurysms at autopsy. Similar lesions have occasionally been described in the middle cerebral artery, and Norman and Urich (1957) recorded an example in an infant.

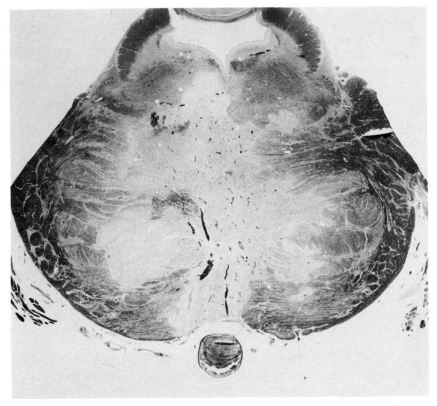

Figure 3.19. Basilar artery thrombosis of four weeks standing in a male, age 18 years. Central softening of pons with loss of myelin. (Myelin stain × 3.5.)

INTRACEREBRAL HAEMORRHAGE

In this consideration of intracerebral haemorrhage we are not concerned with immediate or late effects of trauma, or with haemorrhage occurring in the neonatal period.

The incidence of abnormalities associated with cerebral haemorrhage varies from series to series and, as pointed out by Blackwood (1962), when comparing series from the London Hospital (a large General Hospital) and the specialised National Hospital for Nervous Diseases, the figures in different series reflect very closely the type of hospital in which the series originated.

Dorothy Russell's (1954) series from the London Hospital illustrates the most important aetiological factors associated with intracerebral haemorrhage. The series consisted of 461 cases which came to autopsy. All traumatic and neonatal haemorrhages were excluded and only massive haemorrhages thought likely to be the cause of death were considered. Lesions less than 3 cm in diameter in the cerebral hemisphere, and less than 1.5 cm in diameter in the brainstem, were excluded. Approximately half the cases (229) were not associated with hypertension. Of these, 92 had saccular (berry) aneurysms, 36 had various blood dyscrasias, 28 had mycotic aneurysms, 21 angiomas and arterio-venous malformations, 13 arteritis, 9 neoplasms, and 11 cases showed arterial degeneration and congenital arterial defects without aneurysms. In 16 of the cases, no cause for the haemorrhage was demonstrated. The other 232 cases in Russell's series were associated with hypertension. The specialised National Hospital series contained 73 patients with aneurysms, 32 hypertensive haemorrhages, 8 vascular haematomas, and 7 with haemorrhage into neoplasms. The cause was not found in 4 cases, and one case had a blood dyscrasia and another case a mycotic aneurysm.

Since 1954, other causes and associations of intracerebral heamorrhage have become apparent, for example, spontaneous intracerebral haemorrhage occurring during haemodialysis with heparin anticoagulation (Weber, Reagan and Leeds, 1972).

Hypertensive intracerebral haemorrhage

Massive haemorrhage associated with hypertension occurs most frequently in the cerebral hemispheres. Stehbens (1972) accumulated data from fourteen series and found that primary haemorrhage occurred in the cerebrum in 81.6 per cent of cases, in the brainstem (or pons) in 10.9 per cent, and in the cerebellum in 7.5 per cent. These figures were based on his analysis of 4566 cases of single primary intracerebral haemorrhage. Within the cerebrum the region of the basal ganglia is the commonest site of haemorrhage. In Russell's (1954) series, 151 of 176 hypertensive haemorrhages within the cerebral hemisphere were in the basal ganglia. The region of the putamen/claustrum is the site of most haemorrhages and the vessel supplying this region (the lenticulo-striate artery) has been called 'the artery of cerebral haemorrhage'. Haemorrhages also occur into the central white matter and into the subcortical white matter. In Freytag's (1968) series of 393 fatal hypertensive intracerebral haematomas, 10 per cent occurred in this situation, 42 per cent were in the striate body and 15 per cent in the thalamus.

In massive intracerebral haemorrhage, the brain is acutely swollen and on removing the calvarium the dura is under considerable tension. The affected hemisphere is visibly more swollen than the unaffected one, and the secondary effects of rapidly expanding intracranial lesions may be present (see p. 37). If the brain is sliced fresh, the contents of the cavity have the appearance of fresh blood clot, which has been described as 'red currant jelly'. The walls of the cavity are ragged and the surrounding brain may show numerous petechial haemorrhages (Staemmler's marginal haemorrhages). As the brain often shows acute oedema and is extremely soft, the distribution of haemorrhages is best studied in the fixed specimen (Figures 3.20, 3.21). Direct rupture of a haemorrhage into the subarachnoid space is unusual but haemorrhages frequently rupture into the ventricular system; 75 per cent did so in Freytag's (1968) series. When this occurs there may be subarachnoid haemorrhage from leakage through the foramina of the fourth ventricle.

Primary brain stem haemorrhage usually involves a large part of the pons, usually arises in the midline, and rapidly leads to coma and death. The haema-

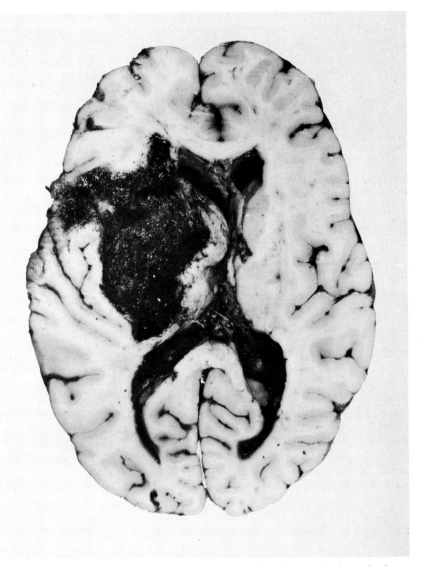

Figure 3.20. Horizontal section of a formalin-fixed brain showing a typical massive hypertensive haemorrhage in the left basal ganglia. The haemorrhage has ruptured into the ventricular system and into the subarachnoid space.

toma often involves the cerebral peduncles and may reach the hypothalamus or thalamus (Dinsdale, 1964). Extension may occur into the cerebellar peduncles but extensive involvement of the medulla is unusual (Stehbens, 1972). Rupture into the fourth ventricle is common. Externally, the pons may be expanded and feel soft, but it may appear unremarkable. Spontaneous rupture into the subarachnoid space is unusual because blood rarely penetrates the superficial transverse fibres of the pons.

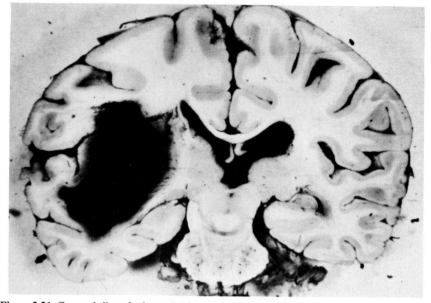

Figure 3.21. Coronal slice of a formalin-fixed brain with a massive external capsular haemorrhage.

Cerebellar haemorrhages tend to arise in the region of the dentate nucleus and are nearly always unilateral. The vermis is an unusual site (Dinsdale, 1964) but can be involved by an extension from one or other hemisphere (Fisher et al, 1965b). Freytag (1968) stated that cerebellar haemorrhages reached the subarachnoid space more often than cerebral haemorrhages but intraventricular extension was less frequent. Cerebellar haemorrhage may be sufficiently large to cause death from medullary pressure cone (Dinsdale, 1964). Supratentorial pressure may be raised because of lateral displacement of the brain stem and occlusion of the cerebral aqueduct (Aronson, Shafey and Gargano, 1965). The possibility of beneficial effects from surgery in acute hypertensive cerebellar haemorrhage prompted Fisher et al (1965b) to suggest that the condition 'should be placed in the same therapeutic category as subdural and extradural haematoma'.

According to Russell (1954), 'malignant' (and 'nephritic') hypertension predominates in primary brain stem haemorrhage (18 of 32 cases), whereas in the cerebellum, benign hypertension predominates. In Dinsdale's (1964) series, 96.7 per cent of the pontine haemorrhages and 89.3 per cent of the cerebellar haemorrhages were associated with hypertension. There were only two cases not associated with hypertension in this series of 82 haemorrhages within the posterior fossa.

In Russell's series, small haemorrhages were excluded. However, smaller haemorrhages are of increasing importance in the understanding of strokes in hypertension. Such lesions (less than 3 cm in diameter in the cerebral hemisphere and less than 1.5 cm in diameter in the brain stem) can occur anywhere within the brain. In the cerebral hemispheres they have a predilection for the junction between grey and white matter. They may occur as subcortical or cortical ball-like haematomas (Figure 3.22), or as slightly larger oval or slit-like lesions involving the subcortical white matter. As these lesions are small they are not lethal and may heal leaving a subcortical slit-like pigmented scar. In very old lesions the pigment may disappear and then the distinction between old haemorrhages and old infarcts is not always possible on pathological grounds.

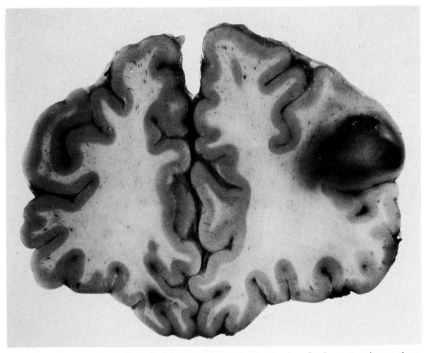

Figure 3.22. Two recent subcortical haemorrhages in the brain of a hypertensive patient.

The importance of haemorrhagic lesions in small strokes in hypertensives was pointed out by Cole and Yates (1968). In 100 hypertensive brains 13 per cent showed small haemorrhagic lesions. There were none in 100 normoten-sives. Approximately twice as many of Cole and Yates's hypertensive patients had cerebral vascular lesions (ischaemic or haemorrhagic) compared with the normotensives. The hypertensives also suffered a greater number of attacks. The question of the underlying cause of recurrent strokes in hyper-tensives was discussed by Marquardsen (1968). He showed that in 23 of 47 cases the fatal recurrence was caused by massive cerebral haemorrhage. Furthermore, in approximately a quarter of the 24 patients with a verified cerebral haemorrhage, an old haemorrhagic lesion was demonstrated. Hudson and Hyland (1958), in a clinico-pathological study of 100 cases with hyper-tensive cerebro-vascular disease, mentioned 10 cases with non-fatal intra-cerebral haemorrhage. Six of these cases eventually died of cerebral haemorrhage. In Chapter 12, the clinical histories and gross post mortem findings of five cases with fatal intracerebral haemorrhage are described. All these cases had previous strokes, some of which were shown to be due to haemorrhagic lesions. It is interesting in this context that Dinsdale (1964) briefly mentions a hypertensive patient who died of a cerebellar haemorrhage while receiving anticoagulants because of 'recurring transient hemiparesis'. At present, it is not possible on clinical grounds to differentiate between an infarct and a localised haemorrhage as a cause of a stroke, even in hypertensive patients. The ability to make this distinction will have to await the results of a planned prospective clinical and pathological study.

PATHOGENESIS OF HYPERTENSIVE INTRACEREBRAL HAEMORRHAGE

Various lesions that could give rise to haemorrhages have been described in the hypertensive brain.

Rouchoux (1844) suggested that haemorrhages arose from an artery that had lost its support because the surrounding brain had undergone softening. This view was supported by Westphal and Bär (1926), who suggested that the ischaemia was the result of spasm. Globus and Strauss (1926) and Globus and Epstein (1953) supported the view that haemorrhage followed softening. In addition to studying human material, Globus and Epstein occluded cerebral arteries in dogs and monkeys. The animals occasionally developed spontaneous haemorrhagic lesions, and haemorrhages resembling human hypertensive haemorrhages were induced by the injection of neosynephrine after the vessel had been occluded. Breutman et al (1963) suggested that infarction followed by haemorrhage was the mechanism of six intracerebral haemorrhages in their series of 900 patients with carotid artery occlusion. The six patients were hypertensive and all had had surgical correction of carotid artery disease.

Disease of cerebral arteries secondary to hypertension is well described (see Blackwood, 1962). In his experience, the vessels of the Circle of Willis and the main branches, show muscular hypertrophy, medial fibrosis, abnormalities of the internal elastica, adventitial fibrosis and intimal fibrosis. The arterioles show thickening of the wall due to medial fibrosis or hyaline change. Medial fibrosis (Figure 3.23) in benign hypertension could predispose to rupture of the arterial wall. In malignant hypertension, fibrinoid necrosis may be widespread in the brain. Russell's series (1954) showed that this change was most marked in the pons, and primary pontine haemorrhage occurred more frequently in malignant hypertension than it did in benign hypertension. Byrom (1954, 1958–59) suggested that vascular necrosis induced by spasm could explain major haemorrhages occurring in experimental hypertension.

Zülch (1971), during a discussion of the pathology of cerebral accidents in hypertension, summarised his findings and conclusions regarding the pathogenesis of massive haemorrhage. He described arteriosclerosis predominantly affecting the proximal segment of the lenticulostriate artery while the distal segments show hyalinosis. With increasing age, the proximal segment shows dilatation and tortuosity. In persisting hypertension, the small distal branches

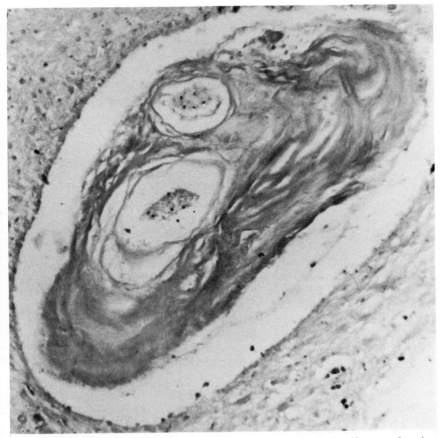

Figure 3.23. Extreme medial fibrosis in an artery adjacent to the lentiform nucleus in a hypertensive. (Elastic van Gieson stain × 145.)

became progressively narrowed and occluded, raising the pressure within the proximal segment. Zülch (1971) suggests that during a hypertensive crisis the thin, sclerotic proximal segment ruptures, giving rise to an acute, massive haemorrhage.

Fisher (1971) suggested that hypertensive lipohyalinosis (hyalinosis) 'might well have been the predisposing vascular disease' in three haemorrhages he studied by means of serial sections. These consisted of two putaminal haemorrhages and one pontine haemorrhage. In each case, multiple bleeding points were identified as consisting of a 'fibrin globe' with a ball of haemorrhage and a central core of platelet material filling the lumen of the artery. He suggested that one artery in the pons (possibly 200 μm in diameter) ruptured and disrupted the brain tissue, causing damage to other vessels, the haemorrhage progressing in 'avalanche fashion' as a result of multiple secondary haemorrhages. In the putaminal haemorrhages, a possible primary origin of the bleeding in the form of a large fibrin globe was identified.

86

Several miliary aneurysms were also present in Fisher's material but he did not consider them to be 'an intermediate stage on the way to a major haemorrhage'. Charcot and Bouchard (1868) investigated cerebral haemorrhage and described saccular and fusiform aneurysms on small cerebral arteries probably 250 to 400 µm in diameter. They described 'periarteritis', which they thought caused the aneurysms and considered that rupture of these lesions resulted in haemorrhage. Such miliary aneurysms were most frequent in the thalami and corpora striata. They were also seen in the pons, grey matter of the convolutions, the claustrum, cerebellum and, least frequently, in the central white matter. Other workers have also demonstrated miliary aneurysms (Green, 1930; Matsuoka, 1952) and Ross Russell (1963b) demonstrated multiple microaneurysms in 14 out of 15 brains from hypertensives. Lesions were demonstrated by microangiography of fixed and cleared slices of brain (Figure 3.24). Microaneurysms were also present in 10 out of 35

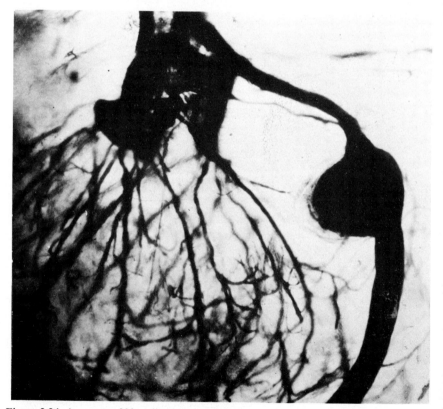

Figure 3.24. Aneurysm 800 µ diameter on long penetrating artery from parietal cortex of 71-year-old hypertensive man. (By kind permission of Dr R. W. Ross Russell and the editor of *Brain*.)

brains from normotensives. The aneurysms were from 300 to 900 µm in diameter and occurred on small arteries 100 to 300 µm in diameter. They were commonly found on the lateral branches of the striate arteries and on perforating vessels from the cortex. Thirteen aneurysms from 9 cases were studied by serial sections. The walls of the aneurysm were composed of connective tissue, and the muscle of the artery terminated abruptly at the origin of the aneurysm. A layer of hyaline material lined the lumen of the aneurysm. Occasionally, aneurysms were thrombosed (Figure 3.25). Evidence of leakage of blood in the form of iron-laden macrophages was found in the tissue outside some aneurysms. Occasionally thin-walled aneurysms ruptured while the contrast medium was being injected. In view of these two observations, Ross Russell argued that microaneurysms could be the source of massive haemorrhage, but no haemorrhages were definitely traced to particular aneurysms.

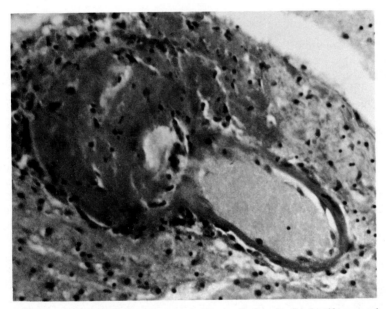

Figure 3.25. Thrombosed microaneurysm. A chance finding in the lentiform nucleus of a hypertensive patient (see Figure 3.26). (Haematoxylin and Eosin × 180.)

Cole and Yates (1967b) applied similar methods to a series of 100 hypertensive and 100 age- and sex-matched normotensive brains. Aneurysms were demonstrated in only 7 of the normotensives, but they were present in 46 hypertensives. They measured up to 2 mm in diameter and most occurred on vessels below 250 μm in diameter but a minority were on the main striate vessels up to 500 μm in diameter. As in Ross Russell's material, aneurysms were usually multiple; there were never less than 9 and usually between 15 and 25. Again, the basal ganglia were mainly affected and some occurred in the subcortical white matter. In Cole and Yates's series the pons was affected in 15 cases and the cerebellum in 4.

'Haemorrhage' of the contrast medium, demonstrating points of weakness in the wall of the aneurysm, was again demonstrated and foci of old and recent haemorrhage was seen adjacent to aneurysm. Subcortical white matter is a frequent site of slit haemorrhages in hypertensives, and 30 per cent of Cole and Yates aneurysms occurred in this site. In one case they traced a haemorrhage to a specific aneurysm.

In both Ross Russell's and Cole and Yates's investigations aneurysms occurred in patients in the age group when hypertensive haemorrhage is most frequent (over the age of 50 years), and were unusual in young patients even when severely hypertensive. The duration of hypertension necessary for the development of these presumably irreversible lesions is not known. From data available at the present, it seems most likely that these microaneurysms are the underlying lesions in both localised and massive intracerebral haemorrhage.

Lacunes

Lacunes are small cavities 0.5 to 1.5 cm in diameter, seen mainly in the basal ganglia, internal capsule, the central white matter, and the pons. There is general agreement that they are closely associated with hypertension but widely differing views are held on their pathogenesis.

Lacunes are regarded as old infarcts by Fisher (1969) and as expanded perivascular spaces by Cole and Yates (1968). Fisher (1969) investigated 50 of these lesions by serial sectioning and in 45 demonstrated occlusions of the artery supplying the area. This was associated with a localised swelling of the artery proximal to the lacune and due to degenerative disorganisation of the entire vessel walls; thrombosis of the vessel was found both proximal and distal to the swelling. Fisher was unwilling to label the lesions aneurysms although he considered this possibility. Cole and Yates (1968), Blackwood (1963) and Hughes (1965) emphasised that they have invariably found an artery traversing the cavities. This vessel usually showed lipohyaline degeneration, which is so common in hypertension, but thrombosis was not seen. They considered the cavities showed clear evidence that they were expanded perivascular spaces with nothing to suggest infarction or that they were the result of haemorrhage. Proponents of this view attribute lacunes to tissue damage due to pulsation of a coiled vessel elongated by hypertension (Hughes, 1965).

Those who accept the 'vascular space' explanation for these lesions consider that they are usually without clinical manifestations. The view that they are infarcts, however, implies their more sudden development and Fisher, together with others who take this view, believe that they may cause little strokes. Fisher, Mohr, and Adams (1974) state that the development of these lesions is often accompanied by the sudden onset of symptoms without any change in consciousness. Pseudo bulbar palsy, pure motor hemiplegia from capsular lesions, and dysarthria with the 'clumsy hand syndrome' from pontine lesions are amongst the syndromes they describe.

Whatever the pathogenesis of lacunes we would agree with Cole and Yates (1968) that they must be distinguished from the small cavities that are recognisably the result of a previous small haemorrhage, for there can be no doubt that small non-fatal haemorrhages do produce symptoms. The distinction does not always appear to have been made. Figure 3.26 shows lesions

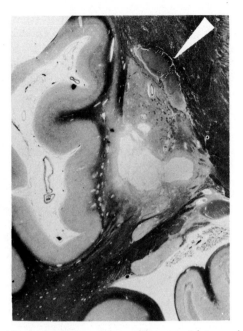

Figure 3.26. 'Lacunes' in the lentiform nucleus with a recent haemorrhage adjacent to the lentiform nucleus (arrowed). Adjacent to the haemorrhage is a microaneurysm (same case as Figure 3.25). (Myelin × 2.4.)

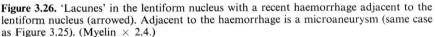

in a lentiform nucleus in a 63-year-old hypertensive man, who died of pulmonary embolism. Macroscopically, the clear lesions appeared to be lacunes, but histological examination showed extensive iron pigmentation of the walls. We believe that these lesions are old haemorrhages. A recent haemorrhage associated with a microaneurysm (Figure 3.25) is present adjacent to the lentiform nucleus. Small haemorrhages of this type could give rise to the older lesions which macroscopically appear to be lacunes.

Berry aneurysms

Stehbens (1972) discussed the aetiology of saccular arterial aneurysms in detail. Of the two main theories, the congenital and the acquired (degenerative) views, Stehbens accepts the latter.

Early aneurysmal changes are probably dependent on such lesions as degenerative changes near arterial forks associated with atherosclerosis and haemodynamic stresses at forks. Failure of compensatory intimal thickening at the apex of forks, and focal failure of tensile strength of branch apices and the origins of daughter branches, are also related to early aneurysmal changes.

There is evidence that hypertension is related to the development and rupture of aneurysms. Hypertension is a feature of coarctation of the aorta and of polycystic disease of the kidneys. Both these conditions are associated with aneurysms. Walton (1956) believed that hypertension probably contributed to the death of patients with subarachnoid haemorrhage. Brewer, Fawcett and Horsfield (1968), in a study of the relationship between heart weight and non-traumatic cerebral haemorrhages and softenings, found a highly significant relationship between increased heart weight and fatal subarachnoid haemorrhage. At least 140 of their 154 cases of primary subarachnoid haemorrhage had aneurysms. Stehbens (1962) investigated the relationship between hypertension and cerebral aneurysms in 251 necropsies where aneurysms (with and without rupture) were demonstrated. The presence of hypertension was assessed critically and conservatively and at least 54 per cent of patients with aneurysms had hypertension. Hypertension was more common in the aneurysm-bearing group than in the 839 controls.

Apart from subarachnoid haemorrhage, intracerebral haematoma is an important consequence of rupture of a berry aneurysm. Such haemorrhages occur in one or both frontal lobes following rupture of an anterior cerebral artery aneurysm (Figure 3.27), the temporal pole from rupture of an aneurysm of arteries in the Sylvian fissure, and the inferior horn of the lateral ventricle and white matter of the temporal lobe from rupture of an aneurysm of the posterior communicating artery. Aneurysms of the bifurcation of the internal carotid artery can cause massive haematomas at the level of the striatum (Figures 3.28, 3.29).

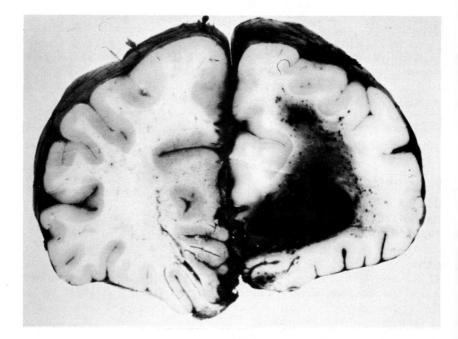

Figure 3.27. Haematoma in the right frontal lobe following rupture of a berry aneurysm of the anterior cerebral artery. Extensive, bilateral subarachnoid haemorrhage is also present.

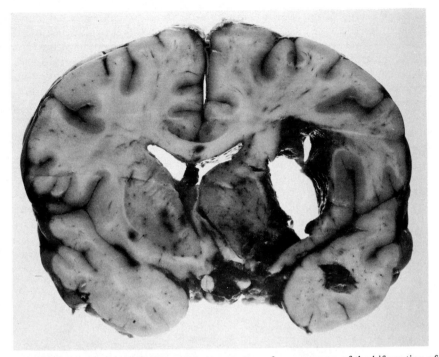

Figure 3.28. Intracerebral haematoma due to rupture of an aneurysm of the bifurcation of the right internal carotid artery. During cutting, part of the haematoma became displaced leaving the clear area (see Figure 3.29).

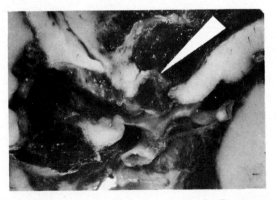

Figure 3.29. Caritod bifurcation with aneurysm (arrowed). (Same case as Figure 3.28.)

In Tomlinson's (1959) series of 32 cases of ruptured intracranial aneurysm there was bleeding into the brain in 17 cases (53 per cent). In 12 of these blood had reached the ventricles. There were 5 cases of intracerebral haematoma without rupture into the ventricles. Three of these were in the basal ganglia and originated via the insular cortex. One ruptured into the temporal lobe and one into the frontal lobe. Tomlinson was careful to separate subarachnoid haematomas from true intracerebral haematomas and the incidence of true intracerebral haemorrhage is consequently somewhat lower than the 75 per cent which had usually been recorded. If the two types of haemorrhage were combined they amounted to 68 per cent of Tomlinson's series. He also pointed out the difference between massive intracerebral bleeding and the linear haemorrhages which are common in the neighbourhood of a ruptured aneurysm. These are perivascular and run at right angles to the cerebral cortex with appearances suggesting that they may result from blood tracking along Virchow-Robin spaces.

Crompton (1962) investigated intracerebral haematomas in 103 consecutively examined cases of ruptured berry aneurysms. There were 62 cases of intracerebral haematoma, 32 of which also showed gross cerebral infarction. Anterior communicating and anterior cerebral artery aneurysms resulted in intracerebral haematomas more frequently than aneurysms elsewhere. These commonly produced haematomas in the frontal lobes and in the cavum of the septum pellucidum (Figure 3.30). The corpus callosum was less often involved. Middle cerebral aneurysms most frequently ruptured into the external capsule.

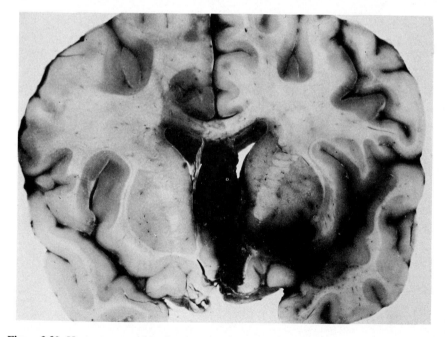

Figure 3.30. Haematoma within the septum pellucidum following rupture of an aneurysm of the anterior communicating artery.

Crompton (1962) compared the situation of hypertensive haemorrhages with those following ruptured aneurysm. The main differences demonstrated were that frontal haemorrhages were more frequent in ruptured aneurysm and external capsule haemorrhages more frequent in hypertensive haemorrhages. Thalamic and caudate haematomas were virtually always due to hypertension, and frontal haemorrhages were due to aneurysms. Previous subarachnoid haemorrhages from a particular aneurysm were more likely to be associated with rupture into the brain.

Intracerebral and intraventricular rupture was more often associated with admission in coma (42 of 62 cases) than rupture with subarachnoid bleeding only (21 of 41 cases). Anterior cerebral aneurysms more often produce coma and intracerebral haemorrhage than aneurysms elsewhere.

Crompton (1963) has also made a detailed study of the hypothalamic lesions after rupture of cerebral artery aneurysm. Sixty-one per cent of 106 aneurysms had hypothalamic lesions. The aneurysms most likely to produce lesions were on the anterior cerebral and posterior communicating arteries. Middle cerebral aneurysms involving the first 1 cm of the artery also produced hypothalamic lesions. The lesions were regions of ischaemic necrosis, small haemorrhages, and massive haemorrhages due to rupture through the hypothalamus into the third ventricle. Pathogenetic mechanisms such as damage to fine hypothalamic arteries in the subarachnoid space and distortion of perforating vessels by blood spreading along perivascular sheaths were discussed.

Cerebral infarction is another important sequel of rupture of berry aneurysms. In Tomlinson's (1959) series 78 per cent of cases showed ischaemic lesions, 40 per cent of which were described as massive. Schneck (1964) demonstrated infarction in 55 per cent of cases and Crompton (1964a) showed that 80 per cent of women, 69 per cent of men with ruptured aneurysms had infarction. The majority of ischaemic lesions occur in the territory of the aneurysm-bearing artery, but they can occur anywhere in the brain. Smith (1963) showed the importance of histological examination in demonstrating lesions following subarachnoid haemorrhage which are not obvious macroscopically.

The pathogenesis of these infarcts has been widely discussed (Tomlinson, 1969; Smith, 1963; Crompton, 1964b; Schneck, 1964; Schneck and Kricheff, 1964). The presence of subarachnoid haematomas causing compression and kinking of various vessels is an important factor. Spasm of vessels, possibly due to irritation of vessels by subarachnoid blood, release of vasoactive amines, or by surgery soon after the haemorrhage, has also been implicated as a cause of infarction following ruptured aneurysm.

Other causes of non-traumatic intracerebral haemorrhage

VASCULAR HAMARTOMAS

In Russell's (1954) series of 461 intracranial haemorrhages, 133 were due to diseases other than hypertension or berry aneurysms; vascular hamartomas were the cause in 21 cases. Twenty of these cases were due to arteriovenous hamartomas. The other case was due to multiple cavernous haemangiomas. Haemorrhages due to such lesions mainly occur in young people. The majority of Russell's cases were in the second decade and none was beyond the fourth decade. Thus, these lesions cause haemorrhages in a younger group of

patients than hypertension of berry aneurysms (Figure 3.31). The hamartomas consist of a collection of abnormal arterial and venous channels (see
Russell and Rubenstein, 1971) and the haemorrhage is probably caused by
rupture of a thin-walled dilated venous channel.

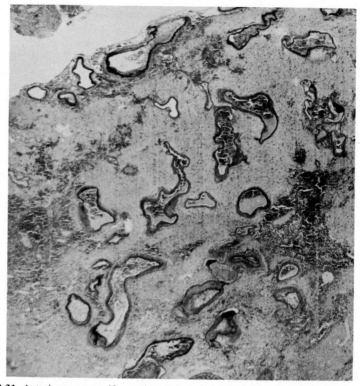

Figure 3.31. Arteriovenous malformation removed surgically from a patient aged 30 years
who presented with an intracerebral haematoma. (Elastic van Gieson × 24.)

Russell (1954) drew attention to small lesions and Crawford and Russell
(1956) described 'cryptic' hamartomatous lesions of the brain in detail.
They discussed 20 cases of spontaneous cerebral and cerebellar haemorrhage
in patients between the age of 3 and 33 years, 7 of whom survived operation.
The haemorrhages were due to small arteriovenous or venous hamartomas
which occurred in three sites in the brain. Cerebral convexities, central
cerebral, and cerebellar tissues were involved. The lesions were described
as 'cryptic' because of the clinical latency, and the fact that they were small.
Despite the presence of a haematoma, the causal lesion was difficult to
demonstrate. Because of the extremely small size of these lesions (one of
Crawford and Russell's lesions was 1.2 cm × 0.7 cm), they can be completely destroyed during haemorrhage and they may be the underlying lesion
in patients who develop haemorrhages for which no cause is demonstrable
even after careful autopsy.

Occasionally, a subcortical haemorrhage occurs in older patients for which no cause is demonstrable. Small 'cryptic' arteriovenous malformations may be responsible. However, Cole and Yates (1967b) demonstrated micro-aneurysms in the subcortical white matter in normotensive patients over the age of 66 years, and it is possible that such lesions may give rise to atypical haemorrhages in non-hypertensive patients.

MISCELLANEOUS CONDITIONS

Rupture of mycotic aneurysms is an unusual cause of intracranial haemorrhage. Roach and Drake (1964) reviewed 191 cases of ruptured intra-cranial aneurysm and found that 2.5 per cent were mycotic. All the patients had infective endocarditis but none had cardiac failure. Intracranial haemor-rhage due to rupture of the aneurysm was the presenting feature in each case.

Intracranial haemorrhage is a rare presenting feature of haemophilia. Adeloye et al (1969) described the case of a three-year-old Nigerian boy who presented with intracranial ventricular haemorrhage due to haemophilia. Kerr (1964) described 19 episodes of intracranial haemorrhage in 15 (13.8 per cent) of 109 haemophiliacs. Five patients died and four patients had residual disability.

Blood dyscrasias, associated with thrombocytopenia, are also rare causes of intracranial haemorrhage (Silverstein, 1961). Thrombocytopenia associated with platelet antibodies was the cause of an intracerebral haemorrhage in the case of infectious mononucleosis described by Goldstein and Porter (1969).

Nine of Russell's (1954) cases had intracerebral haemorrhage associated with primary and secondary neoplasms and one of us (P.J.H.F.) has recently seen a medulloblastoma which presented with a massive, fatal haemorrhage into the cerebellar vermis.

PERSPECTIVE

We have stated the evidence for the view that hypertension is of prime importance in causing cerebral haemorrhage. This is true whether large catastrophic haemorrhages are involved or small lesions causing only temporary disability and clinically indistinguishable from small infarcts. Hypertension is also closely associated with development of the controversial small cavitating lesions discussed under the general heading of 'lacunes', whether these are a consequence of a small infarct, vascular space dilatation, or small haemorrhages.

We think there is good evidence also for believing that hypertension precipitates the rupture of berry aneurysm although, of course, rupture is common in normotensive patients.

When we turn to cerebral infarction the role of hypertension is much less obvious. Cole and Yates (1968) found only a small preponderance of in-farction in 100 hypertensives compared with 100 matched normotensive controls. Torvik and Jörgensen (1964) concluded, with some hesitation, that hypertension might have a role in the occurrence of thrombo-embolic carotid occlusion. Brewer, Fawcett and Horsfield (1968) excluded cases of obvious embolic infarction and concluded that there was an excess of hypertensive patients in the infarcted group that remained.

Data from the Framingham study led Dawber et al (1965) to conclude that the higher the blood pressure the higher the incidence of brain infarction. But the diagnosis of the cerebral lesions was either clinical or derived from death certificates and must have been subject to appreciable error; strokes thought to be embolic were excluded. Since hypertension is certainly a common cause of heart disease and an aggravating cause of coronary disease, it is evident that hypertensives will suffer from cardiac embolic strokes more often than patients free from cardiac disease.

Stehbens (1972) accepts that hypertension accelerates the development of cerebral atherosclerosis. Baker and Resch (1964) came to this conclusion on a study of over 2000 autopsies in which they accepted a heart weight of 450 g as evidence of hypertension. The reliance upon heart weight as an indication of blood pressure during life has been criticised by Mitchell and Schwartz (1965), mainly on the grounds that coronary ischaemia itself is a source of cardiomegaly. Any post-mortem series that relies on heart weight for the diagnosis of hypertension must also include a number of cases of unrecognised congestive cardiomyopathy.

The clinical diagnosis of strokes is, of course, subject to considerable error and non-lethal haemorrhages are indistinguishable from infarctions. The clinical effects of hypertension are discussed in detail in Chapter 7. From autopsy observations our tentative conclusion would be that hypertensives would be expected to be more liable to cerebral infarction than normotensives and that the total evidence suggests this is so, though the effect may be small.

If we accept that hypertension accelerates atherosclerosis in general, and in particular coronary atherosclerosis, we might expect that a number of people would die from cardiac causes before cerebral atherosclerosis developed, and that the statistical effect of hypertension on cerebral atherosclerosis would consequently be diminished. That cerebral atherosclerosis develops later in the cerebral arteries than in the coronary vessels seems to be firmly established by the observations of McGill (1968).

It is often impossible to be certain of the cause of a brain infarct at autopsy and non-occlusive infarcts afford ample opportunity for speculation. Atherosclerosis of the cerebral arteries is clearly very important but we have emphasised the contribution of the extracranial causes of cerebral infarction and especially the need to exclude an embolic lesion at autopsy, and to give this diagnosis prime consideration clinically.

In the matter of cerebral infarction the brain is often more sinned against than sinning, and the recognition of extracranial lesions at least has the merit of widening the field of therapeutic endeavour.

REFERENCES

Adams, J. H. (1967) Patterns of cerebral infarction. *Scottish Medical Journal*, **12**, 335.

Adams, J. H., Brierley, J. B., Connor, R. C. R. & Treip, C. S. (1966) The effects of systemic hypotension on the human brain. Clinical and neuropathological observations on 11 cases. *Brain*, **89**, 235–268.

Adams, R. D. & vander Eecken, H. M. (1953) Vascular diseases of brain. *Annual Review of Medicine*, **4**, 213.

Adams, R. D., Cammermeyer, J. & Fitzgerald, P. J. (1948) Neuropathological aspects of thrombocytic acroangiothrombosis. *Journal of Neurology, Neurosurgery and Psychiatry*, **11**, 27.

Adeloye, A., Seriki, O., Luzzato, L. & Essien, E. M. (1969) Intracranial haemorrhage as a first presentation of haemophilia. *Journal of Neurology, Neurosurgery and Psychiatry*, **32**, 470.

Albutt, T. C. (1921) Discussion on visceral syphilis especially of the central nervous system and cardiovascular system. *British Medical Journal*, **ii**, 177.

Alpers, B. J. & Berry, R. G. (1963) Circle of Willis in cerebral vascular disorders. The anatomical structure. *Archives of Neurology* (Chicago), **8**, 398.

Altschuler, J. H., McLaughlin, R. A. & Neuberger, K. T. (1968) Neurological catastrophe related to oral contraceptives. *Archives of Neurology* (Chicago), **19**, 264.

Arendt, A. & Bachmann, P. (1966) Intracerebrale Gefässwandveränderungen bei hypertonischer Hirnmassenblutung. *Acta Neuropathologica*, **7**, 79.

Arkin, A. (1930) A clinical and pathological study of periarteritis nodosa. *American Journal of Pathology*, **6**, 401.

Aronson, S. M. & Rabiner, A. M. (1958) Studies on vascular encephalomalacia: evaluation of clinical syndromes in five hundred consecutive cases studied pathologically. *Archives of Neurology and Psychiatry*, **80**, 324.

Aronson, H., Shafey, S. & Gargano, F. (1965) Intracerebral haematoma. *Journal of Neurology, Neurosurgery and Psychiatry*, **28**, 442.

Askey, J. M. (1946) Hemiplegia following carotid sinus stimulation. *American Heart Journal*, **31**, 131.

Ask-Upmark, E., Glas, J. & Stenram, U. (1969) Oral contraceptives and cerebral arterial thrombosis. *Acta Medica Scandinavica*, **185**, 479.

Baker, A. B. & Iannone, A. (1959) The small intracerebral arteries. *Neurology* (Minneapolis), **9**, 391.

Baker, A. B., Dahl, E. & Sandler, B. (1963) Cerebrovascular disease; etiologic factors in cerebral infarction. *Neurology* (Minneapolis), **13**, 445.

Baker, A. B. & Resch, J. A. (1964) Hypertension in relationship to cerebroarteriosclerosis. *Minnesota Medical Journal*, **47**, 1202.

Barron, K. D., Siqueira, E. & Hirano, A. (1960) Cerebral embolism caused by non-bacterial endocarditis. *Neurology*, **10**, 391.

Batsakis, J. G. (1968) Cardiac enlargement. In *The Pathology of the Heart and Blood Vessels*, ed. Gould, S. E. Ch. X. Springfield, Ill.: Thomas.

Beattie, W. W. (1925) Paradoxical embolism associated with two types of patent foramen ovale. *Bulletin of the International Association of Medical Museums and Journal of Technical Methods*, **64, 9**, 182.

Berry, R. G. (1971) Lupus erythematosus. In *Pathology of Nervous System*, ed. Minckler, J. Vol. 2. New York: McGraw-Hill. pp. 1482–1488.

Berry, R. G. & Hodges, J. H. (1965) Nervous system involvement in systemic lupus erythematosus. *Transactions of the American Neurological Association*, **90**, 231.

Bhattacharji, S. K. (1965) *The Role of the Extracranial and Intracranial Cerebral Arteries in Cerebral Infarction*. Ph.D. Thesis, University of Birmingham.

Bhattacharji, S. K., Hutchinson, E. C. & McCall, A. J. (1967a) Stenosis and occlusion of vessels in cerebral infarction. *British Medical Journal*, **iii**, 270.

Bhattacharji, S. K., Hutchinson, E. C. & McCall, A. J. (1967b) The circle of Willis. The incidence of developmental abnormalities in normal and infarcted brains. *Brain*, **90**, 747.

Bickerstaff, E. R. (1964) Aetiology of acute hemiplegia in childhood. *British Medical Journal*, **ii**, 82.

Bickerstaff, E. R. (1973) Cerebral embolism and oral contraceptives. *British Medical Journal*, **iii**, 736.

Bickerstaff, E. R. & Holmes, J. M. (1967) Cerebral arterial insufficiency and oral contraceptives. *British Medical Journal*, **i**, 726.

Blackwood, W. (1962) In *Greenfields Neuropathology* by Blackwood, W., McMenemey, W. H., Meyer, A., Norman, R. M. and Russell, D. S. 2nd edition, Ch. 2. Edward Arnold.

Blackwood, W., Hallpike, J. F., Kocen, R. S. & Mair, W. G. P. (1969) Atheromatous disease of the carotid arterial system and embolism from the heart in cerebral infarction: a morbid anatomical study. *Brain*, **92**, 897.

Bladin, P. F. (1964) A radiological and pathological study of embolism of the internal carotid-middle cerebral arterial axis. *Radiology*, **82**, 615.

Bornstein, B., Boss, J. H., Casper, J. & Behar, M. (1960) Thrombotic thrombocytopenic purpura. *Journal of Clinical Pathology*, **13**, 124.

Breutman, M. E., Fields, W. S., Crawford, E. S. & de Bakey, M. E. (1963) Cerebral haemorrhage in carotid artery surgery. *Archives of Neurology* (Chicago), **9**, 458.

Brewer, D. B., Fawcett, F. J. & Horsfield, G. I. (1968) A necropsy series of non-traumatic cerebral haemorrhages and softenings with particular reference to heart weight. *Journal of Pathology and Bacteriology*, **96**, 311.

Brice, J. G., Dowsett, D. J. & Lowe, R. D. (1964) Haemodynamic effects of carotid artery stenosis. *British Medical Journal*, **ii**, 1363.

Brierley, J. B. (1970) Systemic hypotension—Neurological and neuropathological aspects. In *Modern Trends and Neurology*, (Ed.) Williams D. Chapter 9. London: Butterworths. p. 164.

Brierley, J. B., Brown, A. W., Excell, B. J. & Meldrum, B. S. (1969) Brain damage in the Rhesus monkey resulting from profound arterial hypotension. I. Its nature, distribution and general physiological correlates. *Brain Research*, **13**, 68.

Brierley, J. B. & Excell, B. J. (1966) Effects of profound systemic hypotension upon the brain of "M Rhesus". Physiological and pathological observations. *Brain*, **89**, 269–298.

Brihaye, J. F., Retif, J. & Jeanmart, L. (1971) L'obstruction de l'artère basilaire chez le sujet jeune. Aspects cliniques et angiographiques. Reflexions etiopathogeniques. Apropos de trois cas. *Acta Neurochirugica*, **24**, 143.

Brihaye, J., Retif, J., Jeanmart, L. & Flament Durand, J. (1971) Occlusion of the basilar artery in young patients. *Acta Neurochirugica*, **25**, 225.

Brown, G. E. & Giffin, H. Z. (1930) Peripheral artery disease in polycythaemia vera. *Archives of Internal Medicine*, **46**, 705.

Bruetsch, W. L. (1971a) Aortic arch syndrome. In *Pathology of the Nervous System*, ed. Minckler, J. Vol. 2. Chapter XVII. Section 112. New York: McGraw-Hill.

Bruetsch, W. L. (1971b) Cerebral thromboangiitis obliterans. In *Pathology of the Nervous System*, ed. Minckler, J. Vol. 2. Chapter XVII. Section 108. New York: McGraw-Hill.

Burton, A. & Spiegel, P. K. (1968) Foreign body embolus in the middle cerebral artery. *Virginia Medical Monthly*, **95**, 151.

Byrom, F. B. (1954) Pathogenesis of hypertensive encephalopathy and its relation to the malignant phase of hypertension. *Lancet*, **ii**, 201.

Byrom, F. B. (1958–59) The significance of hypertensive encephalopathy. *Lectures on the Scientific Basis of Medicine*, **8**, pp. 256. University of London.

Callow, A. D., Moran, J. M., Kahn, P. C. & Deterling, R. A. (1968) Patterns of atherosclerosis of extracranial cerebral arteries. *Annals of the New York Academy of Science*, **149**, 974.

Calverley, J. R. & Millikan, C. H. (1961) Complications of carotid manipulation. *Neurology* (Minneapolis), **11**, 185.

Cardell, B. S. & Hanley, T. (1951) A fatal case of giant cell or temporal arteritis. *Journal of Pathology and Bacteriology*, **63**, 587.

Carroll, J. D., Leak, D. & Lee, H. A. (1966) Cerebral thrombophlebitis in pregnancy and in the puerperium. *Quarterly Journal of Medicine*, **35**, 347.

Carter, A. B. (1964) *Cerebral Infarction*. London: Pergamon.

Castaigne, P., Lhermitte, F., Gautier, J. C., Escourelle, R. & Derouesné, C. (1970) Internal carotid artery occlusion. *Brain*, **93**, 231.

Castaigne, P., Lhermitte, F., Gautier, J. C., Escourelle, C., Derouesné, C., Agopian, P. & Popa, C. (1973) Arterial occlusions in the vertebrobasilar system. A study of 44 patients with post-mortem data. *Brain*, **96**, 133.

Charcot, J. M. & Bouchard, C. (1868) Nouvelles recherches sur la pathogenie de l'haemorrhagie cerebrale. *Archives de Physiologie* (Paris), **1**, 110, 725.

Chiang, J., Marayoshi, K., Ames, A., Wright, R. & Majuo, G. (1968) Cerebral ischaemia. Vascular changes. *American Journal of Pathology*, **52**, 455.

Chiari, H. (1905) Ueber das Verhalten des Teilungswinkels der Carotis communis bei der Endarteriitis chronica deformans. *Verhandlungen der deutschen Gesellschaft für Pathologie*, **9**, 326.

Churg, J. & Strauss, L. (1951) Allergic granulomatosis, allergic angiitis and periarteritis nodosa. *American Journal of Pathology*, **27**, 277.

Clyne, D. H., Epstein, J., Sloman, G., Andrews, J. T., Hare, W. S. C., Morris, P. J., Marshall, V. C. & Kincaid-Smith, P. (1970) Retrograde cerebral emboli during procedures to clear arterial thrombi from haemodialysis shunts. *Medical Journal of Australia*, **1**, 359.

Cole, F. M. & Yates, P. O. (1967a) Pseudo-aneurysms in relation to massive cerebral haemorrhage. *Journal of Neurology, Neurosurgery and Psychiatry*, **30**, 61.

Cole, F. M. & Yates, P. O. (1967b) The occurrence and significance of intracerebral microaneurysms. *Journal of Pathology and Bacteriology*, **93**, 393.

Cole, F. M. & Yates, P. O. (1968) Comparative incidence of cerebrovascular lesions in normotensive and hypertensive patients. *Neurology*, **18**, 255.

Collaborative Group for the Study of Stroke in Young Women (1973) Oral contraception and increased risk of cerebral ischaemia or thrombosis. *New England Journal of Medicine*, **288**, 871.

Cravioto, H. & Feigin, I. (1959) Non-infectious granulomatous angiitis with predilection for the nervous system. *Neurology*, **9**, 599.

Crawford, T. (1956) The pathological effects of cerebral arteriography. *Journal of Neurology, Neurosurgery and Psychiatry*, **19**, 217.

Crawford, R. & Crompton, M. R. (1968) The pathology of strokes. In *The Management of Cerebrovascular Disease*, by Marshall, J. 2nd edition. Chapter III. London: Churchill.

Crawford, J. V. & Russell, D. S. (1956) Cryptic arterio-venous and venous hamartomas of the brain. *Journal of Neurology, Neurosurgery and Psychiatry*, **19**, 1–11.

Crompton, M. R. (1962) Intracerebral haematoma complicating ruptured cerebral berry aneurysm. *Journal of Neurology, Neurosurgery and Psychiatry*, **25**, 378.

Crompton, M. R. (1963) Hypothalamic lesions after rupture of cerebral artery aneurysms. *Brain*, **86**, 301.

Crompton, M. R. (1964a) Cerebral infarction following rupture of cerebral berry aneurysms. *Brain*, **87**, 263.

Crompton, M. R. (1964b) The pathogenesis of cerebral infarction following rupture of cerebral berry aneurysms. *Brain*, **87**, 491.

Cross, J. N., Castro, P. D. & Jennett, W. B. (1968) Cerebral strokes associated with pregnancy and the puerperium. *British Medical Journal*, **iii**, 214.

Dalal, P. M., Shah, P. M. & Aiyar, R. R. (1965) Arteriographic study of cerebral embolism. *Lancet*, **ii**, 358.

Dalal, P. M., Shah, P. M., Sheth, S. C. & Deshpande, C. K. (1965) Cerebral embolism. Angiographic observations on spontaneous clot lysis. *Lancet*, **i**, 161.

Daley, R., Mattingly, T. W., Holt, L., Bland, E. F. & White, P. D. (1951) Systemic arterial embolism in rheumatic heart disease. *American Heart Journal*, **42**, 566.

Daniel, D. G., Campbell, H. & Turnbull, A. C. (1967) Puerperal thrombo-embolism and the suppression of lactation. *Lancet*, **ii**, 287.

Danta, G. & Williams, P. O. (1969) Multiple emboli from left ventricular myxoma. *British Heart Journal*, **31**, 799.

Davie, J. C. & Coxe, W. (1967) Occlusive disease of the carotid artery in children. *Archives of Neurology*, **17**, 313.

Davis, J. M. & Golinger, D. (1966) Cervical rib, subclavian artery aneurysm, axillary and cerebral emboli. *Proceedings of the Royal Society of Medicine*, **59**, 1002.

Dawber, T. R., Kannell, W. B., McNamara, P. M. & Cohen, M. E. (1965) An epidermiologic study of apoplexy ("Strokes"). *Transaction of the American Neurological Association*, **90**, 237.

Deisenhammer, E., Von, Hammer, B. & Tulzer, W. (1970) Akute kindliche Hemiplegia. *Münchener medizinische Wochenschrift*, **112**, 370.
De Villiers, J. C. (1966) A brachiocephalic vascular syndrome associated with cervical rib. *British Medical Journal*, **ii**, 140.
Digiacinto, G., Cantu, A. B. & Cantu, R. C. (1970) Influence of hypertension on post-ischaemic cerebrovascular obstruction. *Journal of Surgical Research*, **10**, 229.
Dinsdale, H. B. (1964) Spontaneous haemorrhage in the posterior fossa. *Archives of Neurology* (Chicago), **10**, 200.
Dooley, J. M. & Smith, K. R. (1968) Occlusion of the basilar artery in a six year old boy. *Neurology* (Minneapolis), **18**, 1034.
Duguid, J. B. (1949) Pathogenesis of atherosclerosis. *Lancet*, **ii**, 925.
Eastcott, H. H. G., Pickering, G. W. & Rob, C. G. (1954) Reconstruction of internal carotid artery in a patient with intermittent attacks of hemiplegia. *Lancet*, **ii**, 994.
Enzel, K. & Lindelmalm, G. (1973) Cryptogenic cerebral embolism in women taking oral contraceptives. *British Medical Journal*, **14**, 507.
Fessel, W. J. (1965) Odd men out. *Archives of Internal Medicine*, **115**, 736.
Fisher, C. M. (1951) Occlusion of the internal carotid artery. *Archives of Neurology and Psychiatry*, **65**, 346.
Fisher, C. M. (1954) Occlusion of the carotid arteries. *Archives of Neurology and Psychiatry*, **72**, 187.
Fisher, C. M. (1955) The clinical picture of cerebral arteriosclerosis. *Minnesota Medicine*, **38**, 839.
Fisher, C. M. (1957) Cerebral thromboangiitis obliterans. *Medicine* (Baltimore), **36**, 169.
Fisher, C. M. (1967) The non-sudden onset of cerebral embolism. *Neurology* (Minneapolis), **17**, 1025.
Fisher, C. M. (1969) The arterial lesions underlying lacunes. *Acta Neuropathologica* (Berlin), **12**, 1.
Fisher, C. M. (1970) Occlusion of the vertebral arteries. *Archives of Neurology*, **22**, 13.
Fisher, C. M. (1971) Pathological observations in hypertensive cerebral haemorrhage. *Journal of Neuropathology and Experimental Neurology*, **30**, 536.
Fisher, C. M. & Adams, R. D. (1951) Observations on brain embolism with special reference to the mechanism of haemorrhagic infarction. *Journal of Neuropathology and Experimental Neurology*, **10**, 92.
Fisher, C. M., Gore, I., Okabe, N. & White, P. D. (1965a) Atherosclerosis of the carotid and vertebral arteries: extracranial and intracranial. *Journal of Neuropathology and Experimental Neurology*, **24**, 455.
Fisher, C. M., Mohr, J. P. & Adams, R. D. (1974) In *Harrison's Principles of Internal Medicine*. 7th edition. New York: McGraw Hill. p. 1749.
Fisher, C. M., Picard, E. H., Polak, A., Dalai, P. & Ojemann, R. G. (1965b) Acute hypertensive cerebellar haemorrhage. *Journal of Nervous and Mental Disease*, **140**, 38.
Fleming, H. A. & Bailey, S. M. (1971) Mitral valve disease, systemic embolism, and anticoagulants. *Postgraduate Medical Journal*, **47**, 599.
Foix, C., Hillemand, P. & Ley, J. (1927) Relativement au ramollissement cérébral, à sa fréquence et à son siège, et à l'importance relative des oblitérations arterielles, complétes ou incompletès dans sa pathogénie. *Bulletin et Memoires de la Societe de Medécine de Paris*, **51**, 189.
Freytag, E. (1968) Fatal hypertensive intracerebral haematomas: a survey of the pathological anatomy of 393 cases. *Journal of Neurology, Neurosurgery, and Psychiatry*, **31**, 616.
Gaan, D., Mallick, N. P., Brevis, R. A. L., Seedat, Y. K. & Mahoney, M. P. (1969) Cerebral damage from declotting Scribner's shunts. *Lancet*, **ii**, 77.
Garunn, C. F. (1941) Mural thrombus in the heart. *American Heart Journal*, **21**, 713.
Geroulanos, S. (1969) Embolie eines Papillarmuskel Fragmentes in der Arteria cerebri media rechts nach Mitralklappenersatz, durch Beal-Scheibenklappe. *Thoraxochirurgie und Vasculäre Chirurgie*, **17**, 320.
Gilbert, H. S. & Silverstein, A. (1965) Neurogenic polycythaemia. Report of a patient with transient erythrocytosis associated with occlusion of the middle cerebral artery. A review of the literature. *American Journal of Medicine*, **38**, 807.

Gilder, J. C. Van, & Coxe, W. S. (1970) Shotgun pellet embolus of the middle cerebral artery. *Journal of Neurosurgery*, **32**, 711.

Globus, J. H. & Epstein, J. A. (1953) Massive cerebral haemorrhage, spontaneous and experimentally produced. *Journal of Neuropathology and Experimental Neurology*, **12**, 107.

Globus, J. H. & Strauss, I. S. (1926) Massive cerebral haemorrhage. Its relation to cerebral softening. *Archives of Neurology and Psychiatry* (Chicago), **18**, 215.

Goldstein, E. & Porter, D. Y. (1969) Fatal thrombocytopaenia with cerebral haemorrhage in mononucleosis. *Archives of Neurology*, **20**, 533.

Green, F. H. K. (1930) Miliary aneurysms in the brain. *Journal of Pathology and Bacteriology*, **33**, 71–77.

Gunning, A. J., Pickering, G. W., Robb-Smith, A. H. T. & Ross Russell, R. (1964a) Mural thrombosis of the internal carotid artery and subsequent embolism. *Quarterly Journal of Medicine*, **33**, 155.

Gunning, A. J., Pickering, G. W., Robb-Smith, A. H. T. & Ross Russell, R. (1964b) Mural thrombosis of the subclavian artery and subsequent embolism in cervical rib. *Quarterly Journal of Medicine*, **33**, 133.

Harris, L. S. & Kennedy, J. H. (1967) Atheromatous cerebral embolism. A complication of surgery of the thoracic aorta. *Annals of Thoracic Surgery*, **4**, 319.

Heptinstall, R. H., Porter, K. A. & Barkley, H. (1954) Giant cell (temporal) arteritis. *Journal of Pathology and Bacteriology*, **67**, 507.

Hicks, S. P. & Warren, S. (1951) Infarction of the brain without thrombosis. *Archives of Pathology*, **52**, 403.

Hill, N. C., Millikan, C. H., Wakim, H. G. & Sayre, G. P. (1955) Studies in cerebrovascular disease, VII. *Proceedings of the Staff Meeting of the Mayo Clinic*, **30**, 625.

Hoobler, S. W. (1942) The syndrome of cervical rib with subclavian arterial thrombosis and hemiplegia due to cerebral embolism. *New England Journal of Medicine*, **226**, 942.

Huber, R. (1965) Bedeutung der Lungenembolie für gekreuzte Embolien bei offenem Foramen ovale. *Schweizerische medizinische Wochenschrift*, **95**, 964.

Hudson, A. J. & Hyland, H. H. (1958) Hypertensive cerebrovascular disease: A clinical and pathological review of 100 cases. *Annals of Internal Medicine*, **49**, 1049.

Hughes, J. T. & Brownell, B. (1968) Traumatic thrombosis of the internal carotid artery in the neck. *Journal of Neurology, Neurosurgery and Psychiatry*, **31**, 307.

Hughes, W. (1965) Origin of lacunes. *Lancet*, **ii**, 19.

Hultquist, G. T. (1942) *Ueber Thrombose und Embolie der Arteria carotis*. Stockholm: Norstedt.

Hutchinson, E. C. & Yates, P. O. (1956) The cervical portion of the vertebral artery: a clinico-pathological study. *Brain*, **79**, 319.

Hutchinson, E. C. & Yates, P. O. (1957) Carotico-vertebral stenosis. *Lancet*, **i**, 2.

Hymen, A. S. & Parsonnet, A. E. (1932) *The Failing Heart of Middle Life*. Philadelphia: Davis.

Illis, L., Kocen, R. S., McDonald, W. I. & Mandkar, V. P. (1965) Oral contraceptives and carotid artery occlusion. *British Medical Journal*, **ii**, 1164.

Irey, N. S., Marion, W. C. & Taylor, H. B. (1970) Vascular lesions in women taking oral contraceptives. *Archives of Pathology* (Chicago), **89**, 1.

Jennett, W. B. & Cross, J. N. (1967) Influence of pregnancy and oral contraception on the incidence of strokes in women of childbearing age. *Lancet*, **i**, 1019.

Johnson, B. I. (1951) Paradoxical embolism. *Journal of Clinical Pathology*, **4**, 316.

Johnson, R. T. & Richardson, E. P. (1968) The neurological manifestations of systemic lupus erythematosus. *Medicine* (Baltimore), **47**, 337.

Johnson, R. T. & Yates, P. O. (1956) Brainstem haemorrhages in expanding supratentorial conditions. *Acta Radiologica* (Stockholm), **46**, 250.

Jörgensen, L. & Torvik, A. (1966) Ischaemic cerebrovascular diseases in an autopsy series. Part I: Prevalence, location and predisposing factors in verified thrombo-embolic occlusions, and their significance in the pathogenesis of cerebral infarction. *Journal of Neurological Sciences* (Amsterdam), **3**, 490.

Kameyama, M. & Okinaka, S. (1963) Collateral circulation of the brain with special reference to atherosclerosis of the major cervical and cerebral arteries. *Neurology* (Minneapolis), **13**, 279.

Kerr, C. B. (1964) Intracranial haemorrhage in haemophilia. *Journal of Neurology, Neurosurgery and Psychiatry*, **27**, 166.

Kety, S. S. (1950) Circulation and metabolism of the human brain in health and disease. *American Journal of Medicine*, **8**, 205.

Krayenbuhl, H. A. (1968) Cerebral venous and sinus thrombosis. *Clinical Neurosurgery*, **14**, 1.

Kurland, L. T. & Kurtzke, J. F. (1972) Geographic neuropathology. In *Pathology of the Nervous System*, ed. Minckler, J. Vol. 3. Chapter 28. Section 199. New York: McGraw-Hill.

Kutas, M. & Bodosi, M. (1971) Oral Antikonzeptionsmittel und Schadigungen. *Münchener medizinische Wochenschrift*, **13**, 42.

Le Mar, J. D. (1962) Repeated paradoxic embolism. *Lancet*, **82**, 248.

Lesch, R. & Engelhardt, K. (1966) Tödliche Hirnembolie aus umschribener arteriosklerotisch begingter Thrombosierung im Aortenbogen. *Medizinische Welt*, **4**, 201.

Lhermitte, F., Gautier, J. C. & Derousné, C. (1966) Anatomopathologie et physiopathologie des stenoses carotidiennes. *Revue Neurologique* (Paris), **115**, 641.

Lhermitte, F., Gautier, J. C. & Derousné, C. (1970) Nature of occlusion of the middle cerebral artery. *Neurology* (Minneapolis), **20**, 82.

Lorentz, I. T. (1962) Parietal lesion and "Enavid". *British Medical Journal*, **ii**, 1191.

McCall, A. J. (1967) Embolic cerebral infarction. Presidential Address to the Association of Clinical Pathologists. (Unpublished.)

MacDonald, R. A. & Robbins, S. L. (1957) The significance of non-bacterial thrombotic endocarditis: An autopsy and clinical study. *Annals of Internal Medicine*, **46**, 255.

McDonald, W. L. (1967) Recurrent cholesterol embolism as a cause of fluctuating cerebral symptoms. *Journal of Neurology, Neurosurgery and Psychiatry*, **30**, 489.

McGill, H. C. (1968) The geographic pathology of atherosclerosis. *Laboratory Investigation*, **18**, 463.

Marquardsen, J. (1968) The natural history of acute cerebro-vascular disease. *Acta Neurologica Scandinavia*, **45**, Suppl. 38, 160.

Marshall, V. C., Epstein, J. & Kincaid-Smith, P. (1970) Retrograde cerebral arterial embolism due to declotting of arteriovenous shunts. *British Journal of Surgery*, **57**, 382.

Martin, J. P. (1941) Thrombosis in the superior sagittal sinus, following childbirth. *British Medical Journal*, **ii**, 537.

Martin, J. P. & Sheehan, H. L. (1941) Primary thrombosis of the cerebral veins following childbirth. *British Medical Journal*, **i**, 249.

Masi, A. T. & Dugdale, M. (1970) Cerebrovascular disease associated with the use of oral contraceptives. A review of the English language literature. *Annals of Internal Medicine*, **72**, 111.

Matsuoka, S. (1952) Histopathological studies on the blood vessels in apoplexia cerebri. *Proceedings of the First International Congress of Neuropathology* (Rome), **3**, 222.

Maurizi, C. P., Barker, A. E. & Truehart, K. E. (1968) Atheromatous emboli. A postmortem study with special reference to the lower extremities. *Archives of Pathology*, **86**, 528.

Meldrum, B. S. & Brierley, J. B. (1969) Brain damage in the Rhesus monkey resulting from profound arterial hypotension. II. Changes in the spontaneous and evoked electric activity of the neocortex. *Brain Research*, **13**, 101–118.

Meyer, W. W. (1947) Cholesterinkrystallembolie kleiner Organarteries und ihre Folgen. *Virchows Archives für Pathologische Anatomie und Physiologie und für Klinische Medizin*, **314**, 616.

Miller, D. & Adams, J. H. (1972) Pathophysiology and management of increased intracranial pressure. In *Scientific Foundations of Neurology*. (Eds.) Critchley, M., O'Leary, J. L. & Jennett, B. London: William Heinemann.

Millikan, C. H. (1965) The pathogenesis of transient focal cerebral ischaemia. *Circulation*, **32**, 438.

Millikan, C. H., Siekert, R. G. & Whisnant, J. P. (1960) Intermittent carotid and vertebral-basilar insufficiency associated with polycythaemia.

Missen, G. A. K. (1966) Temporal arteritis. *British Medical Journal*, **i**, 419.

Missen, G. A. K. (1974) Personal communication.

Mitchell, J. R. A. & Schwartz, C. J. (1965) *Arterial Disease*. Oxford: Blackwell.

Modan, B. & Modan, M. (1968) Benign erythrocytosis. *British Journal of Haematology*, **14,** 375.

Moossy, J. (1965) Cerebral infarction and intracranial arterial thrombosis; necropsy studies and clinical implications. *Transactions of the American Neurological Association*, **90,** 113.

Morrisson, A. N. & Abitol, M. (1955) Granulomatous arteritis with myocardial infarction. *Annals of Internal Medicine*, **42,** 691.

Mulder, O. G., Evenblij, H. & Endtz, L. J. (1971) Thrombose veineuse cerebral et anticonception orale. *Revue Neurologique* (Paris), **124,** 84.

Norman, R. M. & Urich, H. (1957) Dissecting aneurysm of the middle cerebral artery as a cause of acute infantile hemiplegia. *Journal of Pathology and Bacteriology*, **73,** 580.

Nothnagel, C. W. H. (1877) Anaemia, hyperaemia, haemorrhage, thrombosis and embolism of the brain. In *Encyclopaedia of the Practice of Medicine*. (Ed.) von Ziemmsen, H. Vol. 12. p. 3. London: Samson Low.

Nurick, S., Blackwood, W. & Mair, W. G. P. (1972) Giant-cell granulomatous angiitis of the central nervous system. *Brain*, **95,** 133.

Orbison, J. L. (1952) Morphology of thrombotic thrombocytopenic purpura with demonstration of aneurysms. *American Journal of Pathology*, **28,** 129.

Peters, H. J. & Chandler, A. B. (1971) Thrombotic atherosclerosis of human cerebral arteries. In *Pathology of the Nervous System* (Ed.) Minckler, J. Vol. 2. Chapter XVII. New York: McGraw Hill.

Piazza, G. & Gaist, G. (1960) Occlusion of the middle cerebral artery by foreign body embolus. *Journal of Neurosurgery*, **17,** 172.

Poller, L. (1969) Relation between oral contraceptive hormones and blood clotting. *Journal of Clinical Pathology*, (Supplement 3), **23,** 67.

Poller, L. & Thomson, J. M. (1966) Clotting factors during oral contraception: Further report. *British Medical Journal*, **ii,** 23.

Pribram, H. F. & Courves, C. M. (1965) Retinal embolism as a complication of angiography. *Neurology*, **15,** 188.

Price, D. L. & Harris, J. (1970) Cholesterol emboli in cerebral arteries as a complication of retrograde aortic perfusion during cardiac surgery. *Neurology* (Minneapolis), **20,** 1209.

Pruitt, A. B. & Mole, H. W. (1967) Middle cerebral artery occlusion in pregnancy. *Obstetrics and Gynecology*, **29,** 545.

Retan, J. W. & Miller, R. E. (1966) Microembolic complications of atherosclerosis. *Archives of Internal Medicine*, **118,** 534.

Roach, M. R. & Drake, C. G. (1964) Ruptured cerebral aneurysms caused by micro-organisms. *New England Journal of Medicine*, **273,** 240.

Romanul, F. C. A. (1970) *Examination of the Brain and Spinal Cord in Neuropathology—Methods and Diagnosis*, ed. Tedeschi, C. G. Boston: Little Brown.

Romanul, F. C. A. & Abramowicz, A. (1964) Changes in the brain and pial vessels in arterial border zones. *Archives of Neurology* (Chicago), **11,** 40.

Rouchoux, J. A. (1844) Du ramollissement de cerveau de sa curabilité. *Archives of General Medicine*, **6,** 265. cited by Fawcett, F. J. & Smith, T. W. (1966) Current views on the pathogenesis of "strokes". *Postgraduate Medical Journal*, **42,** 5.

Russell, D. S. (1954) The pathology of spontaneous intracranial haemorrhage. *Proceedings of the Royal Society of Medicine*, **47,** 689.

Russell, D. S. & Rubenstein, L. J. (1971) *Pathology of Tumours of the Nervous System*. (Third Edition) (Chapter 5). London: Edward Arnold.

Russell, R. W. R. (1963a) Atheromatous retinal embolism. *Lancet*, **ii,** 1345.

Russell, R. W. R. (1963b) Observations on intracerebral aneurysms. *Brain*, **86,** 425–442.

Sandok, B. A. & Spiegel, P. K. (1968) Foreign body embolus to middle cerebral artery. *Virginia Medicine*, **95,** 151.

Sauer, H. A. (1955) Paradoxical embolism in pregnancy. Reviews of the literature and report of a case. *Journal of Obstetrics and Gynaecology of the British Empire*, **62,** 906.

Schneck, S. A. (1964) On the relationship between ruptured intracranial aneurysm and cerebral infarction. *Neurology* (Minneapolis), **14,** 691.

Schneck, S. A. & Kricheff, I. I. (1964) Intracranial aneurysm rupture, vasospasm and infarction. *Archives of Neurology*, **11,** 668.

Schoenberg, B. S., Whisnant, J. P., Taylor, W F & Kempers, R. D. (1970) Strokes in women of childbearing age. A population study. *Neurology*, **20**, 181.

Schröter, T. (1967) Zur Ursache des embolischen Gehirninfarktes bei Tuberkulosilikose der Lungen. *Beitraege zur Pathologie*, **135**, 291.

Schwartz, C. J. & Mitchell, J. R. A. (1961) Atheroma of the carotid and vertebral arterial system. *British Medical Journal*, **ii**, 1057.

Shucksmith, H. S. (1963) Cerebral and peripheral emboli caused by cervical ribs. *British Medical Journal*, **ii**, 835.

Silverstein, A. (1961) Intracranial haemorrhage in patients with bleeding tendencies. *Neurology*, **11**, 310–317.

Smith, Barbara (1963) Cerebral pathology in subarachnoid haemorrhage. *Journal of Neurology, Neurosurgery and Psychiatry*, **26**, 535.

Solaway, H. B. & Aronson, S. M. (1964) Atheromatous embolism to central nervous system. *Archives of Neurology*, **11**, 657.

Spain, D. M. (1968) Endocarditis. In *The Pathology of the Heart and Blood Vessels* (Ed.) Gauld, S. E. Chapter 15. Springfield, Ill.: Charles C. Thomas.

Stehbens, W. E. (1962) Hypertension and cerebral aneurysms. *Medical Journal of Australia*, **2**, 8.

Stehbens, W. E. (1972) *Pathology of the Cerebral Blood Vessels*. Chapter 8. St. Louis: C. V. Mosby.

Stevens, H. (1954) Puerperal hemiplegia. *Neurology*, **4**, 723.

Sturgill, B. C. & Netsky, M. G. (1963) Cerebral infarction by atheromatous emboli. *Archives of Pathology*, **76**, 189.

Symonds, C. P. (1927) Two cases of thrombosis of the subclavian artery with contra-lateral hemiplegia of sudden onset, probably embolic. *Brain*, **50**, 259.

Symonds, C. P. & MacKenzie, I. (1957) Loss of vision in cerebral infarction. *Brain*, **80**, 415.

Tapp, E., Geary, C. G. & Dawson, D. W. (1969) Thrombotic microangiopathy with macro-scopic infarction. *Journal of Pathology*, **97**, 711.

Thompson, T. & Evans, W. (1930) Paradoxical embolism. *Quarterly Journal of Medicine*, **23**, 135.

Thomson, J. M. (1970) *A Practical Guide to Blood Coagulation and Haemostasis*. p. 145. London: Churchill.

Tomlinson, B. E. (1959) Brain changes in ruptured intracranial aneurysms. *Journal of Clinical Pathology*, **12**, 391.

Tomlinson, B. E., Blessed, G. & Roth, M. (1968) Observations on the brains of non-demen-ted old people. *Journal of Neurological Sciences*, **7**, 331.

Tomlinson, B. E., Blessed, G. & Roth, M. (1970) Observations of the brains of demented old people. *Journal of Neurological Sciences*, **11**, 205.

Torvik, A. & Jörgensen, L. (1964) Thrombotic and embolic occlusions of the carotid arteries in an autopsy material. Part I: Prevalence, location and associated diseases. *Journal of Neurological Sciences*, **1**, 24.

Torvik, A. & Jörgensen, L. (1966) Thrombotic and embolic occlusions of the carotid arteries in an autopsy series. Part II. Cerebral lesions and clinical course. *Journal of Neurological Sciences*, **3**, 410.

Vessey, M. P. & Doll, R. (1969) Investigation of relation between use of oral contraceptives and thromboembolic disease. A further report. *British Medical Journal*, **ii**, 651.

Veterans Administration (1967) Treatment and survival of patients with cancer of the prostate. Report of the Co-operative Urological Research Group. *Surgery, Gynecology and Obstetrics*, **124**, 1011.

Vost, A., Wolochow, D. A. & Howell, D. A. (1964) Incidence of infarcts of the brain in heart disease. *Journal of Pathology and Bacteriology*, **88**, 463.

Walton, J. M. (1956) *Subarachnoid Haemorrhage*. Edinburgh: Livingstone.

Weber, D. L., Reagan, T. & Leeds, M. (1972) Intracerebral haemorrhage during haemo-dialysis. *New York State Journal of Medicine*, **72**, 1853.

Westphal, K. & Bär, R. (1926) Über die Enstehung des Schlaganfalles. 1. Pathologisch-anatomische Untersuchungen zur Frage der Enstehung des Schlanganfalles. *Deutsche Archiv klinische Medizin*, **1**, 151.

Williams, W. G. (1963) Dilatation of the left atrial appendage. *British Heart Journal*, **25**, 637.

Winkleman, N. W. & Moore, M. T. (1950) Disseminated necrotising panarteritis (peri-arteritis nodosa). *Journal of Neuropathology and Experimental Neurology*, **9**, 60.

Winter, W. J. & Gyari, E. (1960) Pathogenesis of small cerebral infarcts. *Archives of Pathology*, **69**, 224.

Wishoff, H. S. & Rothballer, A. B. (1961) Cerebral arterial thrombosis in children. *Archives of Neurology*, **4**, 258.

Wood, P. (1968) *Diseases of the Heart and Circulation*. Third edition. p. 623. London: Eyre and Spottiswoode.

Yates, P. O. & Hutchinson, E. C. (1961) Cerebral infarction: the role of stenosis of the extracranial cerebral arteries. *Medical Research Council Special Report Series*, No. **300**. London: H.M. Stationery Office.

Zadek, I. (1927) Die Polycythämien. *Ergebnisse der gesamten Medizin*, **10**, 355.

Zatz, L. M., Iannone, A. M., Eckman, P. B. & Hecker, S. P. (1965) Observations concerning intracerebral vascular occlusion. *Neurology*, **15**, 389.

Zülch, K. J. (1971) Pathological aspects of cerebral accidents in arterial hypertension. *Acta Neurologica Belgica*, **71**, 196–220.

Zülch, K. J. & Behrend, R. C. H. (1961) 'The pathogenesis and topography of anoxia, hypoxia and ischaemia of the brain in man'. In *Cerebral Anoxia and the Electro-encephalogram*, Ed. Gastaut, H. & Meyer, J. S. Ch. 14, p. 144. Springfield, Ill.: Thomas.

CHAPTER FOUR

Epidemiology

Before considering in detail the natural history of patients where a clinical diagnosis of cerebral ischaemia has been made it is necessary to examine two important areas relating to this problem. The first is the contribution contained in reports of epidemiological studies which have added certain important facets to our understanding of the natural history. The second is the potential effect of normal ageing and the sex of the patient on the prognosis in cerebrovascular disease. After this introduction we give a description of a group of patients who will be described throughout the monograph as a 'personal series'. This refers to 500 untreated patients where the natural history has been studied prospectively over a period of ten years and the results of the study compared with other published work.

CONTRIBUTION OF EPIDEMIOLOGY

Epidemiology may be defined as a study of the natural history of disease in groups rather than individual patients, but the definition does not exclude the study of results of attempts to alter the course of a disease (Kurtzke, 1969). To the practising clinician, epidemiology has considerable interest in that it provides information, often unexplained, of apparent variations in the incidence of the common types of cerebral vascular disease not only between nations but within nations and often within countries, states, municipalities or whatever term is used for describing the geographical distribution of aggregates of population.

Another important area of knowledge contributed to by epidemiological studies is the evidence that has been adduced to suggest that there is a change in pattern of cerebral vascular disease over the last three decades, particularly with reference to cerebral infarction and cerebral haemorrhage.

A third, and probably the most important contribution epidemiology has made, has been the demonstration that a stroke is basically a disease of senescence and, therefore, many hospital-based studies are really concerned with the fringe of the problem. This is not to diminish the importance of these studies, whether they be medically or surgically orientated, since they are concerned with the considerable problem of management of cerebral vascular disease in patients who are often still in their productive years.

Variations in incidence

There have been many observations which suggest that there is a variation in the relative incidence of cerebral infarction and cerebral haemorrhage, and these are most marked in specific areas such as Japan and the United States. The difference is so striking, and apparently so clearly defined, that it would appear that if the cause for the variation could be determined there would be a fundamental move forward in the understanding of the aetiology of hypertension and possibly atherosclerosis as well.

It has been recognised for some time that in many areas there is no unusual variation in the pattern of cerebral infarction and cerebral haemorrhage. Acheson (1960) published a study of the mortality from the various forms of cerebral vascular disease in Ireland and compared the results in different counties. He examined the figures for 1951 produced by the Registrar General but he could not detect any very strongly defined pattern nor a particularly wide range of variation from county to county. For example, he found the highest death rate from cerebral vascular disease was 369 per 100 000 in County Wicklow which was only three and a half times that for County Longford, where the figure for women was 107 per 100 000.

Kurtzke (1969) examined in considerable detail the evidence supporting a varying incidence of cerebral vascular disease within different countries. He studied the data from Sweden, Denmark, Norway, Ireland and the United States. He chose an arbitrary variation which was a figure of more than 25 per cent on either side of the national mean. He required a variation beyond this national mean of at least several units before he was prepared to concede any biological significance to the differing incidence rates for cerebral infarction, cerebral haemorrhage, and subarachnoid haemorrhage in any particular area. In areas where there were apparently higher frequencies he required a pattern or cluster of increased frequency before the effect of environmental factors could be inferred.

His general conclusion was that the pattern of incidence as judged by the death rate from cerebral vascular disease within the countries specified was more or less uniform. Since the United States was one country which showed an abnormal variation, Kurtzke examined the distribution of physicians in the United States and found a significant inverse relationship between high rates for cerebral vascular disease and reduced medical availability. By the latter he meant a distribution of physicians below 80 per cent of the national mean in that area. From this he reasonably inferred that the high rates of certification of deaths from any form of cerebral vascular disease, since they were associated with an area of reduced medical facilities, really reflected on the adequacy, and thus the accuracy, of medical reporting. If one accepts Kurtzke's interpretation there is no real evidence of significant variation within countries.

Stallones (1965) in a review article on the epidemiology of cerebral vascular disease studied the variations in mortality between countries. He found that between the highest and the lowest reported incidence in terms of death rate there was a seven-fold difference. In countries with a technologically advanced economy the death rate per 100 000 tended to group around the mean. Others showed unusually high figures. This was particularly true in Japan where an incidence of 208.6 per 100 000 was observed for deaths from all vascular lesions of the central nervous system. Clearly this was significantly higher than the figure of 116.2 per 100 000 for England and Wales. When the figures are broken down into diagnostic categories, cerebral haemorrhage was found to be a certified cause of death three and a half times more frequently in Japan than was observed to be the case in England and Wales. Conversely, when the figures for cerebral thrombosis and embolism were compared with cerebral haemorrhage the figures were almost exactly reversed.

Not unnaturally, such a discrepancy inspired further study since at first it seemed clear that there were either genetic or environmental factors operative in Japan which were relevant to the aetiology both of hypertension and cerebral haemorrhage. Gordon (1957) examined the death rates for Japanese nationals in Japan, Hawaii and the United States mainland. He found that the death rate for cerebral vascular disease fell progressively from Japan to the U.S. mainland. Stallones (1965) felt this implied that an environmental influence rather than a genetic factor was responsible. However, he commented that he would not be prepared to exclude the possibility that artefacts may, in fact, be responsible for the difference in the death rates.

Johnson, Yano and Kato (1967) reported a study on the population of Hiroshima between 1958 and 1964 and their conclusions are germane to the present discussion. In their population sample of 9270 subjects they concluded that cerebral thrombosis was under-reported in Japan since they observed it to occur twice as frequently in cerebral haemorrhage. Hospital autopsy findings also suggested that the high incidence of cerebral haemorrhage might very well be an artefact. Johnson, Yano and Kato (1967) quoted a Japanese study of 29 795 autopsies and in these cerebral haemorrhage was found in 2.2 per cent and cerebral thrombosis in 2 per cent. Even allowing for bias in hospital admissions there was no support for the view current at the time that the ratio of cerebral haemorrhage to cerebral thrombosis and embolism was of the order of 12 : 4, figures which were currently accepted as being the normal ratio for Japan. They concluded that to account for a high stroke rate frequency in Japan there was 'no real merit in postulating that a unique or extraordinary disease process other than atherosclerosis is operative'.

Kurtzke (1969) also examined the Japanese figures as well as the oft-reported high rates for cerebral haemorrhage for negroes as compared with the white population in the United States. In respect of Japan he concluded there was clear evidence in the case of cerebral haemorrhage, and probably in all cases of cerebral vascular disease, that the high rates were in fact an artefactual diagnostic finding compounded by a low autopsy rate. The results of examining the evidence for the high incidence of cerebral haemorrhage in the American negro led Kurtzke to conclude that the high death rate reported reflected a scarcity of medical facilities while the evidence from population and hospital based data provided some support of the view that there is, in fact, no excessively high incidence of cerebral haemorrhage in the negro as compared with the white male.

It would seem therefore that as the science of epidemiology extends and refines its techniques, many of the original variations in incidence in the different forms of cerebral vascular disease which appeared to be significant will ultimately prove to have been artefactual.

Change in incidence of cerebral vascular disease

The accuracy of diagnostic information derived from large-scale epidemiological studies based on the death certificate must be treated with some reservation. Kurtzke found evidence from the literature of errors of omission as shown by post-mortem examination to be of the order of 10 to 15 per cent whereas over-reporting gave an error of 10 to 40 per cent of deaths from cerebral vascular disease. Diagnostic customs appeared to be roughly the same in the United States, England and Norway.

Precise information on the incidence of the different types of cerebral vascular disease as determined by live population studies is not easy to obtain. Figures from the Mayo Clinic studies are probably as accurate as any. The reason for this is that the population of Rochester (52 629) is almost unique in medical terms because of the Mayo Clinic's service to the local population, which has been continuing for several decades, and because of the medical index and retrieval system which has been operative there over this time. Whisnant et al (1971) reported a study of the incidence of stroke in the population of Rochester, Minnesota in the years 1945 to 1954. The incidence for all types was 194 per 100 000 per year and of these cerebral infarction represented 146 per 100 000 per year. Cerebral haemorrhage, by contrast, accounted for less than 10 per cent of all strokes. The incidence of cerebral haemorrhage as the cause of death was 15 per cent, which was much lower than the United States mortality statistics. As they point out, the diagnosis of cerebral haemorrhage had been used too loosely and frequently in the past. In a second study of the same population but covering the years 1955 to 1969 (Matsumoto et al, 1973) cerebral infarction was found to account for 79 per cent of all strokes, cerebral haemorrhage for 10 per cent, and subarachnoid haemorrhage for 6 per cent.

The average incidence rate in the 15 years of the study was 164 per 100 000. If, however, the incidence rate in a five-year period was examined, the incidence rate had fallen to 141 for the five-year period 1965 to 1969 inclusive. These figures applied to cerebral infarction only, but the authors could not detect any diminishing incidence in the case of cerebral haemorrhage and subarachnoid haemorrhage. But, as they were careful to point out, the small numbers of cases of the latter two conditions may well have rendered these observations less reliable.

It is pertinent to note that the observed incidence of cerebral haemorrhage in this series was one-fifth of that observed by Wylie (1962) for the United States, England and Wales and only served to underline the unsatisfactory nature of the information obtained for mortality of the different types of cerebral vascular disease within the community.

That there may be a decrease in the number of people dying from cerebral haemorrhage has been suggested by the observations of Yates (1964). When examining the Registrar General's figures for the 30-year period between 1931 and 1969 he found that although there was little change in the overall death rate during this period there was a reversal in the relative positions of cerebral haemorrhage and infarction as a cause of strokes. In the 1930s cerebral haemorrhage was diagnosed twice as frequently as cerebral thrombosis, but in more recent years cerebral thrombosis as a cause of death had been noted as being more common. Yates then turned his attention to the hospital autopsies in three Manchester hospitals. From the results of the findings at autopsy he felt that this confirmed his view of the changing pattern of the relative incidence rates for cerebral haemorrhage and cerebral thrombosis.

Kurtzke (1969) has examined Yates's study in considerable detail. He acknowledged the care and attention to detail in the planning of the study but felt that figures obtained from teaching hospital autopsies, which had been carried out prior to and during the 1939-45 war, may not have been directly comparable to incidence figures obtained in another hospital where, through the advent of the National Health Service, admission policy may have varied. He argued that it was possible that an increase of facilities for the nursing of the chronic sick may have accounted for what may be only an apparent increase in the incidence of cerebral infarction. Kurtzke concluded that the evidence for the falling rate of incidence of cerebral haemorrhage was not proven with certainty. The figures given for the incidence of this condition in the Rochester population quoted by Whisnant et al (1971) would favour Kurtzke's view rather than that of Yates. If Kurtzke is ultimately proved to be correct it will be a somewhat depressing result for the clinician in that there is only one clearly defined area — the treatment of hypertension — where he might hope to influence the course of cerebrovascular disease.

EFFECTS OF AGE

The evidence from epidemiological studies indicates that the incidence rate both for cerebral thrombosis and cerebral haemorrhage rises rapidly in senescence, and this reflects general experience. Three reports, all of which give the age range of the patients, establish this point and all three are drawn from studies of large communities (Table 4.1).

Eisenberg et al (1964) studied a population group of 80 000 in the Middlesex County, Connecticut. The study, carried out in conjunction with a survey of the incidence of coronary artery disease, lasted for twelve months and the information relating to the patients was obtained from general practitioners and from cardiological and hospital records. The constraints of gathering information from such a large group led to certain difficulties of classification of patients, who were finally subdivided into cerebral thrombosis, cerebral haemorrhage and a group which were labelled as 'C.V.A. undetermined'.

Goldner et al (1967), in a similar study, reported on 221 stroke patients who were identified in a mid-Missouri stroke survey and they also relied on multiple sources of information similar to those of Eisenberg et al (1964).

Table 4.1. Average annual incidence of cerebral infarction and cerebral haemorrhage.

(a) Eisenberg et al, 1964 (Middlesex County, Connecticut)

Age groups (years)	Total no. of C.V.As		Cerebral thrombosis		Cerebral haemorrhage		C.V.A. undetermined	
	No.	Rate/1000	No.	Rate/1000	No.	Rate/1000	No.	Rate/1000
55–64	31	4.0	14	1.8	12	1.6	4	0.5
65–74	54	9.4	22	3.8	22	3.8	8	1.4
75–84	58	21.9	31	11.7	18	6.8	8	3.0
85 and over	35	50.7	29	29.0	12	17.4	3	4.3

(b) Goldner et al, 1967 (Missouri)

Age groups (years)	Total population at risk	No. with strokes	No. without strokes	Rate/100 000
55–64	6561	27	6534	411.5
65–74	5408	58	5350	1072.5
75–84	3019	82	2937	2716.1
85 and over	756	44	712	5820.1

(c) Matsumoto et al, 1973 (Rochester, Minnesota)[a]

Age groups	Males		Females		Total	
	No.	Rate/100 000	No.	Rate/100 000	No.	Rate/100 000
55–64	83	407.8	53	184.2	136	276.8
65–74	122	897.7	97	460.6	219	632.0
75 and over	137	2104.5	221	1633.4	358	1786.4

[a]Table 4.1c. refers to cerebral thrombosis only.

112   STROKES

The third report is that of Matsumoto et al (1973), already referred to, which was concerned with the incidence of stroke in Rochester, Minnesota.

Whatever the source, these three reports show clearly that an increase in the incidence of cerebral vascular disease is found with increasing age, whether the cause be cerebral ischaemia or cerebral haemorrhage. It is difficult to accept that any defect of case identification or reporting would account for such a marked increase within the different decades; nor, of course, would one expect that this would be so.

There seems to be no reason to suppose that throughout the Western world figures will differ fundamentally from these which establish the point that the two factors of increasing age and the greater liability to a cerebral vascular episode are associated. It is worth emphasising that the major cause of disability in all series is clearly cerebral infarction.

The demonstration that ageing and an increased stroke incidence are interrelated does not of necessity mean that the survivors should necessarily be subject to a higher mortality than the younger age groups. But it is no surprise that the initial mortality should be related to the age of the patient. Robinson et al (1968) observed that in patients with a stroke in the fifth decade there was a mortality of 9 per cent which rose in a stepwise manner in decades until it reached 63 per cent in the 80 to 90 age group.

The fact that there is a high early mortality in the aged does not itself imply that the survivors should be subject to a worse outcome than younger patients. However, the evidence indicates that this is so. The series from the Mayo Clinic already referred to (Matsumoto et al, 1973) recognised clearly the adverse effects of age as a factor in prognosis. Both Eisenberg et al (1964) and Goldner et al (1967) supported this view both in terms of ultimate morbidity and mortality. Katz et al (1966) also found that in a prospective study of a series of cases observed personally there was a clear association between age, morbidity and mortality from stroke; their experience appears to be a general one.

Howard et al (1963) published a study of survival following stroke where they observed that the subsequent mortality bore a linear relationship to age. In the first six months the mortality was 14 per cent in the 30 to 60-year age groups but this rose to 50 per cent in the 70 to 90 age group. After six months the mortality in the elderly was twice that noted in the younger patients.

Previously, Marshall and Shaw (1959), dealing with a relatively younger population, were able to compare the relationship between the mortality rate and the different age groups. During the period of observation the mortality was 49 per cent in the 50 to 59-year-old group compared with 69 per cent in the 70 to 79-year-old group.

But when dealing with progressively older age groups an increase in mortality might be anticipated from any cause and, therefore, comparisons within the same age group are more revealing. Adams and Merrett (1961), using the Life Tables for Northern Ireland, calculated the median survival for a normal population of 75 or more. The median survival time was found to be 6.6 years for elderly normal patients, which contrasted sharply with their female stroke patient population in the same age group where the survival time after the initial stroke was 3.4 years.

Marquardsen's (1969) study was based on a large general hospital supplying the medical needs of the population of the Municipality of Freidriksberg. It was a retrospective study based on the fate of 769 patients who presented with an acute intracerebral vascular episode, but did not differentiate between cerebral haemorrhage and cerebral infarction. He divided the patients into decades according to the age at onset and he observed that in males below the age of 60 the number of survivors increased at an annual rate of about 10 per cent whereas in males aged 70 to 79 the rate was 25 per cent. As Marquardsen pointed out it came as no surprise to find the mortality increasing with age and so, in a manner similar to Adams and Merrett (1961), he extended his analysis to the important consideration of whether the differing age groups experienced the same excess mortality when compared with normal populations. When examining the Life Survival times, which he expressed as a ratio between the observed death rate and the expected survival, he found there was a lower ratio in the younger males, indicating a better prognosis, and this comparison was affected mainly by a high mortality which was observed in males over 70 in the second year after the stroke. Up to this time, the curves for the older population became nearly parallel, and the curve for patients under 60, when compared with the normal population, tended to assume a horizontal course.

He suggested that this trend, which was observed in both males and females, indicated that the excess mortality between the patient population and the normal population, at least in patients under 60, decreased a few years after the onset of the first vascular episode.

SEX

The reports of studies of the adverse effect of age on a long-term prognosis, whether this be expressed as the comparative mortality between young and old or as survival rates compared with a normal population, are in general agreement; there is not the same agreement on the prognosis when the results in male and female subjects are compared.

Robinson et al (1959) observed a significantly higher initial mortality in females than in males but did not find any persisting difference between the sexes in relation to long-term survival. Eisenberg et al (1964), however, did find a bias in favour of males. When they compared the fate of males under the age of 64 with those over this age they found a statistically significant higher survival rate in the younger age group, but this was not observed in females.

Other reports have given some support to the popular belief that females tolerate vascular disease more readily than males. Marshall and Shaw (1959) and Goldner et al (1967) found that the prognosis in terms of survival was better in females than in males during the period of their follow up studies.

Both Adams and Merrett (1961) and Carter (1964) found that their women patients survived somewhat longer than the men of the same age below the age of 75, but beyond this age the difference appeared to disappear.

Marquardsen (1969) studied the relationship between age and sex and made several interesting observations. The first was that he noted a high mortality at one year after the stroke among the female patients but when examined in decades this observation was restricted only to females between the age of 60 and 69. Another was that between the ages of 70 and 79 the death rate per annum was considerably higher in males than in females, particularly during the second and third year after the stroke. Apart from these two age groups, however, he could find no marked difference between the number of male and female patients surviving at different ages.

PERSONAL SERIES

Throughout the consideration of the natural history of patients afflicted by cerebral ischaemia reference will be made to our personal series. This refers to a group of patients observed over a decade from 1957 to 1967 who were, for practical purposes, untreated. The study was prospective and was designed with two purposes in mind. The first was to detect if possible any recognisable pattern of behaviour in the subsequent clinical history. The second was to determine whether, if such patterns were present, any factors could be defined which could be shown to be causally related to them.

The environment

All the 500 patients entering the study were domiciled in North Staffordshire and the majority came from the City of Stoke-on-Trent or the Borough of Newcastle-under-Lyme. They were predominantly working class, which is shown by the fact that only 66 patients fell into categories 1 or 2 of the Registrar General's classification of social status while the majority fell into categories 3, 4 and 5. The two major industries of the area are pottery manufacture and mining, and a high proportion of the male patients were engaged in one or other of these occupations. Many of the female patients, too, were engaged in the pottery industry. The follow-up rate achieved was 100 per cent and this expressed as much as anything the static nature of the population of the area. Veys (1973), in a study of bladder cancer in relation to occupation in North Staffordshire, out of a total series of 6199 men successfully traced 99.6 per cent. The reason for this high success rate was that between the years 1946 and 1970 over 90 per cent of the population studied were found to be still living within the North Staffordshire area.

The mortality rate due to cerebrovascular disease in males in Great Britain was 1333 per million and the figure for females 1838 in the years 1954-58. The standardised mortality ratio is a ratio between the actual and expected deaths multiplied by 100. The mean for the nation is 100. The North Stafford-shire area shows a 'comparatively high' rate for males with a ratio between 100 and 110. In female patients the figure comes within the category of moder-ately high, with an incidence between 109 and 125. These figures are taken from the *National Atlas of Disease Mortality in the United Kingdom* (Howe, 1963).

Terminology

Terminology in cerebral vascular disease has always been a problem, since it is not always possible to decide the underlying pathological process in any given episode of cerebral ischaemia. In an engaging essay on 'The concepts of stroke before and after Virchow', Schiller (1970) disposes of the term 'cerebral vascular accident'. Apparently, the term appeared in the 16th edition of *Dorlands Medical Dictionary* in 1936 and Schiller observed that this 'pompous piece of nomenclature must have issued from the well-meant tendency to soften the blow to patients and their relatives and also from the desire to replace "stroke" — a pithy term which may sound unscientific'.

In the personal series we deliberately chose the word 'stroke' to categorise patients who presented with an episode that was judged on clinical grounds to be ischaemic, that is, a cerebral infarct. In contrast to this group there were patients who presented with transient cerebral ischaemia, and here the requirements were that the quality of the episode, as judged by the history, indicated that it was ischaemic, it should last less than one hour, and that there should be complete recovery of neural function. It has been general experience that transient cerebral ischaemia usually lasts less than one hour, but many series do accept the diagnosis of transient ischaemia with episodes lasting up to a period of 12 hours.

In the case of transient cerebral ischaemia affecting the vertebro-basilar arterial territory, substantiation of the diagnosis required that two or more symptoms indicating involvement of the brain stem at different levels should be complained of by the patient either in one or in separate episodes. Excluded from the diagnosis of transient vertebro-basilar ischaemia were any patients who consistently related their symptoms to movements of the head since, under these circumstances, it was not possible to exclude vertebral artery compression in association with cervical spondylosis.

In using the term 'stroke' we assumed that cerebral infarction had occurred and accepted from pathological studies over the past two decades that it could very well be due to an embolus from the major neck vessels. But excluded from the study were patients where there was an obvious source of emboli, this for practical purposes referred to evidence of rheumatic heart disease, recent myocardial infarction, or subacute bacterial endocarditis. One of the results of the study was the demonstration at post-mortem examination that the assumption that on clinical grounds one could differentiate between infarction and localised intracerebral haemorrhage was incorrect. This will be discussed later in some detail.

Assessment

The majority of the patients entered the study following referral to the Out-Patient clinic, although in the early part of the study some patients were seen at private consultation. Subsequent follow-up, however, was always conducted under the National Health Service so that no socio-economic factors were operative.

When the patient entered the study, in addition to the routine clinical assessment which involved a detailed clinical history and examination, an x-ray of the chest, ECG, urinary sugar estimation, full blood count and blood Wasserman reaction were carried out. With results of these tests available we were content to accept that we were excluding haematological diseases and neurosyphilis which could obviously simulate closely ischaemic cerebral vascular disease. It was obviously not possible at first assessment to exclude unusual presentations of collagen disease and the like, but we had the opportunity of correcting any such diagnostic errors at subsequent follow up.

In the early part of the study many patients were admitted for investigation, including angiography, and also, at the same time, for studying the behaviour of the blood pressure in cases where it was significantly elevated.

Once patients were fully assessed they were followed up in a special clinic devoted to the purpose. They were seen in the first two years at three-monthly intervals and thereafter at six-monthly intervals and at each consultation any further episodes were recorded and further physical examinations were conducted as required.

Selection

It is important to emphasise that when patients entered the study they were either suffering from transient cerebral ischaemia or were survivors from a stroke episode. This means, of course, that the patients were a selected group, particularly in terms of cerebral infarction. The mean age at onset for both males and females (males 57.0 years, females 58.0 years) is well below the mean age for the incidence of cerebral vascular disease within the community as a whole. This was established during the period of this study by an investigation into the incidence of cerebral ischaemia in general practice, which was carried out and reported on by Acheson, Acheson and Tellwright (1968). This showed that male patients seen in general practice with cerebral ischaemia were nearly seven years older than the hospital series since they presented at a mean age of 64.9 years. The study also showed that in general practice the incidence of minor forms of cerebral ischaemia is very much higher than one would expect to encounter in hospital practice.

It is clear, then, that the series is not representative of cerebral vascular disease as it occurs in the community as a whole, but it certainly is representative of the problems of cerebral vascular disease as they are encountered in hospital practice. There are no great disadvantages in selected series provided that selection is recognised to be present and that the results of the observations are not extrapolated to encompass all age groups. It can, indeed, be argued that studying a selected population who are relatively young in terms of cerebral vascular disease has certain advantages. A major advantage, of course, is that the natural course of the disease is not obscured by the many subsidiary ailments that afflict the aged.

CONCLUSIONS

1. Recent studies cast doubt on the evidence that there is any genuine difference in the incidence rate of cerebral infarction and embolism

when compared with cerebral haemorrhage in different countries.

2. Cerebral haemorrhage is almost certainly over-diagnosed. The long-held belief that the Japanese (domiciled in Japan) and the American Negro have strikingly higher rates for cerebral haemorrhage than other racial groups in other countries may well spring from an artefact of reporting.
3. There is some divergence of opinion upon the apparent fact that cerebral haemorrhage is decreasing as a cause of death.
4. Epidemiological studies indicate that 'stroke' is a disease of the elderly. The usual hospital-based studies are concerned with the 'fringe' of the problem.
5. As anticipated, epidemiological studies indicate that the prognosis both in terms of morbidity and mortality is related in a linear manner to age.

REFERENCES

Acheson, R. M. (1960) Observer error and variation in the interpretation of electrocardiograms in an epidemiology study of coronary heart disease. *British Journal of Preventive Social Medicine*, **14**, 99–122.

Acheson, J., Acheson, H. W. K. & Tellwright, J. M. (1968) The incidence and pattern of cerebrovascular disease in general practice. *Journal of the Royal College of General Practitioners*. **16**, 428–436.

Adams, G. F. & Merrett, J. D. (1961) Prognosis and survival in the aftermath of hemiplegia. *British Medical Journal*, **i**, 309–314.

Carter, A. B. (1961) Anticoagulant treatment in progressing stroke. *British Medical Journal*, **ii**, 70–73.

Carter, A. B. (1964) *Cerebral Infarction*, pp. 115–130. Oxford: Pergamon.

Eisenberg, H., Morrison, J. T., Sullivan, P. & Foote, F. M. (1964) Cerebrovascular accidents. *Journal of the American Medical Association*, **189**, 883–888.

Fisher, C. M. (1961) Anticoagulant therapy in cerebral thrombosis and cerebral embolism: a national cooperative study, interim report. *Neurology*, Minneapolis, **11**, 2, 119–131.

Goldner, J. C., Payne, G. H., Watson, F. R. & Parrish, H. M. (1967) Prognosis after stroke. Original article. *American Journal of the Medical Sciences*, **253**, 129–133.

Goldberg, I. D. & Kurland, L. T. (1962) Mortality in 33 countries from disease of the nervous system. *World Neurology*, **3**, 444–465.

Gordon, T. (1957) Mortality experience among the Japanese in the United States, Hawaii and Japan. *Public Health Report*, Washington, **72**, 543–553.

Howard, F. A., Cohen, P., Hickler, R. B., Locke, S., Newcomb, T. & Tyler, H. R. (1963) Survival following stroke. *Journal of the American Medical Association*, **183**, 921–925.

Howe, G. M. (1963) *National Atlas of Disease Mortality in the United Kingdom*. The Royal Geographical Society. London: Nelson.

Johnson, K. G., Yano, K. & Kato, H. (1967) Cerebral vascular disease in Hiroshima, Japan. *Journal of Chronic Diseases*, **20**, 545–559.

Katz, S., Ford, A. B., Chinn, A. B. & Newill, W. A. (1966) Prognosis after stroke. *Medicine* (Baltimore), **45**, 236–246.

Kurtze, J. F. (1969) *Epidemiology of Cerebrovascular Disease*. Berlin–Heidelberg–New York: Springer-Verlag.

Marquardsen, J. (1969) The natural history of acute cerebrovascular disease. A retrospective study of 769 patients. *Acta Neurologica Scandinavica*, Supplement, **38**.

Marshall, J. & Shaw, D. A. (1959) The natural history of cerebrovascular disease. *British Medical Journal*, **i**, 1614–1617.

Matsumoto, N., Whisnant, J. P., Kurland, L. T. & Okazaki, H. (1973) Natural history of stroke in Rochester, Minnesota, 1955 through 1969. An extension of a previous study, 1945 through 1954. *Stroke*, **4**, 20–29.

Millikan, C. H. (1965) Therapeutic agents—current status: anticoagulant therapy in cerebrovascular disease. In *Cerebral Vascular Diseases*. (Transactions of the Fourth Princeton Conference on Cerebrovascular Disease) (Eds.) Millikan, C. H., Kiekert, R. G. & Whisnant, J. P. pp. 181–184. New York: Grune & Stratton.

Robinson, R. D., Cohen, W. D., Higano, N., Meyer, R., Lukowsky, G., McLaughlin, R. B. & MacGilpin, H. H. (1959) Life-table analysis of survival after cerebral thrombosis. Ten-year experience. *Journal of the American Medical Association*, **169**, 1149–1152.

Robinson, R. W., Demirel, M. & LeBeau, R. J. (1968) Natural history of cerebral thrombosis nine to 19 year follow-up. *Journal of Chronic Diseases*, **21**, 221–230.

Schiller, F. (1970) Concepts of stroke before and after Virchow. In *Medical History*, **24**, 115–131. (Ed.) Poynter, F. N. L. London: British Society for the History of Medicine.

Stallones, R. A. (1965) Epidemiology of cerebrovascular disease. *Journal of Chronic Diseases*, **18**, 859–872.

Veys, C. A. (1973) *A Study on the Incidence of Bladder Tumours in Rubber Workers*. M.D. Thesis. Liverpool University Cohen Library.

Wylie, C. M. (1962) Cerebrovascular accident deaths in the United States and in England and Wales. *Journal of Chronic Diseases*, **15**, 85–90.

Whisnant, J. P., Fitzgibbon, J. P., Kurland, L. T. & Sayre, G. P. (1971) Natural history of stroke in Rochester, Minnesota, 1945 through 1954. *Stroke*, **2**, 11–21.

Yates, P. O. (1964) A change in the pattern of cerebrovascular disease. *Lancet*, **i**, 65–69.

CHAPTER FIVE

Transient Cerebral Ischaemia

A consideration of the natural history of focal cerebral vascular disease, presumed to have an ischaemic aetiology, falls naturally into two parts. The first is the fate of patients presenting with transient ischaemic attacks (TIAs), as defined previously (Chapter 4); the second is the outcome in patients presenting with an acute stroke. It is worth emphasising that the subdivision is a matter of convenience rather than that it implies a fundamentally differing aetiology.

This chapter contains a brief consideration of the clinical syndromes of TIAs and then a review of the available facts on the prognosis of these patients, particular attention being paid to the incidence of stroke and ultimate morbidity.

HISTORICAL NOTE

The ancients were not unfamiliar with the idea that apoplexy may be preceded by transient neurological disturbance. Sorenus of Ephesus (circa 98—238 A.D.) observed that while the onset of apoplexy may certainly be unheralded, dizziness and ringing in the ears were sometimes a precursor of an attack (Drabkin, 1950). Heberden (1802) also commented on the premonitory symptoms, and Kirkland (1792) noted that vertigo may precede the onset of apoplexy but observed that 'it seemed to be the least or lowest symptom of the disease'. Hughlings Jackson (1881) was another to recognise that patients may have attacks of transient paralysis which could be repetitive and similar in pattern. He suggested that such attacks may be due to a small clot or to cerebral softening secondary to the blockage of a small vessel, yet he pointed out that it was often difficult to demonstrate a satisfactory pathological background for such transient episodes.

While these observations have historical interest, a full clinical appreciation of the significance of attacks of transient cerebral ischaemia (TCI) affecting the central nervous system is a development of the past three decades. Two parallel paths in the development of ideas concerning the pathogenesis of the syndrome can be recognised.

The first is the recognition of the importance of major neck vessels in cerebral vascular disease, and in this context Fisher and Cameron (1953) and later Gunning et al (1964) re-emphasised the importance of Chiari's observations published in 1905, in which he firmly established the importance of disease of the origin of the internal carotid artery in the pathogenesis of cerebral infarction. Subsequent developments in the pathological field led to an increasing appreciation of the importance of vascular disease of the major cervical vessels in the pathology of cerebral infarction, and need not be recapitulated here.

The second stage of development directly relevant to the syndrome of TIAs was the concept of dissoluble emboli arising from sites in the major cervical and thoracic vessels which were capable of causing TCI with full resolution and restoration subsequently of normal function.

Millikan, Siekert and Shick (1955), on the basis of clinical observations, put forward a theory on the aetiology of the syndromes they felt would provide a reasonable basis for the observed clinical facts. It ran as follows: a thrombus begins to form on an area of diseased epithelium; this soft material may break from this source, fragment when carried as far as the bifurcation of a vessel, and then break away again, thus causing only transient symptoms.

Clinical observers, such as Fisher (1959) and Ross Russell (1961) were able to witness the process in detail in the retina and the events observed were much as Millikan, Siekert and Shick (1955) had foretold.

Ashby et al (1963) were responsible for an important case report on a patient who had attacks of retinal embolisation that were so frequent that they were able to photograph events within minutes of the onset. They recorded the presence of pearly white material within the retinal vessels and were able to observe and record the intermittent progress of this material through the arterial circulation and its final disappearance. That these were platelet emboli was established by the post-mortem studies of McBrien, Bradley and Ashton (1963).

Gunning et al (1964) published their own clinical and pathological observations on the development of mural thrombus in the subclavian artery adjacent to cervical ribs and in the carotid arteries in association with atheroma. In the latter case their observations led them to the view that repeated emboli were a more satisfactory explanation of recurrent TIAs than the view previously held, namely, that they were clinical expressions of recurrent haemodynamic crises.

As these ideas developed, clinical observers were beginning to appreciate that however trivial the attacks might be there was an under-lying ominous significance and this was, of course, the fact that they might be the precursor of a stroke leading to significant residual disability.

Initially, the information came from retrospective reviews on patients with a clinical diagnosis, usually based on carotid angiography, of internal carotid thrombosis. The interest aroused by these observations led unwittingly to the myth that it was possible on the clinical history to diagnose thrombosis of the internal carotid artery at its origin in the neck. Johnson and Walker

(1951), in a retrospective review of 101 patients with thrombosis of the internal or common carotid arteries which had been demonstrated at angiography, observed that transient neurological disturbances had been noted by about 40 per cent of their patients. Fisher and Cameron (1953) also recognised that transient vascular insufficiency prior to the onset of a stroke was a good deal more common than was generally appreciated at the time but they also indicated that not all patients with the syndrome invariably went on to develop a stroke. Later, Hurwitz et al (1959) observed that in 57 cases of carotid artery occlusion attacks of transient ischaemia were reported in 39 per cent of the patients and these had occurred at widely varying intervals of time, the range being 10 days to nine years before the stroke. They made an attempt at that time to recognise clinical points which would differentiate or identify patients liable to develop a major stroke, but they were unable to do so.

THE SYNDROMES OF TRANSIENT CEREBRAL ISCHAEMIA

Before considering briefly the clinical syndromes of TCI one important point in diagnosis is worth reiterating. This relates to the diagnostic criteria used. Since there has been no universally agreed temporal definition, different authors have applied the clinical diagnosis to attacks that vary in length of time. Some restrict the time of an attack to less than one hour, whereas others will accept attacks of up to 24 hours providing there is subsequent complete resolution of signs. A recent innovation (Ziegler and Hassanein, 1973) has been to accept patients for study with attacks which last less than 24 hours but for more than 15 minutes. The purpose of the latter restriction is not clear and personal experience would indicate that if a period of less than 15 minutes is not accepted this excludes a number of patients where there is no reasonable ground for doubting the diagnosis. These differences based on the duration of the attack obviously have one potentially significant effect and that is that the acceptance of a shorter interval (one hour) as defining a TIA will inevitably lead to a higher incidence of strokes being diagnosed. This is not a major problem as most observers agree that the majority of clinical episodes are short-lived, a point emphasised by Marshall (1964) in his own series.

While the syndromes of TIA are well recognised in the literature, to those unfamiliar with the diagnostic problem they can still present difficulties, and this is particularly true when the vertebrobasilar arterial territory is the site affected. The chance of observing a clinical attack rarely occurs, particularly when these are of short-lived duration, and the diagnosis is therefore based on the subjective symptoms described by the patient. The whole range of vocabulary, experience and intelligence of the patient may either help, or serve to obscure, what is otherwise a straightforward diagnostic problem. A few comments, therefore, on the clinical syndromes of TCI are appropriate.

Transient vertebrobasilar ischaemia

Millikan and Siekert (1955) reviewed 10 cases of intermittent symptoms 'which indicated transitory impairment of function in some portion of the pons, mesencephalon and the occipital lobes'. They suggested that the syndrome be called 'intermittent insufficiency of the basilar arterial system'. Williams and Wilson (1962) studied the clinical syndrome that was associated with vertebrobasilar insufficiency. They suggested that the symptom pattern of fluctuating symptoms which were associated in time but which could not be related on a topographical basis, was the clue to the diagnosis. They particularly instanced bilateral blindness and vertigo which could only be mediated by a common vascular supply, namely, the basilar and the posterior cerebral arteries. They listed in order of frequency the symptoms they encountered in their experience, and these are given in Table 5.1. Marshall (1964) also reported on his own experience with transient symptoms in the carotid and basilar circulation and gave the relative frequency of the individual symptoms noted (Table 5.2).

Table 5.1. Incidence (percentage) of symptoms in vertebrobasilar TCI (Williams & Wilson, 1962).

Symptoms	No.	%
Vertigo	32	48
Visual hallucinations	7	10
Drop attacks or weakness	7	10
Visceral sensations	5	8
Visual field defects	4	6
Diplopia	3	5
Headaches	2	3

Table 5.2. Incidence of symptoms in TCI in carotid and vertebrobasilar territories (Marshall, 1964).

	Carotid	Vertebrobasilar
Vertigo	12	48
Tinnitus	–	1
Visual changes		
Visual field disturbance	14	22
Diplopia	–	7
Dysarthria	3	11
Facial paraesthesiae	4	2
Drop attacks	–	16
Hemiparesis	31	8
Hemianaesthesia	33	9
Confusion	5	1
Dysphasia	20	–
Monoparesis	7	4

VISUAL SYMPTOMS

Visual symptoms are common in vertebrobasilar ischaemia.

Hallucinations, when they occur, are rarely formed but consist of teichopsia, black and white lines, and other unformed images. Coupled with an overall impairment of visual acuity these symptoms are highly suggestive of ischaemia of the occipital lobe. Hemianopia is relatively uncommon as a transient phenomenon, and one reason for its development may be an abnormality at the level of the Circle of Willis where one posterior communicating vessel may arise from the internal carotid supply and thus cause the occipital lobe to share the embolic phenomena originating in that artery. Double vision, however, is much more common, but this type of visual disturbance is not infrequent in clinical practice and needs therefore to be coupled with other symptoms indicating brain-stem ischaemia.

VERTIGO AND TRUNCAL ATAXIA

With a clear-cut history of vertigo and a true hallucination of a sense of movement there is no problem, but there are a number of patients where it is difficult to differentiate between vertigo and acute episodes of truncal ataxia presumably due to ischaemia of the vermis. The origin of vertigo occurring alone cannot usually be identified with certainty by the bedside but when it is coupled with visual symptoms that indicate ischaemia of the occipital lobes, the combination of symptoms is diagnostic. This, of course, is equally true when vertigo is associated with other symptoms of brain-stem ischaemia such as double vision.

DROP ATTACKS

A drop attack, or, in its milder form, a sudden accession of weakness of the lower limbs reminiscent of cataplexy, is not a common feature of transient vertebrobasilar ischaemia, at least in the younger patient, but if present one can assume that it has as much relevance as vertigo in making the final assessment.

SENSORY DISTURBANCES

Sensory disturbances in the face, particularly if they follow the typical pattern so often seen in migraine, with a circumoral distribution and affecting the tip of the tongue, are also uncommon but, if present, and provided there is no previous history of migraine, may be sufficiently diagnostic to raise a high index of suspicion.

ALTERNATING SENSORY AND MOTOR SYMPTOMS

The immediate premonitory signs of basilar artery occlusion, alternating sensory and motor signs are now well recognised but they are less common as a transient phenomenon although they certainly occur in transient vertebrobasilar ischaemia.

AKINETIC MUTISM

Whereas akinetic mutism can be seen not infrequently in basilar artery occlusion, it may also occur as a manifestation of TCI in the same territory but it is of considerable rarity.

Transient ischaemia in carotid artery distribution

MONOCULAR BLINDNESS

Perhaps the most typical of all attacks due to ischaemia in the carotid artery territory is that characterised by monocular blindness. Because of its implication, and because of the dramatic clinical observations that have been made on micro-emboli passing through the retinal circulation, the symptomatology of such episodes has been frequently discussed in the literature.

In monocular blindness the onset of symptoms is usually rapid, taking 10 to 15 seconds or even less to evolve. The patient describes either immediate total blindness or a curtain descending from above or ascending from below. Resolution occurs almost as quickly as the evolution of symptoms.

Monocular visual loss is a dramatic event but is often ignored by the patient as having little relevance to the presenting complaint of, for example, weakness of a limb, and it must therefore be enquired for specifically.

Other visual disturbances are associated with carotid artery ischaemia, but are of central origin and are infrequent. From time to time one encounters patients who give a clear-cut description of transient dyslexia as part of the manifestation of TCI.

HEMIPARESIS AND HEMISENSORY LOSS

Both of these are relatively common and can be seen in isolation or combined together. The differentiation between motor paresis and Jacksonian epilepsy is relatively easy since the paresis rarely, if ever, is followed by myoclonic movements of the limbs. The latter can certainly happen in cerebral infarction and may even justify the appellation 'epilepsia partialis continua' for several days.

Sensory phenomena affecting any part of the limb may present their own peculiar problems. If they occur in isolation and are not combined with other manifestations of ischaemia in that hemisphere, the differentiation from focal sensory epilepsy may be impossible for a time. Usually, with repeated attacks the problem clarifies itself in later episodes. Another occasional area of confusion is the ability of a cortical sensory lesion to stimulate approximately the effects of a peripheral sensory nerve lesion. Certainly, in cases where this mistake has been observed, the strict cutaneous distribution of a given peripheral nerve has been somewhat generously interpreted.

SPEECH

Disturbances of speech as a manifestation of transient cerebral ischaemia in the carotid territory present no diagnostic problem if combined with other elements of dominant hemisphere ischaemia. Occurring in isolation, however, the ability to differentiate between a hemisphere lesion and a cerebellar dysarthria originating in the hind brain may be comprehensively defeated by the patient's descriptive abilities.

EPISODIC CONFUSION

Confusional states are rare manifestations of TIAs if the time is limited to less than one hour. Unless the opportunity occurs to see the patient in an attack, and it rarely does so, the differentiation between TCI and temporal lobe epilepsy of vascular origin may be impossible.

THE NATURAL HISTORY OF TRANSIENT CEREBRAL ISCHAEMIA

The literature on the natural history of TIAs is somewhat limited due to the fact that this is a condition that has been recognised relatively recently. However, sufficient observations have now become available to allow a developing picture to be recognised.

The problem of diagnostic criteria has already been considered, and particularly the variation in the length of time accepted as compatible with an attack of TCI. Accepting this limitation there are still important areas of common ground in the different reported series, and the most important of these are the development of a stroke and the ultimate morbidity.

The studies reported fall into two contrasting categories. One is concerned with the epidemiological studies of the incidence of TCI within the community. The other, drawn from detailed studies of hospital populations, is concerned with the clinical problems associated with the natural history observed in relatively small groups of patients. In particular, the latter type of study has concentrated upon the risk of stroke developing subsequently in such cases.

EPIDEMIOLOGICAL STUDIES

Three epidemiological studies examine the incidence of TCI. Goldner, Whisnant and Taylor (1971) published a study on the long-term prognosis in TCI. The study was concerned with patients diagnosed at the Mayo Clinic and critical criteria were applied before accepting the diagnosis. They observed an incidence rate of 0.3 per 1000 per year among a white population. A not dissimilar figure was reported by Friedman, Wilson and Mosier (1969) who observed an incidence rate of 0.9 per 1000 per year.

A third study reported by Karp et al (1973) also approximated to these figures with an observed incidence rate of 1.3 per 1000 per year. This study was based on a survey of a bi-racial community in Evans County, Georgia, where all persons over 40, and a 50 per cent sample of those between 15 and 39 years of age, were invited to participate in a survey. As a result, 3102 individuals were examined. Five years later the survey was repeated, and after an initial screening process a final assessment was made by two consultant neurologists. The ultimate analysis identified 28 out of 2455 stroke patients with an acceptable diagnosis. The age-adjusted rate for TCI was 15.9 per 1000 per year of the white male population compared with 7.9 per 1000 per year for negroes. This was the lowest possible rate since the study specifically excluded patients who developed a stroke prior to the beginning of the study even though there was a prior history of TCI.

The racial differences in incidence may, the authors believed, have been attributed to the fact that atherosclerosis of the neck vessels—a common aetiological factor in TCI—is less frequent in the negro races than in a white population (Heyman, Fields and Keating, 1972).

TRANSIENT CEREBRAL ISCHAEMIA

In considering the natural history of TIAs it is proposed to examine the following points:

The development of a stroke.
Temporal patterns of attacks and their relevance to prognosis.
The morbidity, mortality and survival times.
The incidence of TCI following a stroke.

The consideration of the post-mortem findings in this group of patients will be deferred until the post-mortem findings in the whole group of cases of cerebral vascular disease are examined.

The development of stroke

The incidence of stroke in patients in different series presenting with TIAs is set out in Table 5.3. The details of age at onset and duration of disease in the present series are shown in Table 5.4.

Marshall (1964) divided 158 cases into three groups and only the first two groups need concern us here. The first of the two groups were 68 patients first seen with a major cerebral vascular episode who had a clear history of TIAs preceding the event. In a second group there were 61 patients seen with TIAs who were subsequently observed for periods ranging from three months to seven years. The average duration of observation was 43.9 months for patients with symptoms in the carotid territory and 49.1 months for attacks in the vertebrobasilar territory. In this second group, only one of the 61 patients went on to develop a stroke. If these two groups were combined, then a figure of just under 50 per cent represented the incidence of a stroke in 129 patients. However, combining the two groups in this way may be quite unjustifiable as there are obvious drawbacks to drawing this conclusion from two groups of patients who presented in entirely different ways.

Baker, Ramseyer and Schwartz (1968) studied a somewhat selected population in that all were male veterans. The average period of follow-up was three years and five months. Of the 79 patients in the study, 26 had had a previous cerebral infarct and complained of TCI after this event. If one excludes these and takes into account only those presenting with TCI the incidence of stroke in this particular series is 20 per cent.

Goldner, Whisnant and Taylor (1971) confined their study to patients

Table 5.3. Incidence and time interval of subsequent stroke in patients with transient cerebral ischaemia.

Author		No. of patients	Length of follow up	Average age (years)	% developing stroke	Average time to stroke
Marshall (1964)	Group 1	68	4 years Range 3–84 months		100	Carotid 14.4 months Vertebro-basilar 23.3 months
	Group 2	61			0.5	–
Goldner et al (1971)		140	15 years	59	31	–
Baker et al (1968)		53	3.5 years (3–104 months)	62.6	20	–
Acheson & Hutchinson (1970)		151	4.8 years	57.3	62	17 months
Zeigler & Hassanein (1973)		109	3 years	M 59.7 F 61.3	15.6	Within 3 years
Fields et al (1970)		147	(42 months) 7–63 months)	62	12.4	–

Table 5.4. Age at onset and duration of follow-up in a personal series of 151 patients presenting with TCI

	Male	Female	Total
Presenting with TCI	118	33	151
Age at onset	55.98 years	58.37 years	
	(S.D. 8.17)	(S.D. 9.29)	
Duration	4.98 years	4.22 years	
	(S.D. 2.58)	(S.D. 1.68)	
History of TCI only	45	12	57
Age at onset	55.95 years	59.22 years	56.63 years
	(S.D. 7.36)	(S.D. 9.35)	(S.D. 7.91)
Duration	4.98 years	3.84 years	4.74 years
	(S.D. 2.51)	(S.D. 1.81)	(S.D. 2.41)
History of TCI with stroke	73	21	94
Age at onset	56.00 years	57.88 years	56.42 years
	(S.D. 8.68)	(S.D. 9.48)	(S.D. 8.85)
Duration	4.98 years	4.44 years	4.86 years
	(S.D. 2.64)	(S.D. 1.59)	(S.D. 2.45)

presenting with TCI and without a previous history of stroke. An important aspect of this report in relation to the prognosis was that the diagnosis was made in the years 1950 to 1954, which allowed a period of follow-up of some 15 years. During this time the incidence of stroke was 37 per cent, and the authors imply that the constraints of their data collection in relation to the incidence of stroke may very well have resulted in an under-estimate of the complication. Due also to these constraints there were no figures available for the duration of TCI before the development of a stroke.

Fields, Maslenikov and Meyer (1970) reported on a controlled study of extracranial arterial disease where the purpose was to examine the potential benefits of surgery as opposed to conservative treatment. Their results are not strictly comparable to other series since the object was to study the potential advantages of surgery, and the patients were therefore assigned to groups on the basis of the arterial lesions demonstrated at angiography. With this proviso the incidence of stroke observed in the patients not subjected to surgery was 12.4 per cent.

Acheson and Hutchinson (1970) give a much higher incidence of the complication of a stroke in that it was observed in 62 per cent of 151 patients. One reason for this higher incidence may lie in the clinical definition, in that episodes of more than one hour were accepted as a stroke; another reason may very well be that personal regular supervision at three to six monthly intervals detected a higher incidence rate of further episodes than other studies.

Repeated stroke episodes

Once a stroke had occurred this did not necessarily indicate that the total natural history of the disorder was then concluded. Baker, Ramseyer and Schwartz (1968) observed further cerebral infarction in 27 per cent of their patients who had a previous history of stroke and TIAs. In the present series it was observed that in the 94 patients who developed a stroke, 26 went on to develop a second stroke, and in 10 of these there were repeated episodes up to as many as five episodes (Table 5.5).

Table 5.5. Frequency of recurrent stroke episodes in 36 patients presenting with TCI who later developed multiple stroke episodes.

	Male	Female	Male + female
Transient cerebral ischaemia going on to:			
2 strokes	22	4	26
3 strokes	3	1	4
4 strokes	4	0	4
5 strokes	2	0	2
	31	5	36

Temporal pattern of transient cerebral ischaemia

The temporal pattern of events in patients presenting with TIAs can be looked at in three ways. The first is the length of time before the stroke occurs. The second represents an effort to determine whether there are any major differences in frequency in attacks, prior to the stroke, that can be detected and, therefore, aid in the recognition of a stroke-prone individual. The third is the continuation of TIAs after the stroke or their development in patients presenting with stroke only.

Duration before stroke

The duration of TIAs before stroke in different series has already been shown in Table 5.3. The majority of the observers have noted that the stroke will occur within three years of the onset of the TIAs. Although Marshall's (1964) figure is given in the table as 0.5 per cent this refers only to those patients presenting with TCI without a complicating stroke. In the further 68 patients who were seen for the first time after an acute intracranial episode, but who had complained of TCI before this episode occurred, the time between the onset of symptoms and the stroke was 14.4 months for transient attacks in the carotid territory and 23.3 months in the vertebrobasilar territory.

Frequency of attacks

In the early days of the recognition of the clinical entity of TCI the view was occasionally expressed that a higher frequency rate of attacks indicated a greater likelihood in these particular patients of developing a stroke. If this were true, the therapeutic implications would be considerable.

Baker, Ramseyer and Schwartz (1968) analysed this point in detail when they made a comparison between patients with relatively few attacks (two to five in total) and found they could not detect any difference at all in the liability to develop a stroke based on the frequency of the preceding attack pattern.

Marshall (1964) also supported this view, which is the reverse of the general belief. He found that in the majority of patients with TCI the episodes were restricted to one or two attacks, and he certainly did not detect an increased frequency to develop a cerebral infarct in patients where the attacks were more frequent.

Acheson and Hutchinson (1964) examined the temporal pattern of attacks in a variety of ways in an attempt to determine a difference in the subsequent behaviour of two groups of patients. The examination included the significance of the frequency of attacks over a short time, the frequency of attacks over months or years, and the significance of an occasional episode only of TCI. None of these was found to give any useful indication that would enable a differentiation to be made in patients who may go on to a stroke and those who do not do so. It is certainly true that in patients with more frequent attacks (this referred to attacks occurring at least at daily intervals and sometimes several times a day) the incidence of subsequent stroke was higher than in the remainder. It is important, however, to emphasise that this observation did not reach statistical significance and the conclusion reached, therefore, was that no prediction was possible based on the attack pattern.

Cessation of attacks

There is a well-recognised tendency in patients with episodes of transient vascular insufficiency for the attacks to cease. Acheson and Hutchinson (1970) observed at the end of three years that 62 per cent of the patients had noted a cessation of attacks. In Marshall's (1964) series only 11 of the 60 patients continued with attacks for more than three years, and Baker, Ramseyer and Schwartz (1968) observed cessation of attacks after 12 months in 52 per cent. In their various sub-groups, which were based upon the arterial findings, Fields, Maslenikov and Meyer (1970) in a follow-up period of 42 months observed cessation of attacks in the non-surgically treated groups in figures ranging from 41.7 per cent to 51.9 per cent (Table 5.6).

Table 5.6. The incidence of cessation of TCI in series of cases previously reported and the time taken for this to occur.

Author	Percentage of cases noting cessation of attacks	Mean duration of TCI before cessation
Marshall, 1964	82	3 years
Baker et al, 1968	52	1 year
Fields et al, 1970	41.7 → 51.9	42 months
Acheson & Hutchinson, 1970	62	3 years

However, this cessation of attacks need not imply that cessation of TCI in over half the observed patients means that inactivity of the disease process commonly develops in most patients. In 1964, Acheson and Hutchinson reported 82 patients who had been followed initially for a mean period of 3.3 years; subsequently they repeated their observations upon the same patients after a mean period of 4.9 years. They found that the number of strokes that had been observed in the series had increased from 51.0 per cent to 62.4 per cent. Again, this increase may have been an expression of selection and unrecognised bias but it suggests at least that the process may continue to be active.

The mortality, survival times and morbidity

The mortality observed by Baker et al (1968) at the end of their study was between 21 per cent and 22 per cent. In the personal series the overall mortality at the end of the observational period was 23.8 per cent. However, in the Mayo Clinic series, with a follow-up period of some 15 years, the mortality rose steadily to 60 per cent (Figure 5.1). But, of course, in an ageing population the mortality need not necessarily be an expression of cerebral vascular disease, a point that will be examined in detail in the post-mortem findings.

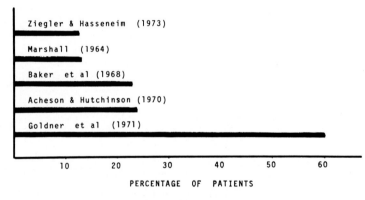

Figure 5.1. Percentage mortality of patients initially presenting with TCI in published series.

It is evident that in populations with a disease beginning at a mean age in the late 50s or early 60s a simple expression of mortality rate has limited value. A complementary assessment is that of comparing the survival time of the population at risk with that of the general population. To do this it is necessary to construct a model population where the age structure is identical with that of the patients in the study.

For the personal series, the details were obtained from English Life Tables No. 12 (1960-62) where the probability of survival per 100 000 of the population for each individual year of life is given. Using the method of Hill (1966), survival rates were then estimated for the 500 patients in the present study, and these are shown in Figure 5.2. Reference to this figure will show that the survival rate in patients with TCI uncomplicated by stroke is not dissimilar from that of the general population, since in the model population used for comparison, 89.8 per cent of the males were alive after a period of 4.5 years, whereas the comparable figure for patients with uncomplicated TCI was 89.3 per cent.

132   STROKES

However, the prognosis is materially altered when the complication of a stroke occurs. This might be anticipated, of course, both from the comparative death rates in the two groups and from clinical experience. The development of the complication of a stroke causes the percentage of patients surviving to fall to 82.2 per cent over a period of 4.5 years. As will be seen later, this figure closely approximates to the figure for patients where the history was that of a single stroke only, without the prior complication of TCI.

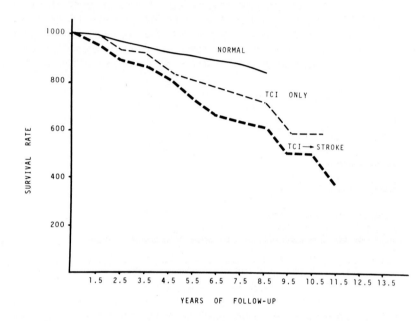

Figure 5.2. Annual survival rates per 1000 compared with normal population in 151 patients presenting with TCI.

Goldner, Whisnant and Taylor (1971), against a background of a 15-year follow-up study, were able to carry the examination of survival times a stage further. Their population at risk sample was matched for age and sex with the West North-Central U.S. Life Tables and they examined the survival times in three age groups. The first age group was of patients beginning with symptoms before the age of 55 years; the second group was of those beginning with symptoms at ages ranging from 55 to 65; the third group was of patients first presenting with symptoms of TCI over the age of 65. They did not, in their examination, differentiate between patients who had a complicating stroke and those who remained free of this complication.

They found that survival was significantly affected in all age groups up to the age of 65 when compared with the general population. However, in patients presenting with TCI at the age of 65 or over the probability of survival was very similar to that of the general population (Figures 5.3 and 5.4).

The observation that patients in both the under 55 and in the 55 to 64 age groups did less well than the patients in the over 65 age group in terms of survival is important. It is for the former groups of patients that therapeutic programmes are designed and in the assessment of these programmes due weight should be given to this observation.

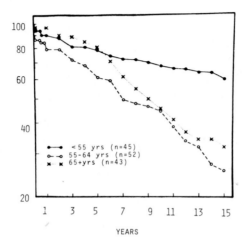

Figure 5.3. Probability of survival after first episode of TCI according to age.

Morbidity

Baker, Ramseyer and Schwartz (1968) assessed in some detail the disability in their patients at the end of the period of observation, and in doing so they expressed the disability as it was observed either at the end of the study or before death. In the present series the clinical state before death is excluded from further consideration, but apart from this the methods of assessing disability in the two series were very similar.

In the series of Baker, Ramseyer and Schwartz (1968), of the patients who presented without previous infarction, 46 of the 53 showed very minimal disability or no disability at all and only 7 were classified as severely disabled and unable to undertake self-care.

In our own series (Table 5.7) 38 per cent of the patients (57) were by definition free of any neurological deficit since they had never developed a major intracranial episode. Eight of the patients, however, had died from unrelated causes and five were disabled from physical defects other than cerebral vascular disease. The remaining 44 patients were either working full time at their own jobs or were enjoying active retirement.

Of the 94 patients presenting with TCI and who later developed either one or more strokes, there were 66 survivors, and of these 67 per cent were capable of working full time (Grade 1) and five were able to work full time but had been reduced to taking a lighter job because of their minimal neurological

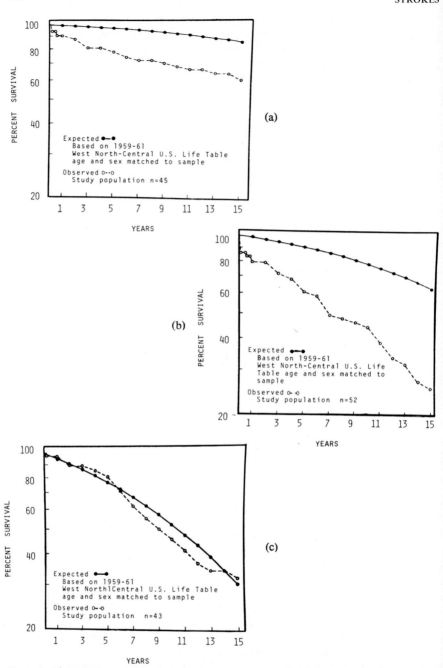

Figure 5.4. Probability of survival after first episode of TCI compared with expected survival in different age groups. a. Less than 55 years at onset; b. 55–64 at onset; c. 65 or more at onset. (Courtesy of Dr J. C. Goldner et al (1971), Long-term prognosis of TCI attacks. *Stroke*, **1**. By permission of The American Heart Association, Inc.)

Table 5.7. Final clinical state at end of study of 151 patients presenting with transient cerebral ischaemia (Reproduced by permission from the *Quarterly Journal of Medicine*, 1971).

	Dead	Alive	Grade 1	Grade 2	Grade 3	Grade 4	Disabled (other causes)	Total
History of TCI only	8 (14.1%)	49 (85.9%)	44 (89.8%)	0	0	0	5 (10.2%)	57
History of TCI with later stroke	28 (29.8%)	66 (70.2%)	44 (66.6%)	5 (7.6%)	9 (13.6%)	2 (3.0%)	6 (9.1%)	94

Grade 1. Complete functional recovery.
Grade 2. Minimal residual disability.
Grade 3. Activity markedly impaired by residual neurological signs.
Grade 4. Confined to chair or bed.

disability (Grade 2). Eleven patients were severely disabled as a direct result of the stroke.

It will be shown later that the history of recurrent episodes of stroke materially alters the prognosis in any group of patients. The same observation appears to apply to patients presenting with transient ischaemia who go on to develop multiple recurrent intracranial episodes. Of the 58 patients who presented with a history of TCI and who subsequently had only one stroke during the period of observation, 28 per cent died but of the survivors 81 per cent were working full time. In contrast, 36 patients went on to develop a varying number of recurrent stroke episodes (Table 5.5). The death rate was very much higher in these patients since 33 per cent died and only 62.5 per cent of the survivors were working full time. However, although the mortality is higher and the morbidity greater in patients with multiple stroke occurring during the period of observation, the difference between the two groups did not reach statistical significance.

Incidence of TCI after stroke

The occurrence for the first time of TCI after an initial stroke was noted by Marshall (1964) in 29 patients. In our personal series this was observed in 31 patients with a single stroke, in 27 with recurrent stroke episodes and in 37 where a stroke complicated a history of preceding TCI.

Baker, Ramseyer and Schwartz (1968) made the interesting observation that whereas TIAs were noted to follow cerebral infarction in 20 per cent, they were observed in 57 per cent where TIAs had preceded the stroke episode. This led them to suggest that 'the transient ischaemic syndrome in some instances may be due to a different pathophysiological process than that which leads to infarction'.

The observation in the present series goes some way to confirm the facts observed by Baker, Ramseyer and Schwartz (1968) (Table 5.8). In patients with a history of a single stroke, TIAs were observed to develop in 18.9

per cent of 164 patients and in 14.5 per cent of patients with a history of recurrent episodes. However, in the 94 patients who had developed a stroke after presenting with a history of TIAs episodes of insufficiency were observed to continue in 39.4 per cent. This figure is clearly much higher than that observed in the single stroke or recurrent episode group of patients.

Table 5.8. Incidence of transient cerebral ischaemia in the personal series of cases following an episode of stroke.

	Single stroke 164 patients			Multiple stroke 185 patients			TCI going on to stroke 94 patients		
	TCI to follow			TCI to follow			TCI to follow		
With 1 or more strokes	164	31	18.9%	185	27	14.5%	94	37	39.4%
With 2 or more strokes				185	24	13.0%	36	11	30.6%
With 3 or more strokes				85	3	1.6%	10	2	20.0%
With 4 or more strokes				29	3	10.3%	6	1	16.7%
With 5 or more strokes				10	0	–	2	0	–
With 6 or more strokes				4	0	–			

CONCLUSION

1. The incidence of transient cerebral ischaemia (TCI) in the community is variously noted as ranging from 0.3 per 1,000 per year to 1.3 per 1,000 per year.
2. Stroke as a complication developing subsequently in patients with TCI is variously described in 12.4 to 62 per cent of cases. This variation in incidence is partly due to definition of stroke. If a 24-hour period of neurological symptoms is accepted as the definition of TCI rather than a 1 hour period, the incidence of subsequent stroke is approximately 30 per cent.
3. Strokes, if they do occur, have been noted after periods ranging from 12 months to 3 years following the onset of TCI.
4. Attacks may cease in at least 50 per cent of patients with TCI after a period of 1 to 3 years.
5. If a stroke does not develop, the prognosis for survival in patients with TCI is normal.
6. Studies have shown that patients below the age of 65 years with TCI have a worse prognosis, in terms of survival, than do those above 65 when compared with populations of similar age.
7. Over 60 per cent of patients who develop a stroke following TCI may eventually be capable of full work.
8. TCI may develop for the first time after a stroke. However, if the stroke has been preceded by TCI the frequency of subsequent TCI is very much higher.

REFERENCES

Acheson, J. & Hutchinson, E. C. (1964) Observations of the natural history of transient cerebral ischaemia. *Lancet*, **ii**, 871–874.

Acheson, J. & Hutchinson, E. C. (1970) The natural history of 'focal cerebral vascular disease.' *Quarterly Journal of Medicine*, **40**, 157, 15–23.

Ashby, M., Oakley, N., Lorentz, I. & Scott, D. (1963) Recurrent transient monocular blindness. *British Medical Journal*, **ii**, 894–897.

Baker, R. N., Ramseyer, J. C. & Schwartz, W. S. (1968) Prognosis in patients with transient cerebral ischaemia. *Neurology*, **18**, 1157–1165.

Drabkin, I. E. (1950) *Acute Diseases and Chronic Diseases.* (Edited and translated) Drabkin, I. E. Chicago, Illinois: University of Chicago Press.

Fields, W. S., Maslenikov, V. & Meyer, J. S. (1970) Joint study of extracranial arterial occlusion. V. Progress report of prognosis following surgery or nonsurgical treatment for transient cerebral attacks and cervical carotid artery lesions. *Journal of the American Medical Association*, **211**, 1993–2003.

Fisher, C. M. & Cameron, D. G. (1953) Case report: concerning cerebral vasospasm. *Neurology*, **3**, 468–473.

Fisher, C. M. (1959) Observations of the fundus oculi in transient monocular blindness. *Neurology*, **9**, 333–347.

Friedman, G. D., Wilson, W. S. & Mosier, J. M. (1969) Transient ischaemic attacks in a community. *Journal of the American Medical Association*, **210**, 1428–1434.

Goldner, J. C., Whisnant, J. P. & Taylor, W. F. (1971) Long term prognosis of transient cerebral ischaemic attacks. *Stroke*, **2**, 160–167.

Gunning, A. J., Pickering, G. W., Robb-Smith, A. H. T. & Russell, R. W. R. (1964) Mural thrombosis of the internal carotid artery and subsequent embolism. *Quarterly Journal of Medicine*, **33**, 155–195.

Heberden, W. (1802) *Commentaries on the History and Cure of Diseases.* Printed for T. Payne, Mews Gate, by S. Hamilton, Falcon Court, Fleet Street, London.

Heyman, A., Fields, W. S. & Keating, R. D. (1972) Joint study of extracranial arterial occlusion. VI. Racial differences in hospitalised patients with ischaemic stroke. *Journal of the American Medical Association*, **222**, 285–289.

Hill, A. B (1966) *Principles of Medical Statistics.* London: Lancet Limited.

Hurwitz, L. J., Groch, S. N., Wright, I. S. & McDowell, F. H. (1959) Carotid artery occlusive syndrome. *Archives of Neurology*, **1**, 491–501.

Jackson, J. Hughlings (1881) On temporary paralysis after epileptiform and epileptic seizures; a contribution to the study of dissolution of the nervous system. *Brain*, **iii**, 433–451.

Johnson, H. C. & Walker, A. E. (1951) The angiographic diagnosis of spontaneous thrombosis of the internal carotid and common carotid arteries. *Journal of Neurosurgery*, **8**, 631–659.

Karp, H. R., Heyman, A., Heyden, S., Bartel, A. G., Tyroler, H. A. & Haymes, C. G. (1973) Transient cerebral ischaemia. Prevalence and prognosis in a biracial rural community. *Journal of the American Medical Association*, **225**, 125–128.

Kirkland, T. (1792) *A Commentary on Apoplectic and Paralytic Affections.* London: William Dawson.

McBrien, D. J., Bradley, R. D. & Ashton, N. (1963) Nature of retinal emboli in stenosis of the internal carotid artery. *Lancet*, **i**, 697–699.

Marshall, J. (1964) The natural history of transient ischaemic cerebro-vascular attacks. *Quarterly Journal of Medicine*, **33**, 309–324.

Millikan, C. H. & Siekert, R. G. (1955) Studies in cerebro-vascular disease. 1. The syndrome of intermittent insufficiency of the basilar arterial system. *Proceedings of the Staff Meetings of the Mayo Clinic*, **30**, 61–68.

Millikan, C. H., Siekert, R. G. & Schick, R. M. (1955) Studies in cerebrovascular disease, 5. Use of anticoagulant drugs in the treatment of intermittent insufficiency of the internal carotid arterial system. *Proceedings of the Staff Meetings of the Mayo Clinic*, **30**, 578–586.

Russell, R. W. R. (1961) Observations on the retinal blood vessels in monocular blindness. *Lancet*, **ii**, 1422–1428.

Williams, D. & Wilson, T. G. (1962) The diagnosis of the major and minor syndromes of basilar insufficiency. *Brain*, **85**, 741–774.

Ziegler, D. K. & Hassanein, R. S. (1973) Prognosis in patients with transient ischaemic attacks. *Stroke*, **4**, 466–673.

CHAPTER SIX

Natural History of Stroke

Early progress in the understanding of the natural history of cerebral vascular disease was slow, and the literature consists largely of personal experience and opinion. Copland (1850) discussed the prognosis of patients with 'apoplexy' and concludes that although complete recovery was rare, patients may live for many years without either recurrence or complication. Some 30 years later, however, Charcot (1881) drew a more depressing picture. He observed that even though the apoplectic attack was not fatal full recovery was rare and ' . . . in the immense majority of cases the patient only retains life at the expense of deplorable infirmities'. Charcot also noted that intellect was commonly affected and that advanced dementia could develop.

Gowers (1888) recognised that there were variations in the subsequent history of patients presenting with stroke and this led him to suggest that the outlook was rather less depressing. He observed that it was rare for the patient to die in the first attack and that the prospects of recovery depended to some extent on the age of the patient and on the history of previous attacks. But Gowers pointed out that there were many difficulties in assessing the prognosis in apoplexy with any accuracy, and this remains true today.

NATURAL HISTORY

The interest in the last 20 years in the prognosis following a stroke is a reflection of the major contribution this type of cerebral vascular disease makes to the morbidity and mortality of the ageing population. A direct comparison between the results recorded by different observers is sometimes difficult and often meaningless. At one end of the spectrum are the relatively young patients represented by the previously fit 55-year-old man or woman with a sudden hemiplegia, and at the other end are the elderly, known to have multiple disabilities, to whom the development of a focal ischaemic lesion is the final straw in a decade of disability. The predominance of one or other group of patients is, of course, simply an expression of the selection that has been imposed on the particular observer by the circumstances of his work. It is only by combining these experiences and recognising selection that a complete picture can be obtained.

There are two aspects to the natural history of stroke. One is the immediate mortality, and the second is the fate of the survivors. In this latter group it is necessary to consider not only long-term survival but the ultimate morbidity shown by the survivors. An important feature of survival is the occurrence of recurrent episodes and the contribution these make to increasing disability.

IMMEDIATE MORTALITY

The definition of immediate mortality is a matter of convenience, and authors vary in assigning arbitrary times up to as long as four weeks after the initial episode. The available evidence comes from two sources. These are population surveys and series of patients studied after admission to acute general hospitals.

Population studies

Eisenberg et al (1964) reported the incidence and survival rates in the population of the Middlesex County, Connecticut. The patients affected were identified over a period of 12 months and were subsequently followed up over a five-year period. During this period of 12 months, 191 people were affected by stroke, and a diagnosis of cerebral thrombosis was made in 48 per cent and cerebral haemorrhage in 36 per cent. In the latter diagnosis no differentiation was made between subarachnoid haemorrhage and cerebral haemorrhage.

Of the patients sustaining an acute 'cerebral vascular episode' for the first time, in the period of the study, there was an initial mortality of 16 per cent in 48 hours in all cases of cerebral thrombosis and cerebral haemorrhage combined. In patients with cerebral thrombosis or cerebral embolism, which were grouped together, a death rate was observed of only 7 per cent in the first two days but the mortality rose rapidly to 30 per cent at the end of seven days and to 36 per cent at 14 days.

Whisnant et al (1971) differentiated between cerebral thrombosis, cerebral embolism and cerebral haemorrhage by traditional methods but indicated that the diagnosis of cerebral infarction included all cases which on clinical grounds did not show evidence of a possible clinical source of a cerebral embolus. In the period 1945 to 1955, 184 patients had suffered a stroke and of these 77 per cent were diagnosed as being due to cerebral infarction.

The importance of this particular study stems from two facts. The first is the acknowledged excellence of the clinical records system of the Mayo Clinic in relation to the local population. The second is that autopsies were carried out in 50 per cent of all patients so that the standard objection to this type of study, namely, the precise cause of death, is readily and accurately answered.

At the end of one month, 27 per cent of the patients with cerebral infarction had died, which is in marked contrast to cerebral haemorrhage where the comparable mortality was 83 per cent. An interesting side-light is that the prognosis for subarachnoid haemorrhage in the general population indicated a 65 per cent mortality in the same period of time.

Even though the comparable mortality rates between the two conditions of cerebral infarction and cerebral haemorrhage are vastly different, they indicate that in their experience the incidence of cerebral haemorrhage is very much over-estimated, the vital statistics for the U.S. giving a ratio of about 2.5:1 of cerebral haemorrhage to infarction whereas in a study of the population in Rochester the ratio was 0.15:1. They found that cerebral infarction was four to six times more frequent in the age group 45 to 64, and 20 times more frequent in the ages over 75 when compared with the incidence of cerebral haemorrhage.

Few studies are available from general practice. Wallace (1964) studied the problem in a general practice in Australia and observed an initial mortality of over 30 per cent but no clear differentiation was made between cerebral haemorrhage and thrombosis due to the circumstances of the study.

General hospital populations

In assessing the initial mortality from studies of general hospital populations three reports seem to give a representative overall picture. They were representative in that, from the description of the source of patients given, they were all admitted to acute general medical wards without prior selection. These are the reports of Robinson et al (1968), Carter (1964) and Marquardsen (1969); (Table 6.1).

The report of Robinson et al (1968) examines the fate of patients admitted to three major hospitals in Worcester, Massachusetts, and in the design of the study all cases of cerebral haemorrhage were excluded by carrying out lumbar punctures and they also excluded all cases which showed a clinically obvious source of embolism such as rheumatic heart disease. They defined the immediate mortality as death occurring within three months of the initial episode and observed a rate of 27 per cent for women and 18 per cent for men, but the difference was not statistically significant.

Carter's (1964) experience in a General Hospital service in England in Ashford, Kent, was of a mortality rate of 26 per cent (159) in a personally observed series of 612 patients admitted who died within four weeks of the onset.

Marquardsen (1969), examining the prognosis in 'cerebral vascular episodes,' conducted a retrospective study of a hospital population in the Municipality of Frederiksberg and accepted into the study all cases with cerebral infarction and cerebral haemorrhage. He defined the immediate fatality rate as that occurring within the first three weeks and observed a fatality rate of 50 per cent for males and 44.8 per cent for females.

If one considers other hospital series where selection is evident one finds that very much lower rates for initial mortality are observed.

Pincock (1957) reported a study of 117 patients who were admitted with acute 'cerebral thrombosis'. All the patients were male but the initial mortality was only 14 per cent in 117 patients. David and Heyman (1960) reported on

Table 6.1. Acute mortality in series where 'acute' was defined in relation to time.

Author	Diagnosis	No. of cases	Age at onset (years)	% Mortality	Definition of 'acute'	Source
Carroll (1962)	Hemiplegia	98	60+	24	14 days	Rehabilitation
Robinson et al (1968)[a]	Cerebral thrombosis	843	M.66.4 F.69.9	23	Less than 3 months	General hospital
Carter (1964)[a]	Cerebral infarction	612	65	26	Within 4 weeks	General hospital
Eisenberg et al (1964)	Thrombosis and embolism	98	74.5	35	14 days	Epidemiology
Matsumoto et al (1973)	Cerebral thrombosis	701	60+	18	30 days	Community
Marquardsen (1969)[a]	Thrombosis and haemorrhage	769	M.67.3 F.69.9	M.54.5 F.44.8	Within 3 weeks	General hospital

[a]Patients from an acute General Hospital.

a study of 100 patients who were admitted to Duke University Hospital or the Veterans' Administration Hospital in Durham, North Carolina. Of the 100 patients, there was a predominance of males since only 10 of the patients were female. In this selected series the initial mortality was only 10 per cent.

It would seem, therefore, on the available evidence relating to cerebral infarction as distinct from other varieties of cerebral vascular disease, that the mortality in the first four weeks after the episode will be between 25 and 35 per cent.

LONG-TERM MORTALITY AND SURVIVAL RATES

In assessing the ultimate outcome in surviving patients it is usual in all but the most recent literature to refer only to mortality rates at the end of a defined period of study. While such figures are valuable in making comparisons with other series it is necessary to take into account the fact that the majority of patients studied are members of an ageing population and, as such, may succumb to other diseases. It is now usual in the literature to construct model populations of the same age and sex structure from available Life Tables and, using this, to compare the outcome in the disease under study with a defined 'normal' population. This gives a more valuable index of the actual effect of the underlying vascular disease.

Late mortality

The late mortality following an acute intracerebral vascular episode is expressed in different ways in different series which obviously relate to the time the individual series of patients is under study. The studies that relate to the mortality at intervals up to five years following an acute stroke are detailed in Figure 6.1.

Clearly, if the survival at the end of the first year is examined there are major differences to be observed (Table 6.2). Marshall and Shaw's (1959) figure of 7 per cent mortality is only a ninth of the mortality observed by Eisenberg et al (1964) with a figure of 65 per cent. The difference can only be explained by the varying method of selecting patients. Eisenberg et al (1964) were studying a county population where all strokes were registered and this series included a large number of elderly people. Marshall's figures are taken

Table 6.2. Number and percentage of patients surviving at 1 year.

Author	Number of survivors	% of series at 1 year
Pincock (1957)	101	99
Marshall and Shaw (1959)	251	93
David and Heyman (1960)	90	75
Carter (1964)	240	63
Eisenberg et al (1964)	83	35
Robinson et al (1959)	737	83
Marquardsen (1969)	407	77

from a study based on a hospital population which was much younger. An initial mortality of only 7 per cent in Marshall's series emphasises the point.

However, it is of interest that when one compares figures for what one would anticipate are broadly similar populations the figures still vary. For example, Carter (1964), working in a large British general hospital observed a 63 per cent survival rate at one year whereas Marquardsen (1969) observed survival in 77 per cent of his patients at the end of the same period of time. Admittedly, the latter author intentionally did not differentiate between haemorrhage and ischaemic stroke but, this being so, he acknowledged that the higher mortality rate in cerebral haemorrhage would result in a higher mortality and, therefore, a lower survival rate.

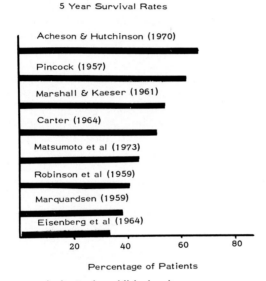

5 Year Survival Rates

Acheson & Hutchinson (1970)

Pincock (1957)

Marshall & Kaeser (1961)

Carter (1964)

Matsumoto et al (1973)

Robinson et al (1959)

Marquardsen (1959)

Eisenberg et al (1964)

20   40   60   80

Percentage of Patients

Figure 6.1. Five-year survival rates in published series.

Adams and Merrett (1961) and Droller (1960), who were both studying patients drawn from a geriatric practice, have a higher survival rate than the general hospital figures mentioned above although the figures probably do not, as in the case of Marquardsen's (1969) series, reach significance.

Marquardsen (1969) also observed a sex variation within the first 12 months in that 25 per cent of the 257 female patients died within this period of time compared with only 14 per cent of females in the second year of study. He observed no such variations in males.

Whatever the reasons for these variations in survival at the end of a year— and one suspects that unavoidable selection due to socio-medical causes has a large responsibility for these—the picture at five years becomes clearer (Figure 6.1).

Three observations stand out from the rest and these are those of Pincock (1957), Marshall and Kaeser (1961) and the present series, all of which show survival rates in excess of 50 per cent. All three are clearly different populations from the remainder, taken as they are from a selected population in hospital practice rather than from a total general hospital practice or from the population at large. All these show figures at five years which range between 34 per cent (Eisenberg et al, 1964) and 46 per cent (Carter, 1964).

Mortality observed beyond a five-year period with a starting age at least in the late fifties, and usually in the early sixties, tends to lose significance and is more appropriately considered in relation to survival and the general population of the same age.

Survival rate

In expressing survival rates it is worth emphasising the obvious, namely, that the observed death rate in patients presenting with cerebral vascular disease does not have any necessary implications in relation to the cause of death. In cerebral infarction, the cause of death may be related only indirectly to intracerebral vascular disease in that death may ultimately be due to manifestations of vascular disease elsewhere, and most commonly in the coronary circulation. This is so in the present series and many other published series and will be considered in some detail later.

Adams and Merrett (1961) were among the early observers to utilise the valuable technique of comparing their results with the general population, which they did by calculating, for the patients studied, the 'half survival time'. This was done in a series of 736 hemiplegics. The 'half survival time' is the number of years after a stroke that half of the given group of observed patients may be expected to live. This could then be compared with the normal average life expectation in various age ranges compiled, in their case, from Life Tables of the Registrar General for Northern Ireland. They arranged their patients and the normal population in three groups. The first contained patients of less than 65 years, the second group were 65 to 75 years of age, and the third group were 75 years or more. They observed that life in the patients under study was greatly foreshortened after a stroke and, indeed, fell below half the period of time that the patient might have been expected to live, given a certain age and being in normal health at the time. This reduction in life expectancy did not apply to the 75 years-and-over age group.

The details of the present series are shown in Table 6.3, which gives the sex and age distribution and, also, the notable difference between the numbers surviving in the patients with a history of one stroke and patients whose history was that of recurring episodes. In parenthesis it should be noted that the mean follow-up time for male patients with a single stroke is significantly shorter than that for the remainder of the group. We believe that this is due to the fact that patients admitted to the study with a history of previous strokes undoubtedly weighted the total duration of disease in favour of this group.

The survival rates (Figure 6.2) are expressed as the number per 1000 surviving at yearly intervals and the 'stroke' patients are compared with a normal population of the same age and sex structure. For ease of comparison the slope of the curve is given also for patients with transient ischaemic

Table 6.3. Classification of age at onset, duration of observation of disease and percentage survivors in 349 patients presenting with stroke.

	Male	Female	% Survivors	Total
Presenting with stroke	250	99		349
Age at onset	57.52 years	57.98 years		
	(S.D. 9.04)	(S.D. 9.70)		
Duration of disease	4.42 years	4.65 years		
	(S.D. 2.93)	(S.D. 2.81)		
Single stroke	112	52	74.4	164
Age at onset	57.17 years	58.34 years		57.54 years
	(S.D. 9.44)	(S.D. 10.18)		(S.D5. 9.66)
Duration of disease	3.94 years[a]	4.44 years		4.1 years[a]
	(S.D. 2.28)	(S.D. 2.34)		(S.D. 2.31)
Multiple strokes	138	47	50.8	185
Age at onset	57.81 years	57.59 years		57.76 years
	(S.D. 8.73)	(S.D. 9.24)		(S.D. 8.84)
Duration of disease	4.80 years	4.88 years		4.82 years
	(S.D. 3.35)	(S.D. 3.26)		(S.D. 3.32)

[a]Significant $P < 0.05$.
(Reproduced by permission from the *Quarterly Journal of Medicine*, **40,** 1971).

attacks going on to a stroke. The trend is obvious. All three groups fare worse in terms of survival than the general population, and worst of all are the patients with multiple stroke episodes who show a survival rate at 5.5 years below 600 per 1000 compared with a normal survival rate at this age of over 900 per 1000 in the general population.

With the exception of the report of Howard et al (1963) previous publications confirm the above findings. Howard et al (1963) reported on 97 patients and observed a mortality rate that declined after six months, but no deaths

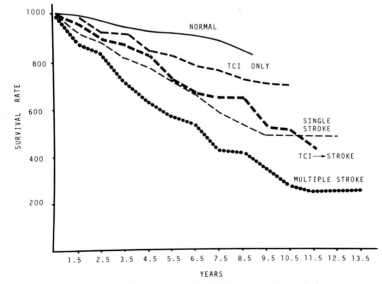

Figure 6.2. Survival rate per 1000 compared with the normal population.

were recorded in the third year. Since only 12 patients were followed for this period it is hardly justifiable to conclude that this represented a recognisable disease pattern in terms of the natural history of the illness.

'Cessation of activity'

The published figures where survival rates have been compared with those in the general population indicate that the occurrence of a stroke affects the ultimate survival as compared with the population at large. However, the slope of the graphs both in the present series (Figure 6.2) and other published data would suggest that the process underlying the development of intra-cerebral lesions is self-limiting after a period of five or more years. At this point there is a tailing off of the curve so they are nearly parallel with the normal population.

If this point could be established beyond doubt it is clearly relevant not only to the management of the individual patient but also to the design of therapeutic trials whether they be medically or surgically orientated.

Ford and Katz (1966), from their own observations, suggest that 'the accelerated rate of death attributed to a stroke appears to have subsided by 24 to 30 months after the stroke'. Matsumoto et al (1973) published the figures obtained from the Mayo Clinic study of the natural history of cerebral vascular disease. This report was an extension of the previous study which had been carried out in 1945-1954 (Whisnant et al, 1971) and is an attempt to identify all patients in the population of Rochester who had a stroke in the period 1955-1969. The study has the many advantages referred to previously. They also observed that as time progressed there was an increased likelihood of survival in patients with cerebral infarction but they were not able so far to identify the reason for this.

Marquardsen (1969) conducted a detailed analysis of his own patients to examine the important point that cessation of activity of vascular disease may occur. If one examines his findings they would certainly suggest that there is a tailing off at the end of the five-year period. Marquardsen, however, believes that this is an artefact, and if the figures are drawn on a logarithmic scale so that each point in the slope is comparable then the resulting straight line indicates the annual probability of dying to be constant. Marquardsen (1969) carried the analysis further by using a ratio, which he termed the average annual probability of dying. This is a ratio between the number of deaths occurring during the period of observation and the number of patient-years at risk. Using this ratio he found that throughout a period of 10 years after the initial episode the number of male and female survivors decreased at an annual rate of 16 per cent and 18 per cent respectively. He found no evidence, therefore, of any indication of cessation of activity.

RECURRENCE RATE

One feature of the natural history of patients with focal cerebral vascular disease, who have been studied, has been a tendency among some patients, having survived the first episode, to have a second and sometimes a third, fourth and fifth episode. The incidence of recurrent episodes in the present series is 53 per cent since such events were observed in 185 out of 349 patients. A brief study of the mortality indicates that the incidence of recurrences is associated with a markedly increased mortality. Clearly, it is relevant to examine this group in detail in an attempt to detect any clue that may differentiate between the two types of behaviour.

Pincock (1957), in the modern literature, commented on the high incidence of death in patients who had recurrent cerebral vascular accidents. He compared them with the survivors of the initial episode and he was surprised, contrary to the view held at that time, at the high number of patients who showed an improvement in neurological function and who were able to lead a reasonable life in spite of the fact that the majority of his patients when they entered the study were at, or just beyond, retirement age. In observing this difference in prognosis between patients who had a single stroke and those who were subject to recurrent episodes he felt that the problem of the subsequent natural history of the stroke patient should be considered under two headings. He suggested that the subdivision should concern 'first, those with recurrence in whom the mortality and morbidity seemed excessively high in comparison to a second group where recurrence is infrequent and functional recovery seems adequate'.

Initially, Marshall and Shaw (1959) were not impressed by the significance of recurrent episodes, as they observed these in only seven out of 102 patients but, as they themselves pointed out, this was a retrospective study with its attendant disadvantages. In a prospective study Marshall and Kaeser (1961) studied 177 patients, and recurrent episodes were observed in 23 patients. They commented that so pronounced is this difference in the two groups that the two groups should be differentiated. They referred to one as the 'inactive group' where no recurrence was observed over a period of many years of observation; and the second was an 'active group' who continued to have cerebral vascular episodes.

The information available from the literature on the incidence of recurrent episodes and their observed effect in various series is contained in Table 6.4.

On *a priori* grounds one would anticipate that recurrent episodes would significantly affect the ultimate prognosis in an adverse manner, and although the percentage incidence of recurrent episodes varies from observer to

Table 6.4. Percentage incidence and influence of recurrent stroke episodes in published series of cases.

Author	No. of cases	Recurrence rate (%)	Effect
David & Heyman (1960)	100	25	Adverse
Goldner et al (1967)	221	33	No effect
Matsumoto et al (1973)	694	27	Adverse
Pincock (1957)	117	30	Adverse
Carter (1964)	612	24	Adverse
Katz et al (1966)	159	13	Adverse
Eisenberg et al (1964)	191	19	No effect
Present series	349	53	Adverse

observer the majority agree that this is so. However, neither Eisenberg et al (1964) nor Goldner et al (1967) could find evidence that recurrent episodes adversely affect the prognosis but both these studies have the disadvantage, for this purpose, of being primarily orientated towards the epidemiological problem rather than the individual's clinical behaviour.

In addition to the observations of Pincock (1957), Marshall and Kaeser (1961), Carter (1964) and Baker, Schwartz and Ramseyer (1968) have observed an association between an adverse prognosis and the occurrence of recurrent episodes.

Temporal pattern

If there were a recognisable form of 'active' cerebral vascular disease in which recurrent episodes of cerebral infarction were a feature, then an examination of the temporal sequence of the history could be revealing. For example, if there were, in any group of patients, two subgroups representing 'active' and 'inactive' disease, a study of the overall temporal pattern of events in the natural history could possibly recognise these.

One could predicate that if there is such an entity then recurrent episodes might be expected to occur over a relatively short period of time. If, however, a recurrence rate simply indicates a greater proclivity to infarction, then episodes might be expected to occur randomly over the years. The greater proclivity referred to would be dictated by the more extensive amount of atheromatous ulceration in the great vessels and, therefore, an increased risk of thrombo-embolism. In this case there would be no justification for drawing crisp lines of distinction between 'active' and 'inactive' varieties of cerebral vascular disease.

To anticipate later results described in this monograph, on causes of death, it is possible to demonstrate that hypertension of significant degree does make a contribution to recurrent episodes by the production of localised intracerebral haematomas which simulate the clinical syndrome of cerebral infarction with precision.

There is no disagreement on the fact that recurrent episodes are not simply confined to one further stroke after the initial episode (Whisnant et al, 1971; Matsumoto et al, 1973; Marquardsen, 1969; and present series). From these results it is clear that the majority of patients have two episodes only, but even so, an appreciable number do go on to further episodes as can be seen in the present series (Table 6.5). It will be seen later that the prognosis is so poor that the history may very well be terminated before the total pattern of the disease can emerge. The higher incidence of recurrence in the present series is no doubt due in part to accepting any episode of more than one hour as representing a stroke, but we believe that equally relevant is the fact that a prospective study with regular examinations resulted in a higher detection rate of further episodes than can be obtained by retrospective surveys using case records.

Where there is disagreement is in the time sequence of events in a patient with a history of recurrent episodes. The results in the present study are shown in Figure 6.3, where the time interval between the initial stroke and the

Table 6.5. Distribution of the number of stroke episodes in 185 patients (M = 138; F = 47) presenting with stroke and going on to multiple stroke episodes.

No. of episodes	Male No. of cases	Male Percent-age	Female No. of cases	Female Percent-age	Male + female No. of cases	Male + female Percent-age
2 episodes	79	57.2	21	44.7	100	54.1
3 episodes	39	28.3	17	36.2	56	30.3
4 episodes	11	8.0	8	17.0	19	10.3
5 episodes	6	4.4	0	–	6	3.2
6 episodes	2	1.4	1	2.1	3	1.6
7 episodes	1	0.7	0	–	1	0.5
	138		47		185	

second episode is indicated; 67.6 per cent of patients had a second episode by the end of the second year, a figure which rose to 76.8 per cent after three years, and 91.4 per cent after five years. Matsumoto et al (1973) reported that 10 per cent had a second stroke within one year and 20 per cent within five years. The difference between the two may, again, be a matter of selection of cases, as the latter study is basically a population survey.

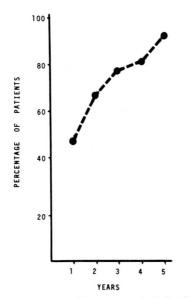

Figure 6.3. Graph showing time interval between an initial episode of stroke and the first recurrent episode.

Marquardsen (1969) examines the problem of recurrent episodes in some detail in his study and his observations are diametrically opposed to the view that there is a temporal pattern recognisable within the natural history. First of all he defines recurrent episodes as a definite worsening of neurological sequelae resulting from the primary stroke and if it occurred abruptly it was accepted as a recurrent attack. He noted that minor episodes (since his was a retrospective study) with transient signs that subsequently recovered may have affected a considerable number of his patients so that these recurrent episodes were unrecorded, but using his criteria he observed recurrent episodes in 56 (37.3 per cent) of the male survivors and in 97 (37.7 per cent) of the female survivors.

As with other observers, he observed that in the majority of patients the history was often one of one further stroke episode, but two or more attacks were recorded in 14 males and 25 females.

Turning to the time interval between the events, Marquardsen (1969) found that the time between the first stroke and the first recurrent episode varied from 'a few weeks to more than 17 years but the average values were 3.7 and 3.4 years for the two sexes'.

He then went on to examine in detail the first 10 years of observation, using the 'patient recurrence rate'. By this, Marquardsen (1969) means the number of patients with recurrences, which is expressed as a percentage of the number of patients who during the interval in question were exposed to the risk of having their first recurrence. In the first year, 8.6 per cent of males and 12.2 per cent of females had a further episode in the first year but the difference between the two sexes did not reach significance. The important point was that in studying the annual recurrence rate this remained constant over the years without a significant upward or downward trend. The annual figure for the recurrence rate for males was 8 per cent and for females 9.9 per cent, and he concluded from his annual risk figures that the incidence of further cerebral vascular episodes appeared to be independent of the length of time that had elapsed since the primary stroke.

Again, the differences in factual observations are so wide that one cannot exclude some form of selection being responsible for such a wide discrepancy. It could possibly be, of course, that the entirely different nature of the two populations where the problem of recurrence has been examined in depth has resulted in the recognition of two differing patterns of behaviour.

MORBIDITY

Although mortality and comparative survival rates are important in assessing the natural history of cerebral vascular disease, of equal importance to the individual is the ultimate morbidity in survivors. The problem can be approached in two ways. The first is to assess the final outcome at the end of a defined period of study; the second is to examine the immediate prognosis in the period following the acute episode.

Final morbidity

In examining and comparing studies in the field of morbidity the results cannot be compared in the same factual way that is possible when considering actual mortality or relative survival. It is, of course, well recognised that there is no standardised way of expressing neurological disability, and this is particularly true of a disease of the central nervous system which may affect varying sites and result not only in different degrees of disability within the same system but also defects in the different systems, which are difficult to compare. Varying degrees of speech disturbance when compared with a permanent visual field defect may be a good example to quote as being impossible to compare quantitatively in terms of the quality of life for survivors.

In the present series we have chosen to express disability in a clinical manner in terms of the presence or absence of residual disability, and when the residual disability remains, to categorise it in terms of three groups that express the degree of that disability. There are reasonable objections to this method and, indeed, the method of assessment of Ford and Katz (1966), where they used as a reference point the patient's own physical abilities before the cerebral episode, is obviously valuable in the aged and infirm, but the patients in the present series were relatively young and were rarely significantly disabled before the initial episode.

The results at the end of the study are shown in Table 6.6, and the figures for mortality are again included to complete the overall picture. The major feature that emerges is the very different outcome in patients where the history is one of repeated episodes in contrast to those where the history is that of one stroke only. It might be anticipated in a selected population that if the patient has survived the acute episode then the ultimate outcome is relatively good. In fact 81 per cent have achieved adequate or complete recovery of function whereas only 10.7 per cent were grossly disabled and in need of some or total care.

Table 6.6. Final clinical state at end of study of 349 patients presenting with stroke. (Reproduced by permission from the *Quarterly Journal of Medicine*, **40**, 1971.)

	Dead	Alive	Grade 1	Grade 2	Grade 3	Grade 4	Disabled other causes	Total
Single stroke	42 (25.6%)	122 (74.4%)	88 (72.1%)	11 (9.0%)	9 (7.4%)	4 (3.3%)	10 (8.2%)	164
Multiple stroke	91 (49.2%)	94 (50.8%)	36 (38.3%)	4 (4.3%)	30 (31.9%)	16 (17.0%)	8 (8.5%)	185

Grade 1. Complete functional recovery.
Grade 2. Minimal residual disability.
Grade 3. Activity markedly impaired by residual neurological signs.
Grade 4. Confined to chair or bed.

The contrast when the history is that of recurrent episodes or multiple strokes is striking. Not only is the mortality nearly twice as high but the number achieving an acceptable existence was only 42.6 per cent, whereas 48.9 per cent were partially or totally disabled.

It has already been indicated that it is difficult to make comparisons with published series but it is possible, in approximate terms, to examine the fate of survivors from the various studies. Allowing for approximation, the information indicates that the prognosis is not universally bad. Again, selection is clearly operative with the present series showing the best prognosis, but once more this may simply be an expression of selection.

Pincock (1957) reviewed 39 patients who were followed for eight years and found that more than half of these were functioning in their normal environment. A similar series, that of David and Heyman (1960) contrasts the effect on the prognosis of recurrent strokes. They observed a death rate of 25 per cent in patients with a single stroke but 61 per cent in those with multiple strokes. Overall, however, only 24 per cent of the survivors were able to return to their premorbid occupation.

Carter's (1964) results probably express, as well as any, what may be expected in terms of recovery in stroke patients admitted to a large general hospital. At five years a figure of 26 per cent recovered, and improvement in 23 per cent offered some hope in a not very optimistic situation. It is again rather odd that somewhat different figures were obtained from another general hospital series, namely, that of Marquardsen (1969), where 407 patients survived for more than three weeks after the acute episode, and of these 52 per cent were restored to independence and self-care; 15 per cent walked unaided but required some help with personal care whereas 33 per cent required total care.

In the population at large, probably the most useful figures for morbidity come from the Mayo Clinic's results in the study of the population of Rochester (Matsumoto et al, 1973). The morbidity was assessed six months after the acute episode and they found that at this time only 4 per cent required total care, 18 per cent were capable of self-care, and 36 per cent were working or able to work. They had not excluded mild strokes from their study, and it was this, they felt, that accounted for the fact that 29 per cent of the survivors were functioning normally.

CONCLUSION

1. Immediate mortality from stroke varies in different series but in population studies it is of the order of 30 per cent in the first month. Abnormally low mortality figures indicate biased case selection.
2. Long-term mortality at 5 years is usually between 35 and 45 per cent. Figures much in excess of these again indicate biased selection.
3. Between 25 and 50 per cent of patients will have further episodes of stroke. This adversely affects the morbidity and mortality; the latter is reflected in the survival rates when compared with the normal population.
4. Cessation of activity of cerebrovascular disease, as judged by survival rates, appears to occur after 5 to 7 years.
5. Views differ on the significance of recurrent episodes. One view would indicate that there is an 'active' form of recurring or progressive cerebral ischaemia to be distinguished from single-stroke episodes with a relatively good prognosis. The other view is that recurrent episodes simply represent more advanced vascular disease.

REFERENCES

Acheson, J. & Hutchinson, E. C. (1970) The natural history of "focal cerebral vascular disease". *Quarterly Journal of Medicine*, **40**, 157, 15–23.

Adams, G. F. & Merrett, J. D. (1961) Prognosis and survival in the aftermath of hemiplegia. *British Medical Journal*, **i**, 309–314.

Baker, R. N., Schwartz, W. S. & Ramseyer, J. C. (1968) Prognosis among survivors of ischaemic strokes. *Neurology*, **18**, 933–941.

Carroll, D. (1962) The disability in hemiplegia caused by cerebrovascular disease. A serial study of 98 cases. *Journal of Chronic Diseases*, **15**, 179–188.

Carter, A. B. (1964) *Cerebral Infarction*. New York: Macmillan Company.

Charcot, J. M. (1881) *Clinical Lectures on Senile and Chronic Diseases*. Translated by William S. Tuke. London: The New Sydenham Society.

Copland, J. (1850) *Causes, Nature and Treatment of Palsy and Apoplexy of Forms, Seats, Complications and Morbid Relations of Paralytic and Apoplectic Diseases*. London: Longman, Brown, Green and Longmans.

David, N. J. & Heyman, A. (1960) Factors influencing the prognosis of cerebral thrombosis and infarction due to atherosclerosis. *Journal of Chronic Diseases*, **11**, 394–404.

Droller, H. (1960) Survival after apoplexy. *Gerontologia Clinica*, **2**, 120–128.

Eisenberg, H., Morrison, J. T., Sullivan, P., & Foote, F. M. (1964) Cerebrovascular accidents. *Journal of the American Medical Association*, **189**, 883–888.

Ford, A. B. & Katz, S. (1966) Prognosis after strokes. Part 1. A critical review. *Medicine*, **45**, 223–244.

Goldner, J. C., Payne, G. H., Watson, F. R. & Parrish, H. M. (1967) Prognosis for survival after stroke (Original articles). *American Journal of Medical Sciences*, **253**, 129–133.

Gowers, W. R. (1888) *Manual of Diseases of the Nervous System*. London: J. & A. Churchill.

Howard, F. A., Cohen, P., Hickler, R. B., Locke, S., Newcomb, T. & Tyler, H. R. (1963) Survival following stroke. *Journal of the American Medical Association*, **183**, 921–925.

Marquardsen, J. (1969) The natural history of cerebrovascular disease. *Acta Neurologica Scandinavica Supplementum*, **45**, 90–188.

Marshall, J. & Shaw, D. A. (1959) The natural history of cerebrovascular disease. *British Medical Journal*, **i**, 1614–1617.

Marshall, J. & Kaeser, A. C. (1961) Survival after non-haemorrhagic cerebrovascular accidents. *British Medical Journal*, **ii**, 73–77.

Matsumoto, N., Whisnant, J. P., Kurland, L. T. & Okazaki, H. (1973) Natural history of stroke in Rochester, Minnesota. 1955 through 1969. An extension of a previous study, 1945 through 1954. *Stroke*, **4**, 20–29.

Pincock, J. G. (1957) The natural history of cerebral thrombosis. *Annals of Internal Medicine*, **46**, 925–930.

Robinson, R. W., Demirel, A. & LeBeau, R. J. (1968) Natural history of cerebral thrombosis nine to nineteen year follow up. *Journal of Chronic Diseases*, **21**, 221–230.

Wallace, D. C. (1964) Cerebral vascular disease in relation to long-term anticoagulant therapy. *Journal of Chronic Diseases*, **17**, 527.

Whisnant, J. P., Fitzgibbons, J. P., Kurland, L. T. & Sayre, G. P. (1971) Natural history of stroke in Rochester, Minnesota, 1945 through 1954. *Stroke*, **2**, 11–21.

CHAPTER SEVEN

Effect of Hypertension on the Natural History of Cerebral Ischaemia

HISTORICAL NOTE

An association between systemic hypertension and the liability to develop a stroke was first suggested in the seventeenth century. Wepfer (1658) was probably the first to suggest that patients with hypertension, obesity or cardiac disease were more prone to develop apoplexy. Burrows (1846) in his Lumleian Lecture also made this suggestion when he reported on 132 cases of apoplexy and seven of hemiplegia; in 84 of these cardiac disease was observed.

Janeway (1913) reported on a series of 458 personal cases seen in private practice throughout the years 1903–1912. He used the systolic pressure only and arbitrarily considered any figure above 160 mm Hg as abnormal. His purpose was to recognise the possible relationship between the abnormalities noted on examination and the subsequent course of the disease. Some of his observations have a familiar ring: 'I always had the impression that the expectancy of life in women with arterial and renal disease is greater than in men. This analysis gives such impressions an objective foundation in fact'.

He did realise clearly that the finding of a systolic pressure above 200 mm Hg in either sex had an adverse prognosis in terms of survival and a much greater probability of death by uraemia or 'apoplexy'. A major conclusion of Janeway's was that his observations indicated that the exact height of the blood pressure does not seem to have much bearing on the expectancy of life. While it is always interesting to read the view of physicians of the past and their frequently penetrating glimpses of the problems as they present today, the difficulties in differentiating between a diagnosis of uraemic and apoplectic fits and a higher prevalence of neurosyphilis all contribute to the difficulties of tracing any smooth progression of ideas up to the present day.

HYPERTENSION

It is, of course, well known that there is no generally accepted figure that specifically defines hypertension as distinct from a normal blood pressure. Some would go further and deny the entity of essential hypertension as a disease, but this monograph is an inappropriate place to examine the arguments that have been advanced by the proponents of the two principal differing views. For practical purposes, the difficulty inherent in the argument can be overcome in a study of the effects of hypertension in cerebral vascular disease by simply stating the observed figures within defined limits. This, however, is rarely done in the literature.

Before considering the evidence that the presence of systemic hypertension may have a significant effect on the natural history of patients presenting with either transient cerebral ischaemia or stroke it is necessary to examine briefly certain selected aspects of hypertension as they relate to the clinical presentation of cerebral vascular disease. The circumstances under which the blood pressure is recorded and the validity of the results obtained are clearly important, for there has been considerable discussion on the relative values of the casual reading of the blood pressure taken in the out-patient clinic or the home as against a basal reading where the patient is at rest. In cerebral vascular disease the mean age of the population studied has commonly fallen within the sixth decade, and clearly, therefore, the effects of physiological ageing on the blood pressure are important. Recently, the hypothesis has been advanced that cerebral vascular disease of the type that is frequently responsible for the clinical syndromes under discussion may cause systemic hypertension; if this hypothesis were substantiated then most of our further discussion would be irrelevant. Finally, it seems that the current evidence indicates that hypertension accentuates the whole process of atheroma, although the precise mechanism of this effect is not entirely clear.

Before considering the evidence that hypertension adversely affects the prognosis in cerebral vascular disease the following points need to be discussed briefly:

1. The possibility that observer error and the use of casual as opposed to basal blood pressure readings may invalidate the results.
2. The effects of physiological ageing on casual blood pressure readings.
3. The evidence that cerebral vascular disease is a significant primary cause of hypertension.
4. The role of systemic hypertension in accentuating the development of atheroma of the cerebral blood supply.

Observer error, 'casual' and 'basal' blood pressure readings

It has been suggested that observer variation can play an important part in blood pressure recordings and that if it does not invalidate the results it certainly reduces the significance of the observations in a given series.

This possibility would appear to be substantiated by Eilertsen and Humerfelt (1968) who conducted an experiment using 19 specially trained nursing staff to survey the blood pressure levels in 70 000 subjects in Bergen, Norway. The majority of the nursing observers showed only insignificant differences but there were, between the extremes of readings obtained, substantial differences and these differences under the conditions of their particular experiment could affect the mean values found in population surveys. Contrary experiences have been recorded under conditions where medical personnel made the observations. A case in point is the report of McKeown, Record and Whitfield (1963) of a study of changes in blood pressure in two populations over a period of time. The populations studied were in Birmingham and in Glamorgan. In Birmingham, the blood pressure was obtained from 883 males in the seventh decade by 11 general practitioners, without any particular precaution being taken at the time of recording of the blood pressure, and therefore was, by definition, a casual reading. In Glamorgan, the blood pressure was recorded by one medical observer in 500 males over 40 years of age with the patients at rest in their home environment. The authors' findings confirmed the known difficulty of attaching significance to one casual reading in an individual patient but, more relevant to the present topic, they doubted whether any refinement such as confining the observations to one observer and taking the blood pressure of the resting patient in familiar surroundings would significantly affect the conclusion drawn from casual readings in a larger population.

Another facet of the significance of a single casual observation is the effect of diurnal variations on the level of arterial blood pressure which are known to occur, and which are distinct from a fall in blood pressure at rest, which is regarded as the 'basal' blood pressure. The problems here have been more clearly understood with the advent of the automatic oscillograph recorders.

When these instruments became available it was possible to monitor the blood pressure throughout a 24 hour period. Richardson et al (1964) studied the diurnal variations of the blood pressure in normal subjects and in subjects with raised arterial pressure. They observed a general tendency for the blood pressure to reach a peak in the early evening and to be followed by a fall which during sleep was often profound. For example, in a patient with a reading of 116/95 it fell to a level of 84/50 during sleep. These considerable variations were not clearly related to age or to the level of the arterial pressure, nor were they related to the presence or absence of the complications of hypertension.

Their informed conclusions are very relevant to the problems of what figures for the blood pressure it is proper to record to relate to cerebral vascular disease. Alam and Smirk (1943) had already reported appreciable differences between the first or casual reading of the blood pressure and the blood pressure after half an hour's rest. From casual to basal levels they recorded a fall of as much as 20 mm in the systolic pressure in their subjects. Richardson et al (1964) certainly did find differences in the basal and casual blood pressure but not of the same order. They went on to express the view that as far as the basal pressure was concerned 'they doubted whether it had any superiority over a single casual blood pressure reading in epidemiological work, providing, of course, that the observer, the circumstances in which he measures the arterial pressure and his attitude to his subject are varied as little as possible'.

Previous to these observations, Hamilton et al (1954) had examined a random sample of the general population and were happy to accept casual blood pressure readings as a representative figure in a large group of patients.

We may conclude that the value of casual blood pressure readings as a reference point is accepted by most workers provided the population is sufficiently large and that no attempt is made to exclude specific groups. This is fortunate when one considers the practical problems involved in obtaining repeated blood pressure readings in a large series of patients attending hospital.

Interrelationship of ageing and hypertension

It is accepted by most observers that the level of the blood pressure tends to rise with age. Hamilton et al (1954) in the study of a normal hospital population, already referred to, found an increase in blood pressure with age, the pressure being higher in males before the age of 30 years and thereafter being higher in females. Harlan, Osborne and Graybiel (1962) re-examined a group of young males previously selected for flight training in America in 1940, and re-examined 785 of these 18 years later. They observed a unimodal increase in the blood pressure over this period of time.

However, Miall and Lovell (1967) take an opposing view. Their data was based on three surveys of two populations in Wales which were carried out over a period of eight-and-a-half to 10 years. They used multiple regression analysis on the changes in pressure, relating them to mean pressure and age. Their conclusion was that changes in pressure over the period of observation were highly significant and were related to the previous mean pressures but only indirectly to age. They believed that the results indicated that ageing plays no direct part in determining the rate of change in pressure.

Kurtzke (1969) re-examined the statistical evidence put forward by Miall and Lovell and did not accept the validity of their conclusions. He believed from their figures that whatever extraneous factors there were, such as age or sex, the final pressures were most often higher than those recorded 10 years earlier.

Evelyn (1970) paints a broader canvas in relation to hypertension and age, and drawing on many sources of information subscribes to the view that 'essential hypertension is basically an asymptomatic disorder of blood pressure homeostasis which gives rise to significant mortality only during the late stages of an average 20-years duration of the disease'. He goes on to indicate that mortality ultimately relates to the failure of the myocardium to compensate, or to arteriolar changes in principal target organs such as the kidney or brain. In a small minority, the final stage is ushered in by an accelerated form of the disease with acute arteriolar changes and potentially fatal sequelae usually mediated by the renal blood supply.

The weight of the evidence therefore indicates that an increase in blood pressure occurs with natural ageing.

Cerebral vascular disease—a primary cause of hypertension?

In most patients with hypertension the aetiology of the raised blood pressure is unknown; as McMichael (1961) observed 'hypertension is no more a disease entity than a skin rash, a fever or an anaemia'.

There are, of course, well-recognised renal, vascular and endocrine causes of hypertension, but there are also well-documented instances of hypertension arising from a primary intracerebral cause. The possibility that hypertension may arise as a direct result of intracranial disease is as old as any view of the pathogenesis of hypertension.

There are established examples of disease of the nervous system which, on the available evidence, indicate that these changes are the cause of significant hypertension. All neurologists are familiar with transient hypertension in subarachnoid haemorrhage and raised intracranial pressure but this is not relevant to the present discussion.

Page (1935) described an entity that he designated as the hypertensive diencephalic syndrome, which he observed in patients with significant hypertension. The essential features of the syndrome were paroxysmal elevations of the blood pressure occurring during stress and accompanied by tachycardia and 'necklace' erythema.

Paroxysmal hypertension may also occur in tabes dorsalis, either in association with typical tabetic crises which in the observed patients are commonly visceral, or are independent of these. In one patient, where the resting pressure rose in an attack from 130/70 to 260/170 mm Hg, the clinical symptoms were so suggestive that an exploratory operation to exclude phaeochromocytoma was carried out (Bennett and Heyman 1948). Patients with cystic tumours of the lateral ventricle have also been observed to develop paroxysmal elevations of the arterial pressure from time to time (Penfield, 1929).

In primary cerebral vascular disease an excellent example of paroxysmal hypertension was described by Montgomery (1961) in three patients. All three patients presented with episodes of paroxysmal hypertension and in two of these at the onset there was no evidence of any neurological lesion.

The rises of blood pressure were quite dramatic and were of the order of 90 mm Hg systolic and 60 mm Hg diastolic. Ultimately, in all patients there appeared the classical symptomatology of transient cerebral ischaemia involving the vertebro-basilar territory and in one patient at post mortem a brain-stem infarct was demonstrated. Although these clinical observations certainly have an intrinsic interest they have not been considered to be anything other than a rare clinical event.

Dickinson and Thomson (1959) put forward a much wider concept. From post-mortem studies they advanced the hypothesis that hypertension may be caused by a reduction in flow through the cerebral blood supply and, particularly, through the vertebral circulation. With constant perfusion pressure they demonstrated a close association between the ante-mortem level of the blood pressure and the fluid-carrying capacity of the vertebral arteries.

Lowe (1961) criticised the application of such data from post-mortem experiments to living patients. His main reasons were that in a survey of the incidence of carotid occlusion in hypertension and of hypertension in patients with carotid artery disease he could find no evidence of an association. Moreover, when plotting retinal artery pressure against brachial artery pressure in patients with hypertension and with strokes he found no evidence of an increased resistance in the carotid arteries.

The hypothesis of Dickinson and Thomson (1959) has not achieved wide acceptance. Dickinson himself (1965) in his introduction to his monograph on neurogenic hypertension wrote 'this hypothesis, once popular, has been abandoned since 1930. In the current climate of opinion it is most unlikely to be accepted'. One can only comment that his forecast has generally proved to be correct but it must be admitted that the hypothesis is as difficult to disprove as it is to prove.

Howard et al (1963), Marshall (1966) and Acheson (1971) have described clinical observations in ischaemic cerebral vascular disease relating to the hypothesis that vertebro-basilar stenosis may cause hypertension. The argument runs that if it is true that a reduction of blood flow through the vertebro-basilar circulation is a major factor in the development of hypertension, then one might reasonably anticipate that the incidence of hypertension will be higher in clinical cases of ischaemia of the hind brain compared with patients presenting with ischaemic symptoms affecting the fore brain. In none of these studies was it possible to establish any relationship between the clinical site of cerebral ischaemia and the level of the blood pressure.

Role of hypertension accentuating the development of atheroma

To the physician or surgeon it is not immediately obvious why the process designated as hypertension should be responsible for the development of atheroma. Indeed, if atheroma is already present it is no more obvious why hypertension should aggravate this process. The problem essentially remains within the sphere of the pathologist, but the contributions from clinical studies of patients are not entirely without significance. The demonstration of a recurring association between hypertension and degenerative vascular disease, where the latter cannot be explained by hypertension alone, must be relevant.

As Evelyn (1970) pointed out, it is difficult these days to find satisfactory evidence in relation to the development of vascular disease accentuated by hypertension because of the world-wide tendency to treat hypertension of a significant degree even though it is unaccompanied by symptoms. Coronary artery disease has been the subject of intensive epidemiological clinical study in all the developed countries but, as Mitchell (1971) pointed out, there is a major drawback within these studies since the majority must of necessity await the development of appropriate symptoms. They are therefore by definition retrospective and the information obtained is only of qualified value because the level of the blood pressure may have been significantly modified by the development of cardiac infarction.

The figures from the large insurance companies indicate that the higher the blood pressure the higher the actuarial risk of developing circulatory disturbance in later life. But there are more satisfactory sources of information than these.

Bechgaard (1946) followed up 1000 patients with hypertension and found that the untreated patients with severe hypertension had a poor prognosis. Mathisen et al (1965), in a study of 290 untreated hypertensive patients aged less than 46 years at the time of entering the study, found that after 10 years 29 per cent of the women and 41 per cent of the men were dead, and after 22 years these figures had risen to 54 per cent and 65 per cent respectively. Hypertension in this report was considered to be present with any figure above 160/90 mm Hg. The causes of death were grouped together according to the predominant organ affected at the time of death. The nature of the investigation limited the precision with which the cause of death could be established but 'cerebral causes' were recognised as the cause of death in 52 per cent, cardiac causes were the next most frequent at 24 per cent, and renal (10 per cent) and miscellaneous causes (14 per cent) were approximately equally represented.

There has always been the suggestion that in patients with a labile blood pressure where the blood pressure falls with rest the prognosis was better and Mathisen et al (1965) concurred with this view.

Perara (1955) was not content to accept this statement without qualification. He studied 50 patients with documented hypertension who were untreated and who were divided into two equal groups depending on whether or not the basal blood pressure fell with rest as compared with casual readings under out-patient conditions. In his view a fall of pressure of the order of 40/20 mm Hg at rest justified the term labile, whereas non-labile hypertension referred to patients with a blood pressure fall of less than 30/15 mm Hg under similar conditions.

He established that the finding of an elevated blood pressure which fell with rest, and was therefore labile, could not simply be ignored. Certainly, the patients with a labile blood pressure lived longer, their mean age at death being 56 years compared with the non-labile group whose mean age at death was 46, a difference that was statistically significant. The other difference was that whereas the non-labile group showed a higher incidence of retinopathy (with haemorrhages, exudates, papilloedema and renal damage), the labile group more frequently developed coronary artery disease and 'cerebral vascular accidents'.

Systemic hypertension in accentuating atheroma

The evidence that hypertension is associated with both an increased morbidity and mortality in cerebral vascular disease can be drawn from the two traditional sources, namely, the reports of pathological studies and of clinical observations. The views of pathologists on the pathogenesis of atheroma and its relation to cerebral infarction, and the mechanisms of cerebral haemorrhage, are included elsewhere in this monograph. Two studies, however, combine clinical and pathological evidence and are therefore relevant to the present theme.

Pathological evidence

Although references to the association between hypertension and an adverse prognosis in cerebral vascular disease go back to the early part of this century it is perhaps with some surprise that one finds that Low-Beer and Phear (1961) were able to quote more recent authorities who stated that cerebral thrombosis was not associated with elevated blood pressure.

Low-Beer and Phear (1961) examined the records of 109 patients with cerebral infarction demonstrated at post mortem from the services of the Middlesex and Central Middlesex Hospitals. 36 per cent of the patients developed complications such as cardiac failure, which invalidated the level of the blood pressure readings, but 72 had died without any such complication. They demonstrated conclusively that hypertension was a common association of cerebral infarction.

Baker, Resch and Loewenson (1969) approached the problem in a different manner. They examined autopsy material in 3924 patients who were 30 years or more at the time of death. A scoring system was developed which expressed the severity and extent of atherosclerosis in the major component vessels of the Circle of Willis. The criteria for hypertension were either the heart weight at post mortem, a clinical diagnosis of hypertension or the known blood pressure during life. They found a clear association between the severity of atherosclerosis and hypertension and, interestingly enough, the association was very much more pronounced if clinical criteria for the diagnosis of hypertension were used for correlation.

Clinical evidence

The evidence that hypertension is associated with an increased risk of cerebral infarction comes from two sources. The first source, which is the most significant and the most difficult from which to obtain reliable figures, is community-based studies, and the second is from clinical observations on patients who present with stroke.

Kuller, Cook and Friedman (1972) reported on a survey of a number of epidemiological studies on stroke and have pointed out the defects that are inherent in them. There are two major problems. The first is that in the United States, whence much of the information is derived, the studies carried out are commonly designed primarily for the study of coronary artery disease. The second is that relatively few cases are identified at the time of the initial event since the majority depend on examination some time after the stroke and the information is then gleaned from hospital records, physicians' reports, and patient interview. Relatively few of the studies involve the neurologist directly. Nevertheless, however crude by clinical standards the methods of gathering information in large populations may be, the information gleaned has considerable value.

None of the criticisms listed relates to the value of the observations made in the Framingham study. The study was designed prospectively, and this is its great value. It set out to examine the relationship between an elevated blood pressure and the development of stroke due to cerebral infarction.

The population studied was a circumscribed community where 5209 men and women between the ages of 30 and 60 years were classified while still symptom-free according to the level of blood pressure. They were subsequently followed up over a period of 14 years.

In an initial survey it was found that the likelihood of hypertensive patients developing a stroke was five times that of the remaining population, and in a later communication Kannel et al (1970) produced further evidence that hypertension was the most potent precursor of the condition they classified as an 'atheroma-thrombotic' brain infarction. They found that whether figures for the systolic, the diastolic or the mean arterial pressure were used it did not affect the results. Moreover, they could detect no diminishing impact of the effects of a raised systolic blood pressure with advancing years and believe that the commonly held view that systolic elevations in the aged are innocent could not be substantiated. The final point was that the authors did not find any critical levels of elevation of blood pressure that could be associated with an increased risk of the development of brain infarction.

Without the type of hard evidence that the Framingham Survey has provided, clinical observations on the presence of hypertension in patients with cerebral vascular disease could easily be criticised on a cause and effect basis. Given the Framingham evidence, however, it is not an unreasonable assumption that there is a direct relationship between the presence of an elevated blood pressure and the development of cerebral vascular disease.

Much of the available literature on the incidence of hypertension in cerebral vascular disease is difficult to compare because of the ways in which the level of the blood pressure are expressed. A selected series is shown (Table 7.1). The lowest figure given is that of Marshall and Kaeser (1961) with an incidence of 36 per cent but equally their criterion for the diagnosis of hypertension, which was a diastolic pressure of more than 110 mm Hg, was the most

Table 7.1. Incidence of hypertension in published series of cases of stroke.

Author	No. of patients	Definition of hyper- tension (mm Hg)	Mean age (years)	Percentage with hypertension
Robinson et al (1968)	843	> 160/90 Mild DBP 90–109 Moderate & severe DBP >110	M 66.4 F 69.9	70
David & Heyman (1960)	100	>160/100 Severe grade 3 or 4 retinopathy	57.3	50
Carroll (1962)	98	Moderate & severe	79% between 51 & 80	70
Howard et al (1963)	97	> 140 systolic	–	75
Marshall & Kaeser (1961)	106	>110 diastolic	–	36
Baker et al (1968)	430	Moderate 140/90 Severe 200/110	–	74

(DBP = Diastolic blood pressure).

stringent of the group. It is clear, however, that in well over half the reported series hypertension has been shown to have a significant association with clinical cerebral vascular disease.

HYPERTENSION AND PROGNOSIS IN CEREBRAL VASCULAR DISEASE

The influence of hypertension on the prognosis in cerebral vascular disease can be examined in a similar manner to the natural history, namely, by considering separately the effect on the early mortality and then its relationship to the prognosis in survivors.

Early mortality

The information on the interrelationship of initial mortality and blood pressure is slender. As most authors stress, blood-pressure readings in patients acutely ill with a stroke can be misleading. Not only are there the general problems of dehydration, heart failure and the like, but also acute cerebral ischaemia, particularly when the vertebrobasilar territory is affected, may very well cause significant elevations of the blood pressure in the acute stage as a direct result of ischaemia without indicating pre-existing hypertension.

It is interesting in this context to refer again to the classical paper by Aring and Merritt (1935) on the differential diagnosis between cerebral haemorrhage and cerebral thrombosis. In 107 cases of haemorrhage and 96 of cerebral thrombosis, where the diagnosis was based on the post-mortem findings, they tabulated the blood pressure by systolic and diastolic levels. Even at the diastolic level of >140 mm Hg no obvious difference could be discerned between the two groups.

Howard et al (1963) examined the relationship of blood pressure to survival in the first six months period after the acute episode. They took an arbitrary level of 140 mm systolic and found a distinctly better prognosis in 25 per cent of the patients below this figure. With systolic readings of 140-190 mm Hg the mortality in the normotensive group at six months was 20 per cent as compared with a figure of 38 per cent in the higher group. They were not, however, able to recognise any variations in the early prognosis correlating with the actual height of the systolic pressure.

Hypertension and prognosis in survivors

With the paucity of effective treatment available for the patient presenting with an acute stroke, knowledge of the state of the blood pressure does not go far beyond the realms of academic interest. This is certainly not true in relation to survivors and the anticipated prognosis in terms of both disability and death.

The observations of Marshall and Shaw (1959) and Marshall and Kaeser (1961) on the effects of hypertension in survivors were early contributions in the field. In the first paper (Marshall and Shaw, 1959) they traced 251 patients who had been admitted to the National Hospital for Nervous Diseases and in whom a firm diagnosis of cerebral vascular disease was made. Although the study was retrospective, with all the attendant disadvantages this implies, they demonstrated an increased mortality in both sexes when the observed diastolic blood pressure was above 110 mm Hg. The second report (Marshall and Kaeser, 1961) was prospective. In this they referred to the effect of high blood pressure as 'most striking'. Again, they subdivided the patients into two groups using an arbitrary level of a diastolic blood pressure of 110 mm Hg. At one year the percentage for survival for patients with blood pressures below this figure was 96 per cent whereas above this figure it was 90 per cent. At two years the same comparison showed a widening of the gap. The figure for survival was again 96 per cent for the group below 110 mm Hg but was 75 per cent for patients with blood pressures above this figure. Analysed at 117 weeks, the figures achieved statistical significance.

Both Howard et al (1963) and David and Heyman (1960) concurred with the view that hypertension adversely affected the prognosis. The first study is not altogether satisfactory since the arbitrary division for comparison of patients was set at 140 mm Hg systolic. David and Heyman (1960), although dealing with relatively small numbers (100 patients), accepted a reading of 150/100 as significant, and by this criterion 50 per cent of their patients were hypertensive. Of this group, 15 patients were described as being 'severe hypertensives', based on retinal changes. At the end of two years' observation only 28 per cent of the normotensive patients died whereas 31 per cent of the moderate hypertensives and 53 per cent of the severe hypertensives had succumbed at the end of this period.

Carter's (1964) experience emphasises as strongly as any the significance of the prognosis in relation to survival. His definition of hypertension was a systolic blood pressure greater than 200 mm Hg and/or a diastolic of 110 mm Hg or more. In male patients, at the end of five years 75 per cent of hypertensives had died whereas in normotensive patients only 8 per cent had died over the same period of time. The figures for females indicated to Carter that 'women stand hypertension better than men', basing this on the fact that the female mortality was only about half that observed in hypertensive males.

Baker, Schwartz and Ramseyer (1968) conducted a long-term prospective survey on 430 patients. They defined hypertension as moderate when the recorded blood pressure was 140/90 mm Hg and severe when the blood pressure was 200/110. During the period of the study 74 per cent had hypertension as defined by the above figures. Of these 43 per cent died compared with 32 per cent of the normotensives and they concluded that 'as measured by the occurrence of a new stroke or death the prognosis is better among the non-hypertensive patients'. They could not detect, however, any significant difference between the different levels of blood pressure. This is an important feature of this paper because it is uncommon to find the term hypertension defined so precisely.

Marquardsen (1969) does define hypertension precisely. He points out that any division between normal and abnormal levels must be arbitrary, and this is so whether one subscribes or not to Pickering's (1955) view that figures for blood pressure which are called hypertension simply represent the upper end of a frequency scale. Another point, which has been considered earlier in this chapter, is the evidence indicating an increase of blood pressure with ageing.

To overcome these difficulties, Marquardsen divided his patients according to the level of the systolic and diastolic blood pressures, separating the patients into groups according to increments of blood pressure of 20 mm Hg. Thus, all patients with a blood pressure of less than 179 mm Hg were grouped together as were all patients with a systolic reading between 180-199 and all patients with pressures above 200 mm Hg. He treated the diastolic blood pressures in a similar way.

His first important observation was that an assessment could be made using either the systolic or diastolic pressures as their effects ran in parallel.

Marquardsen then examined the question of a relationship of hypertension to the ultimate prognosis in some detail. He found that if the systolic blood pressure was taken alone there was no discernible difference in prognosis in patients with blood pressures up to and including 180 mm Hg. Over this figure, particularly those with over 200 mm Hg, there was an unfavourable prognosis in terms of survival. There was, however, an odd variation with age. Under the age of 70 years the mortality rose steadily with an increasing blood pressure but over the age of 70 he found that the mortality rose when the blood pressure exceeded 180 mm Hg but there was no further increase and perhaps even an apparent decline with values over 200 mm Hg. As far as the diastolic blood pressure was concerned in the under 70 age group the mortality increased with a diastolic blood pressure over 100 mm Hg, whereas beyond the age of 70 the trend was only apparent in males.

Because of these findings he classified as hypertensive, patients with a blood pressure of over 180 mm Hg systolic and/or an average diastolic blood pressure over 100 mm Hg. Using this definition of hypertension, patients with readings above this figure fared worse than those with a pressure lower than this. In males, the six-year survival rate was only 28 per cent in the hypertensive group as against 54 per cent in the non-hypertensive group, a difference he thought was probably significant.

Marquardsen (1969) finally went on to examine survival curves in the two groups. In male patients the survival curve of the hypertensive and non-hypertensive diverged from the onset even though in the first year after the episode the difference in mortality was small. In strange contrast, female patients with 'normal' pressures fared rather worse in the first year than their male counterparts but thereafter the curve diverged in a manner similar to males. After the age of 70, the presence of an elevated blood pressure affected males adversely but not females, although by this time the number of the male population surviving was so small as to render its significance dubious.

Thus, it would appear true that there is general agreement that the presence of hypertension adversely affects the prognosis in cerebral vascular disease, but there are exceptions. Adams (1965), in patients observed in geriatric practice, failed to demonstrate any substantial influence of high blood pressure on long-term survival after cerebral infarction, and a more detailed analysis (Merrett and Adams, 1966) confirmed this result. Goldner et al (1967), also studying a geriatric population in terms of age, also could not find any statistical evidence that an elevated blood pressure adversely affected the outcome.

The only factor that would appear to be operative in these two reports was the age of the population studied, and the difference again may be an expression of selection induced by the type of clinical practice rather than by any genuine divergence of fact.

PERSONAL SERIES

Before the results of examining the potential effects of an elevated blood pressure in our personal series are examined it is worth re-emphasising the point that compared with many series the patients under study are very definitely selected. Their mean age at onset (57.3 years) would alone indicate this. Since the patients were drawn in the main from an out-patient source, they are, by definition, survivors from the initial episode and they represent the younger age group with cerebral vascular disease. This may, of course, be an advantage, since they are not subject to the many other ailments that afflict the elderly and thus may present a clearer picture in relation to the problems of an elevated blood pressure.

In assessing the relationship between blood pressure and the clinical patterns of the disease the initial diastolic blood pressure (IDBP) was used. This was a casual reading and therefore it was established that familiarity with clinic routine and visits on a three-monthly basis did not produce a significant fall in the blood pressure between the first and subsequent visits. The blood pressure was read to the nearest 5 mm Hg and in the statistical assessment patients with an IDBP below 90 mm Hg were grouped together as were all patients with an IDBP of 120 mm Hg or more. Between these figures the patients were grouped together in increments of 10 mm of mercury.

There are several aspects of the relationship between the elevation of the systemic blood pressure and the prognosis in transient cerebral ischaemia and in strokes which invite examination.

Since there is a discernible pattern of behaviour in the type of cerebral vascular disease under consideration, it would be important, if it were possible, to establish a relationship between hypertension and subsequent clinical behaviour, since this would have obvious therapeutic implications. Related to this is the obvious question of the significance of blood pressure levels in both survival rates and overall mortality. There is, too, the possibility that the presence of hypertension may affect, for better or for worse, the quality of recovery, as Prineas and Marshall (1966) observed. Finally, and this applies only to the important group of patients with recurrent episodes of stroke, there is a possibility that the presence of hypertension may play some role in the speed with which further episodes occur.

Blood pressure and clinical categories

The clinical categories for this purpose were obtained, as before, by separating the patients with a single stroke from those patients with recurrent episodes, the latter being designated multiple stroke. Also subdivided were the patients presenting with transient cerebral ischaemia on the basis of a history of a complicating stroke. This done, the mean initial diastolic blood pressure (IDBP) was then used as an index of the level of the systemic pressure.

Table 7.2. Mean initial diastolic blood pressure in clinical groups in our personal series.

Clinical groups	Number		mm Hg	
	Male	Female	Male	Female
Single stroke	111	51	100.4[a] (S.D. 18.42)	99.9 (S.D. 16.36)
Multiple strokes	138	46	110.1[a] (S.D. 21.24)	106.2 (S.D. 22.34)
Transient vascular insufficiency	45	12	103.4 (S.D. 16.91)	110.0 (S.D. 16.50)
Transient vascular insufficiency going on to stroke	73	21	105.4 (S.D. 17.85)	107.9 (S.D. 22.03)
All groups	367	130	105.4 (S.D. 19.62)	104.3 (S.D. 19.77)

[a]Significant $P < 0.05$
(Reproduced from *Quarterly Journal of Medicine* by permission, 1972).

The results are shown on Table 7.2. It is immediately apparent, in common with the findings of other observers, that an appreciable degree of hypertension is evident in the whole series, the mean IDBP being 105.4 mm Hg for males and 104.3 mm Hg for females. If individual categories are then examined further positive information emerges.

Blood pressure and transient cerebral ischaemia

Male patients presenting with transient cerebral ischaemia showed the tendency shown by all patients in the series, which was to have an elevated blood pressure that was nearly identical with the mean for the whole group (Figure 7.1 and Table 7.2). In women, the mean IDBP was 110 mm Hg compared with 104.38 mm Hg for all females. However, the figures gave no support for the hope that the level of the blood pressure may be effective in predicting the later recurrence of a stroke. In males, the patients going on to develop a stroke showed a moderate difference of 2 mm Hg only, whereas the female group going on to have a stroke had IDBPs only 3 mm Hg lower than the patients who continued without this complication.

Blood pressure and stroke

If the levels for the IDBP of the stroke patients are examined, an immediate difference is seen (Table 7.2). It is apparent that in male patients in the multiple stroke group the IDBP is significantly raised when compared with that recorded in the whole group of patients. In contrast, in the single stroke group the male patients had a mean IDBP of 100.4 mm Hg which was significantly lower than the figure recorded in all other patients. The differences were even more striking when the distribution of the patients according to the level of the IDBP was compared in the two groups (Table 7.3 and Figure 7.2). In the single stroke group the numbers of patients for each 10 mm Hg increment remained in the range of 20 to 25 whereas in the multiple stroke group the number of patients rose sharply with an increasing diastolic blood pressure, reaching statistical significance at 120 mm Hg or above.

It has been emphasised that these results apply only to the males. The females, although smaller in total numbers, showed none of the trends observed in the male patients, thus offering considerable support for the view that is often expressed in relation to uncomplicated hypertension that women appear to tolerate hypertension better than males. This would appear to be true, even in the face of established cerebral vascular disease.

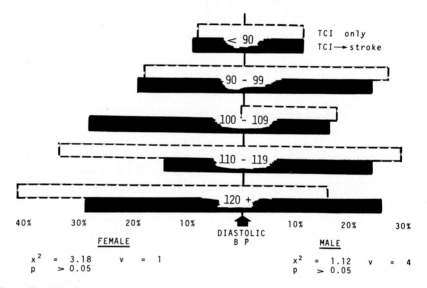

Figure 7.1. Distribution of initial diastolic blood pressure in 151 patients presenting with transient cerebral ischaemia (TCI).

Table 7.3. Distribution of mean IDBP in patients with a history of single stroke compared with those suffering multiple strokes.

IDBP (mm Hg)	Males		Females	
	Single stroke	Multiple strokes	Single stroke	Multiple strokes
89 or less	24	13	10	9
90–99	25	30	7	6
100–109	22	15	14	10
110–119	20	32	12	6
120 or more	20	48	8	15
Total	111	138	51	46
	$\chi^2=16.63$; $v=4$; $P<0.005$		$\chi^2=4.67$; $v=4$; $P>0.05$	

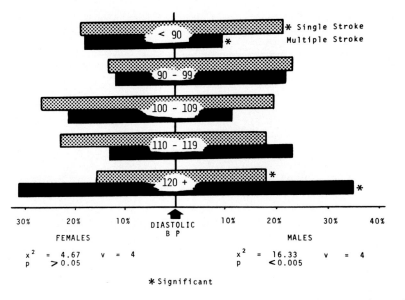

Figure 7.2. Distribution of initial diastolic blood pressure (in mm Hg) in patients with single and multiple strokes.

BLOOD PRESSURE, MORTALITY AND SURVIVAL RATE

Mortality

In view of the above findings, and particularly the close relationship between hypertension and the liability to recurrent episodes, it would be surprising if the level of blood pressure bore no relationship to mortality. In fact, the results indicate a relationship that is as close as that detailed for the clinical categories.

Since the patients suffering only from transient cerebral ischaemia were excluded, 440 patients (male 322; female 118) were available for analysis. The details are given for both sexes in Table 7.4. Again, there is a clear relationship in male patients only between the level of the IDBP and mortality. Significantly more patients died with an IDBP of 120 mm Hg or more, and the group of survivors showed significantly more patients who entered the study with an IDBP of 90 mm or less.

That women show no such difference would support the suggestion that is inherent in the observations in relation to clinical categories which indicated a genuine difference in the response to hypertension between the sexes.

If the individual clinical groups were examined in more detail, certain points emerged in the patients with transient cerebral ischaemia. First of all, there was no obvious relationship between the IDBP and mortality in all of the patients with transient cerebral ischaemia who developed a stroke, and this remained true even when males and females were combined (Table 7.5).

Table 7.4. Initial diastolic blood pressure (IDBP) and mortality in 440 patients(M = 322; F = 118) with cerebral vascular disease (transient cerebral ischaemia going on to stroke(s), single stroke and multiple stroke).

IDBP (mm Hg)	Males			..	Females		
	Total	Alive	Dead		Total	Alive	Dead
89 or less	45	36	9		21	14	7
90–99	73	52	21		17	14	3
100–109	49	31	18		30	19	11
110–119	70	39	31		21	14	7
120 or more	85	43	42		29	19	10
	322	201	121		118	80	38
	$\chi^2 = 14.52$; $v = 4$; $P < 0.01$				$\chi^2 = 2.02$; $v = 4$; $P > 0.05$		

Table 7.5. Initial diastolic blood pressure (IDBP) and mortality in 94 patients (M = 73; F = 21) with transient cerebral ischaemia going on to stroke.

IDBP (mm Hg)	Total	Males and females Alive	Dead
89 or less	10	7	3
90–99	22	17	5
100–109	18	13	5
110–119	21	14	7
120 or more	23	15	8
	94	66	28
	$\chi^2 = 0.77$; $v = 3$; $P > 0.05$		

When the history was complicated by the subsequent development of multiple strokes, however, a different picture emerged. There were only 36 patients (31 male and five female) who developed multiple strokes following the initial presentation with transient cerebral ischaemia. The number was insufficient for analysis and the distribution of the patients is shown in Table 7.6. It will be observed that there is a clear trend for patients with an IDBP of 110 mm or more to have a worse prognosis. Nine of the 12 who died had a reading of 110 mg Hg or more whereas of the 24 survivors 16 had an IDBP of 109 mm or less.

Table 7.6. The mortality and mean IDBP in 36 patients presenting with transient cerebral ischaemia and then developing recurrent stroke episodes.

IDBP (mm Hg)	Total	Male and female Alive	Dead
89 or less	2	1	1
90–99	10	10	0
100–109	7	5	2
110–119	7	3	4
120 or more	10	5	5
	36	24	12

Survival rates

It is now generally agreed that the full significance of mortality rates can only be appreciated when compared with the general population of the same age and sex. This is particularly true, of course, when one is dealing with an ageing group of patients. Life Tables have been constructed in the manner previously described, and the patients under observation are then grouped according to the IDBP.

The implications are obvious (Figure 7.3). With an IDBP of less than 90 mm the curve for the normal population and for the patient group is virtually the same in the first year and, indeed, up to the eighth year the divergence of the two curves is not remarkable. In the patients with an IDBP reading between 90 mm Hg and 109 mm Hg there is an obvious difference when both are compared with the general population. The difference, however, between these two groups is not great in the first three-and-a-half years.

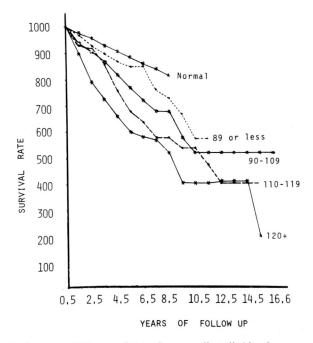

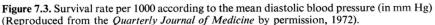

Figure 7.3. Survival rate per 1000 according to the mean diastolic blood pressure (in mm Hg) (Reproduced from the *Quarterly Journal of Medicine* by permission, 1972).

Patients with a diastolic pressure of 120 mm Hg or more stand out. The survival curve falls sharply away even in the first six months, confirming the implications of the simple mortality rate. Within this group the percentages are interesting in that, again, the difference between the sexes shows up. At four-and-a-half years after the onset of symptoms of cerebral vascular disease 63 per cent of males were alive as compared with 73 per cent of females.

Blood pressure and morbidity

Prineas and Marshall (1966) made the observation that in patients present-ing with a stroke there were no immediate clinical differences at the onset of the ictus but the surviving patients with a diastolic blood pressure of 110 mm or more achieved a better quality of recovery than those with a diastolic blood pressure below this level. Thus, if one postulates that a high diastolic blood pressure would be more likely to be associated with an intracerebral haematoma in the traditional sites one would forecast a better recovery for this group than for patients who had sustained an extensive cortical infarct.

This observation, and the fact that there is a clear association between progressive disability due to recurring stroke episodes and hypertension, prompted an examination of the possibility that it may be possible on clinical grounds to detect a different clinical pattern of recovery in the two groups of patients and thus to confirm the observations of Prineas and Marshall (1966). Since the patients were being observed at three-monthly intervals it was possible to assess the clinical state at three, six, and twelve months after the ictus. Because of deaths and the incidence of recurrent stroke the number of patients available for analysis gradually fell. At three months, 391 patients were available for study; at six months, the disability in 363 patients was available, and in 324 disability after twelve months was known. With these facts available, the neurological disability at stated intervals of time following the stroke episode was then related to the level of the diastolic blood pressure (Table 7.7). If reference is made to the results in male patients (and the female patients were identical with these) there was no evidence to show any associa-tion between the level of the IDBP and the speed of functional recovery at these intervals of time following the first stroke episode. The state of recovery at three months and at twelve months is shown (Table 7.7). We could not, therefore, confirm the observations of Prineas and Marshall (1966). However, their patients were of a slightly younger age group and, once again, the problem of selection may have affected the results.

In view of the fact that there was a close relationship between the IDBP and mortality it might be anticipated that when the study was complete there would be a demonstrable association between the blood pressure and the functional state. Our results, however, show no evidence of any association along these lines and this statement applies to 201 surviving males and 80 females who had either single or multiple strokes or presented with transient cerebral ischaemia, going on to develop the complication of a stroke.

It is believed that this apparent anomaly can be explained only by the fact that patients with an elevated diastolic blood pressure did not survive in the same numbers as normotensive patients and therefore are not contributing to this aspect of the analysis.

Blood pressure and temporal pattern

By temporal pattern is meant the time interval in patients with recurrent episodes between the first and the second stroke. It has already been demon-strated that at one year 46 per cent of the patients had had a second episode

Table 7.7. The distribution of the initial diastolic blood pressure (IDBP) and degree of neurological disability at three months and one year following the first stroke in males.

IDBP (mm Hg)	Total	Neurological disability at 3 months				Total	Neurological disability at 1 year			
		Grade 1	Grade 2	Grade 3	Grade 4		Grade 1	Grade 2	Grade 3	Grade 4
89 or less	42	13	17	10	2	40	26	4	8	2
90–99	60	20	18	14	8	47	25	10	11	1
100–109	45	14	14	12	5	38	21	5	9	3
110–119	67	22	23	21	1	51	29	10	11	1
120 or more	70	23	25	20	2	56	30	17	9	0
	284	92	97	77	18	232	131	46	48	7

$\chi^2 = 1.88; v = 8; P > 0.05$

$\chi^2 = 9.15; v = 8; P > 0.05$

Grade 1 — Complete functional recovery
Grade 2 — Moderate disability
Grade 3 — Residual marked disability
Grade 4 — Bedridden

Table 7.8. The distribution of the initial diastolic blood pressure (IDBP) and the time interval between the first and second stroke in 169 male and 51 female patients (multiple stroke = 184; transient cerebral ischaemia → stroke = 36).

Mean IDBP	Total	Up to 3 months	4 months to 6 months	7 months to one year	one year one month to 2 years	2 years one month to 5 years	More than 5 years
Males							
89 or less	15	2	0	4	4	2	3
90–99	39	11	6	6	2	12	2
100–109	20	4	2	1	4	7	2
110–119	38	6	7	5	8	8	4
120 or more	57	13	8	5	18	11	2
	169	36	23	21	36	40	13

$\chi^2 = 5.58; \nu = 3; P > 0.05$

Mean IDBP	Total	Up to 3 months	4 months to 6 months	7 months to one year	one year one month to 2 years	2 years one month to 5 years	More than 5 years
Females							
89 or less	10	3	2	1	1	2	1
90–99	6	2	0	1	0	3	0
100–109	12	3	2	2	2	3	0
110–119	7	0	0	0	4	2	1
120 or more	16	2	2	6	3	1	2
	51	10	6	10	10	11	4

$\chi^2 = 0.23; \nu = 1; P > 0.05$

and at the end of five years 91.4 per cent of patients had suffered a similar episode.

An analysis was carried out to determine whether or not there was any evidence of the presence of hypertension that could influence the time interval between the first and second stroke. To do this, the distribution of the IDBP in 169 male patients and 51 female patients was examined, and of these patients 184 went on to suffer further stroke episodes. The remaining 36 presented with transient cerebral ischaemia, going on to multiple strokes.

In order to achieve adequate group size it was necessary in this case to combine male patients who had their second stroke episode within a year and, also, to group together female patients who had their second stroke episode within two years. These were then compared with the remaining male and female patients. Patients with an IDBP of 109 mm Hg or less and patients with 110 mm Hg or more were grouped together.

It will be seen from the results that there was no evidence at all that the level of the IDBP had any contribution to make to the length of time that elapsed between the first and second stroke episode (Table 7.8).

CONCLUSION

1. There is evidence that arterial hypertension will accentuate the process of atheroma and that the presence of hypertension is an important precursor of a stroke.
2. Most observers agree that the prognosis in stroke is adversely affected by the presence of hypertension.
3. The blood pressure is elevated in 35 to 75 per cent of patients with stroke. The variations are usually an expression of the definition of what constitutes a significantly elevated blood pressure.
4. The tendency to suffer recurrent episodes of stroke is significantly associated with hypertension. This applies to males only.
5. Long-term mortality is significantly associated with the level of blood pressure. The higher it is, the worse the prognosis. Again, this applies only to males.
6. Although the presence of an elevated B.P. is important in relation to the incidence of recurrent episodes there is no evidence that it affects the time when the second stroke episode is likely to occur.

REFERENCES

Acheson, J. (1971) Factors affecting the natural history of 'focal cerebral vascular disease'. *Quarterly Journal of Medicine*, **40**, 25–46.
Adams, G. F. (1965) Prospects for patients with strokes with special reference to the hypertensive hemiplegic. *British Medical Journal*, **i**, 253–259.
Alam, M. & Smirk, F. H. (1943) Casual and basal blood pressures in British and Egyptian men. *British Heart Journal*, **5**, 152.
Aring, C. D. & Merritt, H. H. (1935) Differential diagnosis between cerebral haemorrhage and cerebral thrombosis. A clinical and pathological study of 245 cases. *Archives of Internal Medicine*, **56**, 435–456.

Baker, A. B., Resch, J. A. & Loewenson, R. B. (1969) Hypertension and cerebral athero-sclerosis. *Circulation*, **39**, 701–710.

Baker, R. N., Schwartz, W. S. & Ramseyer, J. C. (1968) Prognosis among survivors of ischaemic strokes. *Neurology*, **18**, 933–941.

Bechgaard, P. (1946) Arterial hypertension. A follow up study of 1000 hypotonics. *Acta Scandinavica*, Supplement **172**.

Bennett, I. L. & Heyman, A. (1948) Paroxysmal hypertension associated with tabes dorsalis. *American Journal of Medicine*, **5**, 729–735.

Burrows, G. (1846) *Disorders of Cerebral Circulation and the Connection Between Affections of the Brain and Heart Disease*. London: Longman, Brown, Green, Longmans.

Carter, B. (1964) *Hypertension—Monograph Cerebral Infarction*. pp. 125–127. Oxford: Pergamon.

David, N. J. & Heyman, A. (1960) Factors influencing the prognosis of cerebral thrombosis and infarction due to atherosclerosis. *Journal of Chronic Diseases*, **11**, 394–404.

Dickinson, C. J. (1965) *Neurogenic Hypertension*. Oxford: Blackwell Scientific Publication.

Dickinson, C. J. & Thomson, A. D. (1959) Vertebral and internal carotid arteries in relation to hypertension and cerebrovascular disease. *Lancet*, **ii**, 46–48.

Eilersten, E. & Humerfelt, S. (1968) Objective method for evaluation of observer variation in blood pressure reading. *Acta Medica Scandinavica*, **184**, 145–157.

Evelyn, J. A. (1970) The natural history of hypertension. *Transactions of the Association of Life Insurance, Medical Directors of America*, **53**, 84–112.

Goldner, J. C., Payne, G. H., Watson, F. R. & Parrish, H. M. (1967) Prognosis for survival after stroke. *American Journal of the Medical Sciences*, **253**, 129–133.

Hamilton, M., Pickering, G. W., Roberts, F. & Sowry, G. S. C. (1954) The aetiology of essential hypertension: (1) The arterial pressure in the general population. *Clinical Science*, **13**, 11–35.

Harlan, M. R., Osborne, R. K. & Graybiel, A. (1962) Longitudinal study of blood pressure. *Circulation*, **26**, 530–543.

Howard, F. A., Cohen, P., Hickler, R. B., Locke, S., Newcombe, T. & Tyler, H. R. (1963) Survival following stroke. *Journal of the American Medical Association*, **183**, 921–925.

Janeway, T. C. (1913) Clinical study of hypertensive cardiovascular disease. *Archives of Internal Medicine*, **12**, 755–798.

Kannel, W. B., Wolf, P. A., Verter, J. & McNamara, P. M. (1970) Epidemiological assessment of blood pressure in stroke. The Framingham Study. *Journal of the American Medical Association* **214**, 301–310.

Kuller L. H., Cook, L. P. & Friedman, G. D. (1972) Survey of stroke epidemiology studies. *Stroke*, **3**, 579–585.

Kurtzke, J. F. (1969) *Epidemiology of Cerebro-Vascular Disease*. pp. 90–95. Berlin, Heidelberg and New York: Springer-Verlag.

Lowe, R. D. (1961) Resistance of carotid arteries in hypertension and stroke. *Clinical Science*, **21**, 409–417.

Low-Beer, T. and Phear, D. (1961) Cerebral infarction and hypertension. *Lancet*, **i**, 1303–1305.

McKeown, T., Record, R. G. & Whitfield, A. G. W. (1963) Variations in casual measurement of arterial pressure in two populations (Birmingham and South Wales) re-examined after interval of 3–4½ years. *Clinical Science*, **24**, 437–450.

McMichael, J. (1961) Reorientations in hypertensive disorders. *British Medical Journal*, **ii**, 1239–1244.

Marquardsen, J. (1969) *The Natural History of Acute Cerebrovascular Disease. A Retrospective Study of 769 Patients*. Copenhagen: Munksgaard.

Marshall, J. (1966) Evidence upon the neurogenic theory of hypertension. *Lancet*, **ii**, 410–412.

Marshall, J. & Kaeser, A. C. (1961) Survival of the non-haemorrhagic cerebrovascular accidents. A prospective study. *British Medical Journal*, **ii**, 73–77.

Marshall, J. & Shaw, D. A. (1959) The natural history of cerebrovascular disease. *British Medical Journal*, **i**, 1614–1617.

Mathisen, H. S., Loken, H., Brox, D. & Stokke, H. (1965) The prognosis in essential hypertension. *Scandinavian Journal of Clinical and Laboratory Investigation*, **17**, 257–261.

Merrett, J. D. & Adams, G. D. (1966) Comparison of mortality rates in elderly hypertensive and normotensive hemiplegic patients. *British Medical Journal*, **ii**, 802–805.

Miall, W. E. & Lovell, H. G. (1967) Relation between change of blood pressure and age. *British Medical Journal*, **ii**, 660–664.

Mitchell, J. R. A. (1971) Hypertension and arterial disease. *British Heart Journal*, **33**, 122–126.

Montgomery, B. M. (1961) Basilar hypertensive syndrome. *Archives of Internal Medicine*, **108**, 559–569.

Page, I. H. (1935) A syndrome simulating diencephalic stimulation occurring in patients with essential hypertension. *Journal of Medical Science*, **190**, 9–14.

Penfield, W. (1929) Diencephalic: Autonomic epilepsy. *Archives of Neurology and Psychiatry*, **22**, 358–374.

Perara, G. A. (1955) Relation of blood pressure lability to prognosis in hypertensive vascular disease. *Journal of Chronic Diseases*, **1**, 121–126.

Pickering, G. W. (1955) High blood pressure. *British Medical Journal*, **i**, 244–247.

Prineas, J. & Marshall, J. (1966) Hypertension and cerebral infarction. *British Medical Journal*, **i**, 14–17.

Richardson, D. W., Honour, A. J., Fenton, G. W., Stott, F. H. & Pickering, G. W. (1964) Variation in arterial pressure throughout the day and night. *Clinical Science*, **26.** 445–460.

Wepfer, J. J. (1658) Observationes anatomicae ex cadaveribus eorum quos sustulit apoplexia (cum exercitatione de eious loco affecto). Schaffussii: J. C. Suteri.

CHAPTER EIGHT

The Electrocardiogram, Heart Size and Prognosis

A relationship between brain infarction and heart disease is not a new concept. Dozzi (1937) when examining the incidence of cerebral embolism as a complication of cardiac infarction concluded that it was wise to suspect the heart in all cases of cerebral embolism and, indeed, observed that hemiplegia may as a result be the first indication of cardiac infarction. Subsequently, the main source of information about the role of heart disease in relation to cerebral ischaemia has come from pathologists, and this has been discussed in detail elsewhere in this monograph.

In considering the factors that may influence the prognosis in ischaemic cerebral vascular disease, we are not here concerned with the now familiar picture of sudden hemiplegia developing in a patient with a history of myocardial infarction in the recent past, or with focal neurological signs developing in the setting of a patient suffering from advanced degenerative heart disease. This is not to deny, of course, the fact that, in the analysis of any patient presenting with transient ischaemia or a stroke, it is obviously important to exclude the possibility of a recent myocardial infarction.

In both transient cerebral ischaemia (TCI) and cerebral infarction several investigators have drawn attention to the importance not only of a previous history of angina or cardiac infarction but also to the finding of abnormalities in the electrocardiogram (ECG). Attempts have also been made to differentiate between the importance of hypertension and atheroma in the development of cardiac abnormalities.

As in previous chapters, the two related problems of TCI and stroke are examined separately.

Transient cerebral ischaemia and the ECG

There are now a number of studies in the literature with clinical or ECG evidence of significant cardiac abnormality observed in association with the syndrome of TCI.

Baker, Ramseyer and Schwartz (1968) in a prospective study of 79 patients with TCI attacks found that 29 per cent (23) had evidence of previous myocardial infarction. In an analysis of their observations they could find no evidence that prior coronary artery disease influenced the development of further episodes of TCI or, for that matter, episodes of cerebral or myocardial infarction. However, if the patients were sub-divided into two groups on the basis of a previous history of myocardial infarction, it was found that just over 50 per cent in both groups had further TCI attacks but 28 per cent of the group with a history of myocardial infarction had a later history of cerebral infarction compared with only 20 per cent of the patients presenting with no such previous history.

Friedman et al (1969) made some interesting observations on a community of retired persons in California. The description of the medical and social facilities available to this community would seem to indicate that they were a group selected on economic grounds alone. The study reported has two great merits. The first is that it was prospective and involved a relatively static population, and the second is that the community was relatively large (10 500) and 90 per cent of the population were registered with a single medical centre.

In an elderly population, where the average age was 68.8 years, the incidence of all cerebral vascular events was 9.7 per 1000 persons per year. The rate for TCI as an initial episode without a history of previous cerebral infarction was 1.1 per 1000 per year. In all, there were 60 patients who met the strict clinical criteria laid down and these were observed for an average period of 28.6 months.

The findings in this group were compared with a healthy population of similar age structure who were available as controls. Hypertension was defined as a diastolic blood pressure of more than 90 mm Hg and it was observed that this was only slightly more frequent in patients with a history of transient ischaemic attacks (TIAs) (48 versus 46 per cent); cardiac enlargement was present in 15 per cent of the patients studied but was also present in 13 per cent of the controls. However, the incidence of an abnormal ECG was very much higher in the transient ischaemic group, where it was observed in no less than 48 per cent as compared with 24 per cent of the controls.

Ziegler and Hassanein (1973) found that out of 109 patients with TIAs more than 50 per cent had an abnormal ECG on the initial examination. The abnormalities observed were not described in detail but were listed as 'myocardial ischaemia, arrhythmia or conduction defects'.

Marshall and Wilkinson (1971) reported a study of the outcome in patients with TIAs who also had normal angiograms. 54 of the patients had ECGs and 40 of these were normal, but even so, 20 (50 per cent) had further cerebral vascular episodes; 14 patients had abnormal ECGs, and of these nine (71 per cent) had further episodes. Although the difference did not achieve the 1-in-20 level of statistical significance, they did find that ECG evidence of 'severe' ischaemia was more frequently associated with further cardiac and cerebral vascular episodes.

THE PRESENT SERIES

In the present series, routine enquiries were made of all patients for a clinical history of myocardial infarction and angina of effort, and in the initial clinical assessment the majority had a routine ECG taken. Reporting on the ECG records was carried out by an independent observer, a consultant cardiologist who was an acknowledged authority in the interpretation of ECGs.* The observer was not aware at the time of reporting, the records of either the clinical history or the chest x-rays in the individual patients. In a final analysis the ECG records were classified as normal or abnormal and the abnormal records were further subdivided in the following manner:

1. Ventricular hypertrophy.
2. Evidence of old or recent myocardial infarction.
3. Evidence of myocardial ischaemia.

In addition to the ECG examination, standard x-rays of the chest were available in over 400 patients but these, unlike the ECG, were reported upon routinely in the x-ray service of the Hospital Centre. Since we were only interested in the question of heart size, cardiac enlargement in excess of 50 per cent of the cardio-thoracic ratio was considered to be abnormal.

Myocardial infarction and angina

The clinical history of myocardial infarction was elicited in relatively few patients since there were only 27 males (7.3 per cent) and 2 females (1.5 per cent) with such a history. A further 26 males (7.1 per cent) and 10 females (7.6 per cent) gave a history of angina of effort (Table 8.1). In this small group of patients there was no particular distribution of ECG abnormalities within the different clinical groups nor could the incidence of myocardial infarction or angina of effort be related to the mean initial diastolic blood pressure. However, the numbers are so small that no particular significance is attached to this observation.

Table 8.1. Incidence of angina and myocardial infarction in personal series.

Clinical group	Total in group		Clinical myocardial infarction				Angina of effort			
	Male	Female	Male	%	Female	%	Male	%	Female	%
Single stroke	112	52	7	6.3	0	0	6	5.4	2	3.8
Multiple stroke	138	47	10	7.2	2	4.3	12	8.7	2	4.3
TCI only	45	12	3	6.7	0	0	4	8.9	3	25.0
TCI → stroke	73	21	7	9.6	0	0	4	5.5	3	14.3
	368	132	27	7.3	2	1.5	26	7.1	10	7.6

*The late Dr J. P. P. Stock, author of *Diagnosis and Treatment of Cardiac Arrhythmias.* London: Butterworth.

In contrast to the clinical evidence of coronary artery disease the incidence of abnormal ECGs was very much higher. Attention was therefore concentrated on this aspect, as there were sufficient numbers to relate statistically the ECG findings to prognosis in the statistical sense.

In all, 430 patients had an ECG record and 416 patients a routine x-ray of the chest.

TRANSIENT CEREBRAL ISCHAEMIA

One hundred and forty one patients presenting with TCI had an ECG record available for analysis and 45 of these (33 male and 12 female) had an abnormal ECG (Table 8.2).

Table 8.2. Distribution of normal and abnormal ECG's within the clinical groups in 141 patients (110 male, 31 female) presenting with transient cerebral ischaemia.

Clinical groups	Males			Females		
	Total	Normal	Abnormal	Total	Normal	Abnormal
TCI only	44	33	11	12	7	5
TCI → stroke	66	44	22	19	12	7
	110	77	33	31	19	12
	$\chi^2 = 0.87; v = 1; P > 0.05$			$\chi^2 = 0.08; v = 1; P > 0.05$		

In the analysis, no association could be found in either the male or female patients, between the finding of an abnormal ECG and a subsequent liability to develop stroke. It was true, however, that in the patients with the best prognosis, namely, those with a history of TCI only, there was a lower incidence of abnormal ECGs.

On examining the type of ECG abnormality, that is whether it reflected hypertensive changes alone or coronary artery disease presumed to be due to atheroma, no relationship could be established between the three categories of ECG abnormality and the clinical behaviour of the patients (Table 8.3).

Table 8.3. Distribution of the type of ECG abnormality in 45 patients (33 male, 12 female) presenting with transient cerebral ischaemia.

Clinical groups	Total	Left ventricular hypertrophy	Myocardial infarct (old and recent)	Myocardial ischaemia
TCI only	16	5	1	10
TCI → stroke	29	12	3	14
	45	17	4	24
	$\chi^2 = 0.45; v = 1; P > 0.05$			

Cardiac enlargement

Examination of the relationship between heart size and ultimate prognosis was no more rewarding. The cardio-thoracic ratio was known in 136 patients

182

presenting with TCI, and of these 25 male and 10 females had an enlarged heart on x-ray. No relationship between the presence of an enlarged heart and the development of a later stroke could be detected (Table 8.4).

Table 8.4. Distribution of cardio-thoracic ratio within the clinical groups in 136 patients (107 male, 29 female) presenting with TCI.

Clinical groups	Males Heart size			Females Heart size		
	Total	Normal	Enlarged	Total	Normal	Enlarged
TCI only	42	35	7	12	8	4
TCI → Stroke	65	47	18	17	11	6
	107	82	25	29	19	10
	$\chi^2 = 1.74; v = 1; P > 0.05$			$\chi^2 = 0.00; v = 1; P > 0.05$		

Both the ECG findings and the cardio-thoracic ratio were available in each of the 130 patients presenting with TCI, and 97 with a normal heart size showed an incidence of 25.8 per cent abnormal ECGs. The incidence of ECG abnormality was much higher (60.6 per cent) in patients with an enlarged heart. Even so, no statistical association could be found in either group between the ECG findings and the likelihood of a cerebral infarct developing (Table 8.5).

Table 8.5. Distribution of ECG findings within the clinical groups in 130 patients presenting with TCI (97 heart size normal, 33 heart enlarged).

Clinical groups	Heart size—normal ECG			Heart enlarged ECG		
	Total	Normal	Abnormal	Total	Normal	Abnormal
TCI only	43	32	11	11	6	5
TCI → Stroke	54	40	14	22	7	15
	97	72	25	33	13	20
	$\chi^2 = 0.00; v = 1; P > 0.05$			$\chi^2 = 1.59; v = 1; P > 0.05$		

STROKE

Tnere is good evidence from epidemiological studies, actuarial figures and studies of hospital populations, of an association between heart disease and the development of a stroke.

The findings of Berkson and Stamler (1965) led them to suggest that individuals with an abnormal ECG were more likely to develop a stroke than those with a normal tracing. This was also emphasised in the Framingham study where a marked relationship was found between the initial finding of an abnormal ECG and the development of a stroke. The observations on hypertension have already been referred to in the Framingham study and, as a corollary of these observations, they found that patients with cardiac enlargement and ECG evidence of left ventricular hypertrophy had three times as high a risk of developing stroke as a normal population (Kannel, 1971).

In another study, designed to select risk factors, Gertler, Rosenberger and Leetma (1972) observed that the presence of an abnormal ECG would help to identify stroke-prone individuals.

David and Heyman (1960), in a study of 100 patients, found an abnormal ECG in 44 per cent (37) of the 85 patients, where the record was available. When they examined the mortality data, death was found to have occurred in 46 per cent of patients with definite ECG changes as compared with 29 per cent of patients found to have a normal or borderline record. The patients who were to die from myocardial disease and coronary thrombosis were among those with definite ECG changes when they were first assessed.

Howard et al (1963), in a prospective study of the survival of 97 patients, observed a high incidence of coronary artery disease in the whole group and many patients gave a history of myocardial infarction prior to the stroke. This was also observed by Silverstein and Doniger (1963), who found that 41 out of 100 patients with a stroke had definite evidence of cardiac disease.

Baker, Schwartz and Ramseyer (1968), in their prospective study of 430 patients, found that 30 per cent had evidence of coronary artery disease either prior to or at the time of the onset of the stroke. They also commented that the presence of coronary artery disease adversely affects the incidence of further cerebral vascular episodes.

The association between an abnormal ECG and the prognosis is not confined to the relatively young hospital population with a stroke but is also present in the elderly.

Droller (1965) examined 275 elderly patients and found that 25 per cent of men and 30 per cent of women had angina on exertion and that the ECG was abnormal in 29 per cent (79) of the patients. He drew the obvious conclusion that certain abnormal ECG patterns may indicate a poor prognosis. Cutler (1967), questioned 863 patients about symptoms of cerebral vascular disease, and the patients were also examined for signs thought to be premonitory indications of the liability to a stroke. They found that the patients who had had strokes previously had significantly more abnormal ECGs than the patients without such a history.

Friedman, Loveland and Ehrlich (1968) reported on a study of a retired population with a mean age of 71 years. The medical records of 117 patients who had developed their first stroke were examined and compared with the records of 234 controls. The analysis showed that 41.9 per cent of the stroke patients and 24.4 per cent of the controls had coronary artery disease. Of patients with a stroke, 26.5 per cent and 19.2 per cent of controls also had an enlarged heart prior to the development of a stroke.

Finally, Marquardsen (1969), in a retrospective study of 769 patients with cerebral vascular disease, found that the presence of auricular fibrillation or of other ECG abnormalities was associated with a tendency to develop recurrent episodes.

PRESENT SERIES

ECGs were available for analysis in 289 patients who first presented with a stroke, and an abnormal record was noted in 148 patients (109 male and 39 female).

Table 8.6. Distribution of ECG findings within the clinical groups in 289 patients (209 male, 80 female) presenting with stroke

Clinical groups	Total	Males Normal	Abnormal	Total	Females Normal	Abnormal
Single stroke	95	55 ↑	40	39	24	15
Multiple strokes	114	45 ↓	69	41	17	24
	209	100	109	80	41	39
	$\chi^2 = 7.05$; $v = 1$; $P < 0.005$			$\chi^2 = 3.22$; $v = 1$; $P > 0.05$		

It will be seen from the results presented in Table 8.6 that just as the number of normal ECGs is significantly higher in patients where the history is ultimately confined to that of a single stroke episode, so does the number of normal ECGs fall to a significant degree in the patients where the history is ultimately that of recurrent stroke episodes. This applies only in male patients, for in the females, just as in hypertension, no statistical association could be demonstrated between an abnormal ECG and a tendency to recurrent episodes. This, of course, may be simply a reflection of their ability to withstand hypertension better than males.

When the type of ECG abnormality was considered, there was no significant association between the abnormality observed and the ultimate prognosis. In order to obtain adequate numbers (Table 8.7) it was necessary to combine male and female patients, but again no significant association could be found.

Table 8.7. Distribution of the type of ECG abnormality in 148 patients (109 male, 39 female) presenting with a stroke.

Clinical groups	Total in group	Left ventricular hypertrophy	Myocardial infarct (old or recent)	Myocardial ischaemia
Males				
Single stroke	40	14	7	19
Multiple strokes	69	27	9	33
Total	109	41	16	52
	$\chi^2 = 0.46$; $v = 2$; $P > 0.05$			
Females				
Single stroke	15	5	0	10
Multiple strokes	24	4	4	16
Total	39	9	4	26
	Numbers too small for analysis			

As a final exercise, the records of 430 patients were examined as a group. A total of 193 patients had abnormal records and, when analysed statistically, there was a significant association between male patients with a history of recurrent strokes associated with an abnormal ECG (Table 8.8). This is in contrast to the lack of association between normal and abnormal ECGs and a history of single stroke or TCI.

Table 8.8. Distribution of ECG findings within the clinical groups (430 patients, 319 male, 111 female).

Clinical groups	Males ECG			Females ECG		
	Total	Normal	Abnormal	Total	Normal	Abnormal
Single stroke	95	55	40	39	24	15
Multiple strokes	114	45	69 ↑	41	17	24
TCI only	44	33	11 ↓	12	7	5
TCI → stroke	66	44	22	19	12	7
	319	177	142	111	60	51
	$\chi^2 = 22.17; v = 3; P < 0.001$			$\chi^2 = 4.21; v = 3; P > 0.05$		

ECG and initial diastolic blood pressure

In the knowledge that hypertension had a significant association with a history of recurrent episodes, and by definition therefore a poor prognosis, it was obviously necessary to examine the association between hypertension and ECG abnormalities.

The initial diastolic blood pressure was known for all patients with an ECG abnormality (Table 8.9) and, as might have been anticipated, there was a definite correlation between the finding of an abnormal ECG and the level of the diastolic blood pressure. The correlation emerges when one considers male patients with an initial diastolic blood pressure of 120 mm Hg or more, for in this group the number of abnormal ECGs was significantly elevated. Once more the association fails to appear in female patients, although here the numbers are very much smaller (Table 8.9).

Table 8.9. Distribution of ECG findings and initial diastolic blood pressure in 319 male and 111 female patients.

Initial diastolic BP	Males ECG			Females ECG		
	Total	Normal	Abnormal	Total	Normal	Abnormal
89 or less	44	31	13	18	12	6
90–99	75	52	23	17	10	7
100–109	51	32	19	25	16	9
110–119	67	37	30	22	10	12
120 or more	82	25	57	29	12	17
	319	177	142	111	60	51
	$\chi^2 = 31.64; v = 4; P < 0.001$			$\chi^2 = 4.82; v = 4; P > 0.05$		

Table 8.10. Distribution of the type of ECG abnormality and the level of initial diastolic blood pressure in 152 male and 51 female patients.

Initial diastolic BP	Males				Females			
	Total	Left ventricular hypertrophy	Myocardial infarct	Myocardial ischaemia	Total	Left ventricular hypertrophy	Myocardial infarct	Myocardial ischaemia
89 or less	13	2	3	8	6	1	1	4
90–99	23	5	8	10	7	0	1	6
100–109	19	7	2	10	9	1	1	7
110–119	30	12	4	14	12	6	0	6
120 or more	57	29 ↑	3 ↓	25	17	4	1	12
	142	55	20	67	51	12	4	35

$\chi^2 = 16.04$; $\nu = 4$; $P < 0.01$

Numbers too small

Finally, the relationship between the initial diastolic blood pressure and the type of ECG abnormalities was examined (Table 8.10). In order to achieve adequate group size it was necessary to combine patients with a diastolic pressure of 99 mm Hg or less, patients with a diastolic pressure between 100 mm Hg and 119 mm Hg, and, finally, patients with 120 mm Hg or more. It was evident that at a level of 120 mm Hg or more there were significantly less patients with evidence of previous myocardial infarction; there were also significantly more patients with such evidence in the group observed to have a diastolic blood pressure at or below 99 mm of mercury.

As might have been forecast, male patients with ECG evidence of left ventricular hypertrophy showed a significantly greater number of patients with a diastolic blood pressure of 120 mm or more.

Cardiac enlargement

In considering the cardio-thoracic ratio in patients presenting with stroke it was observed that 48 (23.6 per cent) males and 30 (38.9 per cent) females had an enlarged heart, but again no significant association could be found in either male or female patients between the history of a stroke and the size of the heart as observed on the x-ray (Table 8.11).

Table 8.11. Distribution of cardio-thoracic ratio within the clinical groups in 203 male and 77 female patients presenting with stroke.

Clinical groups	Males Total	Heart size Normal	Enlarged	Females Total	Heart size Normal	Enlarged
Single stroke	93	74	19	39	23	16
Multiple strokes	110	81	29	38	24	14
	203	155	48	77	47	30
	$\chi^2 = 0.99; v = 1; P > 0.05$			$\chi^2 = 0.16; v = 1; P > 0.05$		

However, a difference begins to appear when the relationship of the cardio-thoracic ratio and ECG record were examined in 255 patients. There were 186 patients with a heart size that was considered to be normal and of these, 76 (40.8 per cent) had an abnormal ECG compared with 53 (76.8 per cent) of the 69 patients with enlarged hearts (Table 8.12). In the patients with a

Table 8.12. Distribution of electrocardiographic findings within the clinical groups in 255 patients presenting with stroke (186 heart size—normal, 69 heart enlarged).

Clinical groups	Heart size—normal Total	ECG Normal	Abnormal	Heart enlarged Total	ECG Normal	Abnormal
Single stroke	89	62	27	30	10	20
Multiple strokes	97	48	49	49	6	33
	186	110	76	69	16	53
	$\chi^2 = 7.83; v = 1; P < 0.01$			$\chi^2 = 3.06; v = 1; P > 0.05$		

normal heart size the abnormal ECG was observed significantly less frequently in patients with a single stroke and, in contrast, significantly more patients with a history of multiple stroke had an abnormal ECG. In patients with an enlarged heart, however, no association could be found between the clinical groups and the ECG findings.

CONCLUSIONS

1. An abnormal ECG is commonly present both in patients with TCI and in the 'stroke' patient. The abnormalities comprise left ventricular hypertrophy, evidence of past myocardial infarction and/or myocardial ischaemia. No one abnormality is associated with any particular clinical group.
2. No relationship can be found between an abnormal ECG and enlarged heart, on the one hand, and the likelihood of developing a stroke in patients presenting with TCI on the other.
3. In recurrent strokes in male patients there is a significant association with an abnormal ECG.
4. With a diastolic blood pressure of 120 mm Hg or more there are significantly less patients with evidence of previous myocardial infarction.

REFERENCES

Baker, R. N., Ramseyer, J. C. & Schwartz, W. S. (1968) Prognosis in patients with transient cerebral ischaemic attacks. *Neurology*, **18**, 1157–1165.
Baker, R. N., Schwartz, W. S., Ramseyer, J. C. (1968) Prognosis among survivors of ischaemic stroke. *Neurology*, **18**, 933–941.
Berkson, D. M. & Stamler, J. (1965) Epidemiological findings on cerebrovascular disease and their implications. *Journal of Atherosclerosis Research*, **5**, 189–202.
Cutler, J. L. (1967) Cerebrovascular disease in an elderly population. *Circulation*, **36**, 394–399.
David, N. J. & Heyman, A. (1960) Factors influencing the prognosis of cerebral thrombosis and infarction due to atherosclerosis. *Journal of Chronic Diseases*, **11**, 394–404.
Dozzi, D. L. (1937) Cerebral embolism as a complication of coronary thrombosis. *American Journal of the Medical Sciences (new series)*, **194**, 824–830.
Droller, H. (1965) The outlook in hemiplegia. *Geriatrics*, **20**, 630–636.
Friedman, G. D., Wilson, W. S., Mosier, J. M. & Nichaman, M. Z. (1969) Transient ischaemic attacks in a community. *Journal of the American Medical Association*, **210**, 1428–1434.
Friedman, G. D., Loveland, D. B. & Ehrlich, S. P. (1968) Relationship of stroke to other cardiovascular disease. *Circulation*, **38**, 533–541.
Gertler, M. M., Rosenberger, J. L. & Leetma, H. E. (1972) Identification of individuals with covert ischaemic thrombotic cerebrovascular disease: A discriminate function analysis. *Stroke*, **3**, 764–771.
Howard, F. A., Cohen, P., Hickler, R. B., Newcomb, T. & Tyler, H. R. (1963) Survival following stroke. *Journal of the American Medical Association*, **183**, 921–925.
Kannel, W. B. (1971) Current status of the epedemiology of brain infarction associated with occlusive arterial disease. *Stroke*, **2**, 295–318.
Marquardsen, J. (1969) The natural history of acute cerebrovascular disease. A retrospective study of 769 patients. *Acta Neurologica Scandinavica Supplementum*, **38**, 45. Copenhagen: Munksgaard.

Marshall, J. & Wilkinson, I. M. S. (1971) The prognosis of carotid transient ischaemic attacks in patients with normal angiograms. *Brain*, **94**, 395–402.
Silverstein, A. & Doniger, D. E. (1963) Systemic and local conditions predisposing to ischaemic and occlusive cerebrovascular disease. *Journal of the Mount Sinai Hospital, New York*, **30**, 435–450.
Stock, J. P. P. (1969) *Diagnosis and Treatment of Cardiac Arrhythmias*. London: Butterworth.
Ziegler, D. K. & Hassanein, R. S. (1973) Prognosis in patients with transient ischaemic attacks. *Stroke*, **4**, 666–673.

CHAPTER NINE

Relevance of Site of Ischaemia to Prognosis

Diffuse vascular disease consequent on atheroma is the main factor in determining the ultimate outcome in patients presenting with symptoms of cerebral ischaemia. In addition, it is clear that hypertension, whatever the precise mechanism of its effect may be, has an important role in dictating the prognosis in these patients in terms of both morbidity and mortality. The main index of hypertension is, of course, the record of the blood pressure but a subsidiary one may be the presence of an abnormal ECG although this, in its turn, may also be an expression of diffuse vascular disease based on atheroma.

Minor roles have been assigned in the literature to other facets of the clinical picture. Three of these are the stroke pattern in the individual patient, the relevance of the anatomical site of brain ischaemia to prognosis and, finally, the information as to future prognosis that can be gained by cerebral angiography.

STROKE PATTERN

The term 'stroke pattern' covers two aspects of the clinical picture. The first is the temporal profile, and by this is meant the speed at which an individual patient notes the onset of disability, for it has been observed that a neurological deficit which is maximal either at or soon after the onset implies an increased morbidity and mortality. This statement relates only to the initial episode, for the majority of observers now agree that recurrent episodes are almost invariably associated with progressive morbidity and mortality. This latter fact also raises a point already considered in relation to hypertension, and that is the possibility that the quality of the episodes in recurrent stroke may differ from those seen in single stroke and thus explain the adverse effect on prognosis.

Temporal profile and prognosis

Some years ago, it was common teaching that the mode of onset of neuro-logical deficit in the stroke syndrome was all-important in differentiating between cerebral embolisation and cerebral thrombosis. Since the latter rarely occurs as a primary event, and the former, where the emboli arise from the major thoracic and cervical vessels, is responsible for many examples of what would previously have been regarded as cerebral thrombosis, this clinical point has tended to be neglected.

Millikan and Moersch (1953) were interested in the mode of onset of an episode and they observed a significant difference in the morbidity and mortality in two groups of patients who were classified according to the speed with which they developed symptoms. In 37 patients in whom the hemiplegia developed within three hours after the onset of symptoms, 33 died or remained hemiplegic two weeks later. By contrast, half the patients where the hemiplegia evolved in a period longer than six hours were found to be improved within two weeks.

It is clear from the literature that there is no consistent pattern of evolution where observations have been made on the mode of onset of stroke. David and Heyman (1960), for example, observed in 64 patients that the onset was sudden in 86 per cent of them but 'stepwise' in 8 per cent. They did not, however, relate the mode of onset to the outcome. Wallace (1967) recorded that the onset was stuttering in 17 per cent of his series of 158 patients. Olivares et al (1973) in a study of 206 patients with a stroke secondary to cerebral haemorrhage, cerebral thrombosis or cerebral emboli, found that the onset was gradual in 37 per cent; this is a higher proportion than that noted by either Wallace or David and Heyman. It seems highly probable that the variations noted were due to differences in the patients selected for study.

Another traditional belief was that cerebral thrombosis was more likely to occur during sleep than during the waking hours. Since most of the population studied have a sleep pattern that involves devoting 25 to 30 per cent of the day to sleep, one would anticipate that a greater proportion of patients than this would awake with the signs of a developing or developed stroke if this old belief were true. To explain the higher proportion one would presumably have to subscribe to the view that the fall in blood pressure during sleep is the main contributory factor. Certainly, the figures of Hamilton et al (1954), which give an example of a fall in systolic blood pressure of 32 mm Hg during sleep, would suggest that if such fluctuations were relevant a sig-nificant number of patients would develop a stroke during the hours of sleep. Certainly, Olivares et al (1973) observed cerebral haemorrhage to develop during sleep in only 20 per cent of their patients as compared with the develop-ment of a stroke due to 'thrombosis' while the patient was at rest in 66 per cent. However, they were concerned with only small numbers.

The most convincing evidence on this point comes from Aring and Merritt (1935) in their study of the clinical differentiation between cerebral haemor-rhage and cerebral thrombosis. In 245 patients who came to post mortem they found that the time of onset was evenly distributed throughout the 24 hours.

Prineas and Marshall (1966) examined the possible role of hypertension affecting the mode of onset of symptoms. In 134 patients they could detect no significant difference in the mode of onset of stroke whether the patient was hypertensive or not.

By no means all observers subscribe to the view that the mode of onset is relevant to the long-term prognosis. Lindgren (1958), Lascelles and Burrows (1965) and Baker, Schwartz and Ramseyer (1968) all examined this point and could find no evidence that this was so. However, both Lindgren (1958) and Carter (1964) felt that a rapid onset did affect the early prognosis in terms of the immediate disability.

In *the present series* details of the mode of onset were known for 164 patients with a history of a single stroke only and for 185 patients with a history of recurrent episodes. The details contrasting the mode of onset within each group and the potential effect of the mode of onset, and the ultimate mortality are shown in Table 9.1.

Table 9.1. Relationship of mode of onset of first episode to mortality in 349 patients with a stroke.

Clinical group	Total	Rapid onset		Slow onset	
			6–24 hours	24–48 hours	48 hours +
Single stroke	164	77%	11%	9%	3%
% Incidence in deceased		(79%)			
% Incidence in living		(76%)			
Recurrent stroke	185	83%	13%	2%	3%
% Incidence in deceased		(88%)			
% Incidence in living		(80%)			

Clearly, both groups are similar in that the majority of patients, regardless of the subsequent history, noted a rapid evolution of the initial stroke. Equally clearly, the speed of evolution had no apparent effect on the ultimate prognosis. It is worth emphasising again that these patients are survivors from the first acute episode and, therefore, these observations do not directly conflict with the observations originally made by Millikan and Moersch (1953).

The histories of patients who had clinical symptoms of transient cerebral ischaemia (TCI) preceding the stroke were also examined in a similar manner but they did not contribute any further relevant information.

Severity of initial episode and prognosis

In considering the differences in outcome of the single stroke group and those with recurrent episodes the quality of the individual episodes may be important. This has already been considered in relation to the level of the systemic blood pressure but, unlike Prineas and Marshall (1966), we found no evidence of any significant difference in the medium-term prognosis that could relate to the level of the blood pressure. Regardless of the blood pressure, if it is postulated that there is a different pathological substrate in a significant number of patients with recurrent episodes, then it might be possible to detect this by comparing the first episode in patients with a single stroke and those with recurrent episodes.

It appears, however, that it is the actual repetition rather than the quality of each individual episode that is important. This statement is based on a study of recovery of function following an initial episode after a period of three months (Table 9.2). At the end of this time, the respective outcomes in the single stroke cases and in patients who had a history that was ultimately that of recurrent episodes were compared, because it was felt that this period of time was sufficient to allow significant comparison between the two. For practical purposes the outcome at three months was the same.

Table 9.2. Degree of neurological disability at three months after the acute episode in 159 patients with a history of single stroke, and 156 patients with a history of multiple strokes.

	Total	Grade 1	Grade 2	Grade 3	Grade 4	Unknown
Single stroke	159	40	61	44	14	5
Multiple strokes	156	50	48	48	10	29
	315	90	109	92	24	34

$\chi^2 = 0.02; v = 1; P > 0.05$

For definition of grades see Table 5.7, p. 135.

With this point established, the state of recovery in all patients who presented with a stroke were examined at intervals of three, six, nine and twelve months. The numbers available for analysis gradually fall because of the occurrence of further stroke episodes. The analysis simply makes the point that there is a trend towards improving function over the subsequent year.

ANATOMICAL SITE

For many years the anatomical site of the stroke has been thought to be of considerable importance in terms of prognosis. When considering this point it is common practice in the literature, and a practice followed in the analysis of the present series, to classify the patients according to the three major arterial territories involved; that is, the right and left carotid circulations and the vertebro-basilar circulation. This it is usually possible to do with a fair degree of accuracy although, admittedly, there are difficulties. For example, in the syndrome of TCI, differentiation between the fore brain and the hind brain vascular territories is not always easy. A good example is transient hemiparesis without any other distinctive characteristics. However, it is the usual experience that the later evolution of clinical symptoms, even in this particular clinical example, usually enables assignment to a particular territory with a fair degree of confidence. In other cases the unfortunate later development of a stroke frequently clarifies the original site of ischaemia.

In the modern literature, the recognition of involvement of a specific

intracerebral terminal artery is rarely attempted. Current views on pathogenesis make this exercise hardly rewarding. Perhaps a classical example of
this is occlusion of the posterior inferior cerebellar artery. There is no doubt
that the results of occlusion of this particular artery achieved undue prominence over many years and the prominence was out of all proportion to its
frequency in clinical practice. There is equally little doubt that the reason
for this prominence was the very precise anatomical correlation which could
be achieved with demonstrable physical signs. Lesions in this particular area
of the brain stem are now more properly characterised in the broader context
of the lateral medullary syndrome, due mainly to the work of Fisher (1960).
Fisher emphasised the numerous variations in the anatomical distributions of
the arteries in this territory and for this reason alone preferred the broader
categorisation. Moreover, recent clinico-pathological correlations by
Castaigne et al (1973) have demonstrated that the majority, if not all, of
these cases are in fact the expression of occlusions of the vertebral artery.

Transient ischaemic attacks and site

The distribution of transient ischaemic attacks as observed by several
authors is set out in Table 9.3. Both Marshall (1964) and Baker, Ramseyer
and Schwartz (1968) found the syndrome to occur with approximately equal
frequency in the carotid and vertebro-basilar circulation. Ziegler and
Hassanein (1973) added to the traditional fore-brain and hind-brain circulation figures a mixed group where they thought it was not justifiable on clinical
grounds to allocate firmly to the carotid or vertebro-basilar circulation. While
acknowledging that complete precision is not always possible, most observers
would not be content to go so far as Ziegler and Hassanein (1973) in
allocating as many as 40 per cent to this mixed group.

Table 9.3. Anatomical site of TCI in reported series.

Author		Carotid (per cent)	Vertebro-basilar (per cent)	Mixed (per cent)
Baker, Ramseyer and Schwartz (1968)		53	44	–
Personal series (1971)		28.4	71.4	–
Marshall (1964)	Group 1	50	50	
	Group 2	42.6	57.4	
Ziegler & Hassanein (1973)		17.4	40.4	42.2

In the present series, the ratio of vertebral to carotid involvement in TCI
is significantly higher than in any other series. We have no absolute explanation for this discrepancy. If we accept the pathological evidence that thrombo-
embolism is the commonest mechanism for TCI then it is possibly not correct
to compare two carotid circulations with one vertebro-basilar circulation.
The vertebro-basilar circulation is ultimately a single anatomical entity, but
it derives from both subclavian arteries and these are a frequent site of
atheromatous ulceration and, by implication, the source of emboli to the
vertebro-basilar circulation. This, however, would do no more than equalise
the incidence of TCI in the fore-brain and the hind-brain circulations. We

believe the true reason for the high incidence of vertebro-basilar ischaemia in this series is that the majority of patients with symptoms of TCI were referred initially to the routine diagnostic neurological clinic, which resulted in a higher proportion of diagnostic problems and, therefore, a higher proportion of patients with vertebro-basilar ischaemia being represented.

Relationship of transient cerebral ischaemia to infarct

If micro-embolism is a common mechanism accounting for TCI then it would be reasonable to predict first of all that the pattern of TCI would be stereotyped in individual patients. It would also be reasonable to expect that the stroke, when it develops, would occur within the same arterial territory as that involved in TCI.

It is undoubtedly true that patients with TCI give a clinical history in which the episodes mimic the previous one down to the smallest detail. Why this should be so is uncertain, since the underlying proposition suggests that small emboli from a remote site of arterial disease are capable of retracing the route of their predecessors with monotonous regularity. This concept has been so difficult for some to accept that doubt has been expressed about the validity of the concept of micro-embolism in this particular group of patients. It is, of course, equally true that many patients describe episodes that indicate that the emboli are restricted to a major arterial territory but do vary from episode to episode in their clinical content.

The fact that most observers are content to classify patients presenting with TCI according to the arterial territory affected as judged by the clinical symptoms would argue that the pattern of attacks in the majority of patients is basically stereotyped. Both in Marshall's (1964) series and in the present one the clinical diagnosis indicating the arterial site of TCI has been compared with the clinical features of the ultimate stroke. If these results are examined, a clear result emerges (Table 9.4). In a total of 126 patients in which the pattern was for practical purposes identical, in only 29 patients (23 per cent) did the

Table 9.4. Arterial site of stroke in relation to territory previously affected by TCI.

Site of TIA	Total no.	Stroke same territory	Stroke other territory
Marshall (1964)			
R. carotid	16	16	0
L. carotid	17	13	4
V. basilar	33	25	8
Generalised	2	0	2
Personal series			
R. carotid	6	3	3
L. carotid	9	9	0
V. basilar	43	31	12
Total	126	97	29

first stroke observed occur in a territory other than that which would have been predicted by the original episode of TCI. Ziegler and Hassanein (1973) also noted the constancy of pattern in the clinical attack where only 16 per cent of the total number of patients observed complained of a change of symptomatology, indicating involvement of a different arterial territory during the period of observation.

Since it seems clear from the facts outlined that a stroke will usually occur in the same territory as that involved by prior TCI, it is no surprise to find that in the personal series an apparently disproportionate number of strokes should have occurred due to infarction in the vertebro-basilar territory. The fact that involvement of the left and right carotid territories is observed significantly less frequently as the site of the first episode of TCI is also controlled by this factor.

TCI attacks after stroke

Marshall (1964) studied the site of TIAs which followed the stroke and found the same trend that was noted in TIAs before stroke. In nine strokes in the right carotid artery territory, TIAs occurred in the same territory in seven. In seven strokes in the vertebro-basilar territory, TIAs followed in the vertebro-basilar territory in all. However, in the left carotid territory, in 13 cases the pattern was inconsistent and only 5 followed in the same territory. A different but complementary analysis was carried out on the personal series, and the results are depicted in Figure 9.1. It demonstrates not only that TIAs in one territory are followed by strokes in the same territory at a frequency which reached statistical significance, but also that TIAs following the first stroke tended to affect the same territory. In the case of the second stroke, the occurrence of transient attacks in the same territory reached statistical significance only in the vertebro-basilar circulation.

Strokes

In patients presenting with a stroke, the relative frequency of involvement of the arterial sites appeared to vary from study to study. Wright and Millikan (1958) found a predominance of right hemiplegia in chronic hospital wards. Lascelles and Burrows (1965), studying an entirely different population, which in terms of cerebral vascular disease was highly selected, reported results on 59 patients with angiographic confirmation of occlusion of the middle cerebral artery; they found 33 occlusions in the territory of the left middle cerebral artery as compared with 26 in the territory of the right.

In a clinical and radiological study, Fogelholm and Vuolio (1967) examined the distribution of occlusions of the internal carotid artery. In a series of 77 patients there was no significant difference between the two sides since 39 were occluded on the right and 38 on the left. Wallace (1967), in a study of an elderly population in general practice could find no significant difference in the site of the stroke, since 65 occurred in the left hemisphere and 61 affected the right hemisphere. Moskowitz, Lightbody and Freitag (1972) in a long-term follow up of elderly patients found on the basis of the clinical signs that the right and left hemispheres were equally involved.

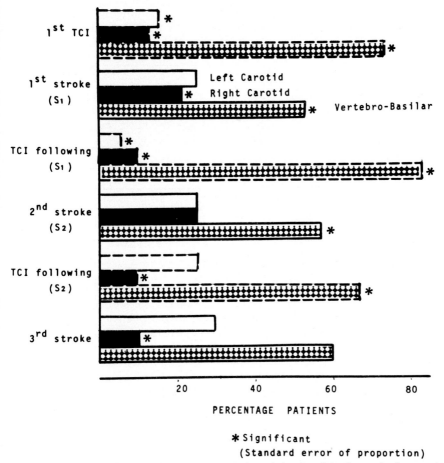

Figure 9.1. Comparison of site of transient ischaemia and the site of the first and subsequent strokes (*significant, i.e. more than twice the standard error from a mean proportion of 0.33).

SINGLE STROKE

In the present series, in 164 patients (112 male and 52 female) where the history throughout was confined to a single stroke there was no evidence that one territory was involved more frequently than the remainder (Table 9.5). These figures do show that there is an obvious disproportion between

Table 9.5. Distribution of the site of the vascular lesion in 164 patients with single stroke (112 male, 52 female).

	Total in group	Left carotid		Right carotid		Vertebro-basilar	
Male	112	40	35.7%	29	25.9%	43	38.4%
Female	52	22	42.3%	14	26.9%	16	30.8%
Male plus female	164	62	37.8%	43	26.2%	59	36.0%

involvement of the left and right carotid arteries in different patients, in that 62 had signs indicating involvement of the left carotid as compared with 43 of the right carotid, but this difference did not achieve statistical significance.

MULTIPLE STROKES (Table 9.6)

In patients with recurrent episodes the information on 185 patients was available for analysis. In the first episode it was observed that in 42 per cent (58) of the male patients the left carotid was the most frequently involved, and this achieved statistical significance. As a corollary, the territory of the

Table 9.6. Distribution of the site of the first episode of vascular disturbance in 185 patients with multiple strokes (138 male, 47 female).

	Total in group	Left carotid		Right carotid		Vertebro-basilar	
Male	138	58[a]	42.0%	31[a]	22.5%	49	35.5%
Female	47	10	21.3%	16	34.0%	21	44.7%
Male plus female	185	68	36.8%	47[a]	25.4%	70	37.8%

[a]Significant (S.E. of the proportion)

right carotid artery was significantly less often involved, being affected in only 31 male patients. How much significance one should attach to this finding is uncertain and the uncertainty is increased when no such discrepancy was observed in 47 female patients. A similar reserve applies to the fact that when the male and female patients were combined, the territory of the right carotid artery was significantly the least often involved.

In considering recurrent episodes it is of interest to examine the distribution of the subsequent strokes in relation to the presenting site in a manner similar to that we have employed in TCI (*see* p. 195). On the basis of a proposition that the thrombo-embolic mechanism is the commonest operative factor one might anticipate that if the carotid or subclavian vessels are the main source of emboli this would be reflected in the pattern of subsequent infarction. One would expect that infarction of an area of brain supplied by a single major artery would be followed by recurrent episodes in that same arterial territory. It is true from the analysis that the majority of recurrent episodes (59 per cent) occurred in the same area of arterial supply as the initial one but, on the other hand, there were a large proportion of these episodes (41 per cent) occurring in a territory other than that which was the site of the first stroke (Table 9.7).

This interesting variation prompted an examination of a possible relationship between the level of the blood pressure, on the one hand, and the incidence of recurrent episodes in single and multiple sites, on the other. As will be demonstrated later, we failed on clinical grounds to differentiate with any confidence between cerebral ischaemia and localised intracerebral haematoma, and in the latter there is no reason why the pathological lesions should be confined to the vascular territory of one major artery. The results of the examination indicate that the number of patients with involvement of multiple arterial sites is higher in patients with a diastolic pressure of 110 mm Hg or more and, conversely, a significantly higher number of patients with involvement

Table 9.7. The incidence of multiple strokes confined to a single arterial territory compared with multiple strokes involving different arterial territories.

	Male	Female		Total
Single site				
L. carotid only	31	5		36
R. carotid only	21	6		27
Vertebro-basilar only	30	16		46
			Total	109 (59%)
Multiple site				
L. & R. carotid	11	11		22
Vertebro-basilar & L. carotid	30	6		36
Vertebro-basilar & R. carotid	15	3		18
			Total	76 (41%)
Single territory = 109 = 59%				
Multiple territory = 76 = 41%				

of a single territory with a diastolic pressure below 110 mm Hg (Table 9.8). This observation has obvious clinical implications but would need to be confirmed by further observations.

Another factor that emerged from the analysis of the group of patients with recurrent episodes was found when the site of the second, third and fourth episodes of stroke were examined. For the analysis there were a sufficient number of patients who went on to two, three, and four episodes

Table 9.8. Single or multiple sites of recurrent episodes compared with the level of initial diastolic blood pressure in 157 patients with multiple strokes.

	Total in group	Initial diastolic blood pressure less than 110 mm Hg	Initial diastolic blood pressure 110 mm Hg or more
Stroke episodes confined to one major vascular territory	76	43*	33
Stroke episodes involving more than one major vascular territory	81	33	48*
	157	76	81
	$\chi^2 = 3.92; v = 1; P < 0.05$ *Significant		

(Reproduced from the *Quarterly Journal of Medicine*, 1972, by permission).

to examine the point statistically. It was found that the vertebro-basilar circulation was significantly the most frequent site of subsequent stroke and the right carotid was significantly the least involved in multiple stroke episodes of the major vessels (Figure 9.2).

The reason for this is again uncertain but, as was discussed in TCI (and this possibly applies with even more force in the stroke syndrome), the incidence of episodes attributed to the vertebro-basilar circulation should probably be halved, thus obtaining a more appropriate apportionment between the responsibility of the two subclavian and carotid arteries in the pathogenesis of strokes.

In the 36 patients who presented with TCI and subsequently went on to suffer recurrent strokes, 30 showed the trend already referred to, namely, that recurrent episodes continued in the territory initially affected and that

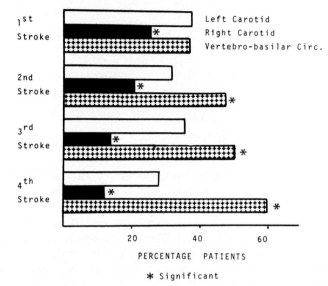

Figure 9.2. Distribution of anatomical site of stroke episodes up to and including the fourth in 185 patients with multiple strokes (*significant, i.e. more than twice the standard error from a mean proportion of 0.33).

this was irrespective of the number of episodes observed. In contrast 6 patients showed a more diffuse pattern with more than one vascular territory being involved. The numbers of patients available for analysis were too small to make a statistical assessment, but even so no recognisable trend was noted.

ARTERIAL SITE, MORBIDITY AND MORTALITY

Transient cerebral ischaemia

MORBIDITY

Marshall (1964), in 68 patients with a history of TCI found that the prognosis of TCI occurring in the vertebro-basilar territory was relatively better than that in the carotid distribution in relation to the length of time before the stroke occurred. His analysis showed that in the vertebro-basilar territory, symptoms were present for some 23 months before the onset of stroke, whereas in the carotid territory the period of time was only 14 months and this difference achieved significance at a 1 per cent level.

Baker, Ramseyer and Schwartz (1968) studied 79 patients with TCI and 53 of these were seen before the stroke occurred. The remainder gave a history of TCI prior to the stroke which had occurred before they came under observation. The final disability was assessed at the end of a two-year period of study. The outcome in patients with involvement of the vertebro-basilar circulation was certainly better than patients with carotid territory involvement. Of the patients in the vertebro-basilar group 85 per cent had achieved a state the authors classified as 'none or minimal disability', which indicated that they were fully active. This compared favourably with the figure of 64 per cent for patients who achieved this level of improvement when the carotid territory was the original site of involvement. Similar observations were made by Ziegler and Hassanein (1973) in their study of 109 patients.

In the present series, the question of morbidity at the end of the study applies only to 66 surviving patients, who were the residuum of the 94 who presented with TCI and subsequently developed a stroke.

Six of the patients were disabled from causes unrelated to vascular disease, leaving 60 available for analysis. Of these, 49 (80 per cent), were working full time either at their old job or at a lighter job. These were subdivided according to the site of the first episode of TCI and a subsequent stroke, and then the degree of disability in these subgroups was compared. Of the patients with symptoms indicating involvement of the vertebro-basilar circulation only, 90 per cent were working full time as compared with 82 per cent of the whole group. The numbers, however, were too small for analysis.

Twenty-one patients who presented with TCI went on to multiple strokes, and 71.4 per cent of these were working full time at the end of the period of observation. Again, although it cannot be established statistically, patients with involvement in the vertebro-basilar circulation apparently had a better prognosis than those affecting the carotid, since 83 per cent of the former group were working full time.

MORTALITY

The mortality in patients who presented with TCI was clearly related in part, at any rate, to the development of a complicating stroke. An analysis was made, therefore, of patients where TCI in the carotid artery territory was compared with TCI in the vertebro-basilar circulation. There was no evidence, however, of any connection between mortality and the anatomical site of the symptoms.

Stroke

In patients presenting with a stroke, it has been stated that the prognosis may relate in part to the anatomical site in that lesions in the vertebro-basilar territory carry a worse prognosis than patients presenting with a lesion in the carotid territory. The evidence now available indicates that this is not necessarily true but opinion on the true state of affairs remains divided.

Marshall and Shaw (1959) examined this proposition but in their observations they found that vascular lesions of the hemisphere carried a prognosis that was certainly as bad and probably worse than that found in patients with lesions of the vertebro-basilar territory. McDowell, Potes and Groch (1961) also could find no support for the view that vertebro-basilar ischaemia carried a worse prognosis. They studied 57 patients with clinical and angiographic evidence of carotid artery disease and compared them with 50 patients with clinical evidence of vertebro-basilar ischaemia. They concluded that disabilities were less in survivors with symptoms indicating involvement of the vertebro-basilar arteries.

Baker, Schwartz and Ramseyer (1968) studied the prognosis of 430 patients with stroke and found that in 80 per cent of the patients the carotid territory was involved as compared with 20 per cent who had involvement of the vertebro-basilar territory. They observed, however, that in the patients in the latter group not only was the initial disability less but significant recovery was more rapid and complete.

David and Heyman (1960), in a study of 100 patients with cerebral infarction, found that 40 per cent of the patients died when the infarction was in the carotid territory; this compared unfavourably with the death rate of 28 per cent in patients who died with a lesion of the vertebro-basilar circulation.

In spite of these reports there is still no general agreement on this point. Marshall and Kaeser (1961), in a prospective study of 177 patients, were unable to demonstrate any clear relationship between the site of the lesion and the ultimate survival. Carter (1964) also failed to demonstrate any difference in terms of survival when he analysed cases according to the original site of involvement, although he did observe, and had, of course, anticipated, that patients with bilateral diffuse hemisphere lesions carried a bad prognosis. Finally, Adams and Merrett (1961) could find no evidence that the anatomical site of the stroke was relevant to survival.

Considering the morbidity in *the present series*, in patients presenting with stroke, they were again subdivided into two groups on the basis of the history of a single stroke or recurrent episodes. Admittedly, the excellent prognosis in the single stroke group must have been an expression of selection, nevertheless it did afford an interesting contrast to patients with a history of subsequent recurrent episodes since these latter originally presented in an identical way. It is this contrast between the two groups that is important.

Of the 122 survivors, physical disability from other causes was present in 10, leaving 112 patients for consideration. Of these 88 (78.6 per cent) were working full time. There is a suggestion, but no more than that, that the patients with a stroke in the vertebro-basilar circulation did rather better than those in whom the carotid territory was involved. Of the former, 95.6 per cent were working full time as compared with 83.6 per cent of the patients in the latter category (Table 9.9).

In patients who ultimately went on to recurrent episodes in the course of the study, there were only 94 survivors and of these 8 were disabled from other causes.

To make any comparison between the arterial sites it was necessary, in order to achieve adequate group size, to combine patients showing complete functional recovery with those who showed a moderate disability at the end of the study. Also grouped together for the puipose of comparison were

Table 9.9. Site of vascular disturbance and disability in 112 surviving patients with a history of a single stroke

	Total alive and disabled from cerebral vascular disease	Grade 1	Grade 2	Grade 3	Grade 4	Disabled other causes
Left carotid	41	29 70.7%	5 12.2%	4 9.8%	3 7.3%	4
Right carotid	26	20 76.9%	2 7.7%	4 15.4%	0 –	4
Vertebro-basilar	45	39 86.7%	4 8.9%	1 2.2%	1 2.2%	2
	112	88 78.6%	11 9.8%	9 8.0%	4 3.6%	10

patients with marked disability and those who were bedridden.

It was also necessary to group together patients where the ischaemic lesion was in the vertebro-basilar circulation, and these were compared with a group of cases with involvement of the left and right carotid territories. No significant association could be found between a history of recurring episodes, morbidity and anatomical site.

In view of these findings and the observations recorded from the literature, the effect of the arterial site on survival is marginal if it is relevant at all.

ANGIOGRAPHY

The contribution of cerebral angiography to the progressive understanding of cerebral vascular disease has been considerable. Not the least of its contributions has been the evidence produced that it is not possible, in the majority of patients, to make a diagnosis of internal carotid occlusion on the basis of the evolution of signs. Bull, Marshall and Shaw (1960) examined the angiographic findings in 80 patients where a diagnosis of internal carotid artery occlusion had been made on clinical grounds. They demonstrated that even the most expert observers cannot differentiate with certainty between carotid artery disease in the neck and occlusion of the intracranial portion of the middle cerebral artery. Sutton and Davies (1966) studied arch aortograms carried out in cases of TCI and were unable to correlate the angiographic abnormalities and the clinical syndromes.

It would not be expected that angiography would make any major contribution to the understanding of the natural history of ischaemic cerebral vascular disease. The reason for this, or course, is that patients submitted for angiography will be a highly selected group, many of whom are potential candidates for vascular surgery. This will exclude, and it is proper that it should do so, the majority of patients suffering from cerebral vascular disease of ischaemic type. Nevertheless, provided selection is borne in mind, some useful information is available.

Lindgren (1958) studied 65 angiographically proven examples of internal carotid artery occlusion in the neck and patients with intracerebral arterial occlusion. The average age was only 42.7 years but the survival rate did not appear to be very much different from that in other series. At the end of two years, 24 per cent had died and 60 per cent were either working or were capable of full self-care.

Acheson et al (1969) reported observations which related the angiographic findings to the type of clinical presentation and to the outcome in 149 patients observed for a mean period of 58 months. They confirmed previous observations on the lack of correlation between angiography and the clinical symptomatology. They did, however, observe a highly significant association between a normal angiogram, on the one hand, and an abnormal angiogram, on the other, and the prognosis. As might be expected, the patients with normal angiograms showed better functional recovery over the period of observation than those with an abnormal angiogram, and this was particularly true if the abnormality consisted of a total arterial occlusion. A previous communication by Shenkin, Haft and Somach (1965) had reached broadly similar conclusions.

These findings do not infer that normal angiography in the face of clinical symptoms of TCI carries a good prognosis. Marshall and Wilkinson (1971) specifically examined the prognosis in TCI in 64 patients who showed normal angiograms. Patients were followed for a mean time of 5.4 years. Although 20 per cent had further TCI episodes only, 16 per cent had serious cerebral vascular episodes and 17 per cent significant cardiovascular lesions. The overall mortality rate from causes related to vascular disease in the series was 11 per cent.

CONCLUSIONS

1. The mode of onset of the first stroke has no effect on the ultimate prognosis in survivors.
2. In patients with recurrent episodes the neurological deficit and subsequent recovery after the first stroke are identical with those observed in patients who have a single stroke only.
3. If TCI is complicated by the subsequent development of a stroke, the stroke commonly occurs in the territory affected by prior TCI.
4. Patients who have recurrent episodes and a diastolic blood pressure of 110 mm Hg or more are more likely to have strokes in multiple arterial sites when compared with other patients with recurrent attacks but with a diastolic blood pressure below this level. The reason for this finding awaits clarification.
5. There is only minimal evidence that the arterial site of ischaemia affects the prognosis in survivors from stroke. The patient with a vertebro-basilar 'stroke' does marginally better in terms of the recovery of function than does a patient with a carotid stroke.

REFERENCES

Acheson, J., Boyd, W. N , Hugh, A. E. & Hutchinson, E. C. (1969) Cerebral angiography in ischaemic cerebro-vascular disease. *Archives of Neurology*, **20**, 527–532.

Adams, G. F. & Merrett, J. D. (1961) Prognosis and survival in the aftermath of hemiplegia. *British Medical Journal*, **i**, 309–314.

Aring, C. D. & Merritt, H. H. (1935) Differential diagnosis between cerebral haemorrhage and cerebral thrombosis. A clinical and pathological study of 245 cases. *Archives of Internal Medicine*, **56**, 435–456.

Baker, R. N., Ramseyer, J. C. & Schwartz, W. S. (1968) Prognosis in patients with transient cerebral ischaemic attacks. *Neurology*, **18**, 1157–1165.

Baker, R. N., Schwartz, W. S. & Ramseyer, J. C. (1968) Prognosis among survivors of ischaemic stroke. *Neurology*, **18**, 933–941.

Bull, J. W. D., Marshall, J. & Shaw, D. A. (1960) Cerebral angiography in the diagnosis of the acute stroke. *Lancet*, **i**, 562–565.

Carter, B. (1964) *Cerebral Infarction*. Oxford–New York: Pergamon.

Castaigne, P., Lhermitte, F., Gautier, J. C., Escourolle, R., Derouesné, C., Der Agopian, P. & Popa, C. (1973) Arterial occlusions in the vertebro-basilar system. A study of 44 patients with post-mortem data. *Brain*, **96**, 133–154.

David, N. J. & Heyman, A. (1960) Factors influencing the prognosis of cerebral thrombosis and infarction due to atherosclerosis. *Journal of Chronic Diseases*, **11**, 394–404.

Fisher, C. M. (1960) *Pathogenesis of Cerebrovascular Disease*. Illinois: Thomas.

Fogelholm, R. & Vuolio, M. (1967) A clinical and radiological analysis of 77 patients with internal carotid artery thrombosis. *Acta Neurologica Scandinavica*, **43**, 120–121.

Hamilton, M., Pickering, G. W., Roberts, F. & Sowry, G. S. C. (1954) The aetiology of essential hypertension (1) The arterial pressure in the general population. *Clinical Science*, **13**, 11–35.

Lascelles, R. G. & Burrows, E. H. (1965) Occlusion of the middle cerebral artery. *Brain*, **88**, 85–96.

Lindgren, S. O. (1958) Course and prognosis in spontaneous occlusions of cerebral arteries. *Acta Psychiatrica and Neurologica Scandinavica*, **33**, 343–358.

McDowell, F. H., Potes, J. & Groch, S. (1961) The natural history of internal carotid and vertebro-basilar artery occlusion. *Neurology*, **11**, 153–157.

Marshall, J. & Shaw, D. A. (1959) The natural history of cerebro-vascular disease. *British Medical Journal*, **i**, 1614–1617.

Marshall, J. & Kaeser, A. C. (1961) Survival of the non-haemorrhagic cerebrovascular accidents. A prospective study. *British Medical Journal*, **ii**, 73–77.

Marshall, J. & Wilkinson, I. M. S. (1971) The prognosis of carotid transient ischaemic attacks in patients with normal angiograms. *Brain*, **94**, 395–402.

Marshall, J. (1964) The natural history of transient ischaemic cerebrovascular attacks. *Quarterly Journal of Medicine*, **33**, 309–324.

Millikan, C. H. & Moersch, F. P. (1953) Factors that influence prognosis in acute focal cerebrovascular lesions. *Archives of Neurology and Psychiatry* (Chicago), **70**, 558–562.

Moskowitz, E., Lightbody, F. E. H. & Freitag, N. S. (1972) Long term follow-up of the post-stroke patient. *Archives of Physical Medicine and Rehabilitation*, **53**, 167–172.

Olivares, L., Castaneda, E., Grifé, A. & Alter, M. (1973) Risk factors in stroke: A clinical study in Mexican patients. *Stroke*, **4**, 773–781.

Prineas, J. & Marshall, J. (1966) Hypertension and cerebral infarction. *British Medical Journal*, **i**, 14–17.

Shenkin, H. A., Haft, H. & Somach, F. M. (1965) Prognostic significance of arteriography in non-haemorrhagic strokes. *Journal of American Medical Association*, **194**, 612–616.

Sutton, D. & Davies, E. R. (1966) Arch aortography and cerebrovascular insufficiency. *Clinical Radiology*, **17**, 330–345.

Wallace, D. C. (1967) A study of the natural history of cerebral vascular disease. *Medical Journal of Australia*, **1**, 90–95.

Wright, I. S. & Millikan, C. H. (1958) *Cerebral Vascular Diseases* (Second Conference). New York and London: Grune and Stratton.

Ziegler, D. K. & Hassanein, R. S. (1973) Prognosis in patients with transient ischaemic attacks. *Stroke*, **4**, 466–673.

CHAPTER TEN

Other Risk Factors: Cholesterol, Diabetes Mellitus, Intermittent Claudication and Epilepsy

While the significance of atheroma and hypertension in the prognosis of cerebral ischaemia can be appreciated, there are other factors that have been reported in the literature where an association with cerebral vascular disease has been noted. Two conditions, namely diabetes mellitus and hypercholesterolaemia, are variously believed to contribute to the development of atheroma and are, therefore, relevant not only to the diagnosis in patients with presumed cerebral ischaemia but also to the prognosis. Two others, namely, intermittent claudication and epilepsy, are, as in the case of the ECG, indices of more widespread vascular disease and therefore need to be examined when considering the natural history.

CHOLESTEROL

It is acknowledged that the attempts to relate the level of serum cholesterol and other lipids to the development of atheromatous vascular disease, whether it be in the coronary or cerebral vascular circulation, present considerable problems. It is self-evident that the finding of an elevated level of serum cholesterol—elevated that is according to an arbitrary figure expressing the normal—in a patient with established vascular disease demonstrably due to atheroma does not prove a direct association. Nor does it disprove a significant role for abnormal cholesterol levels in the development of atheroma in the years anteceding the development of clinical symptoms.

Other difficulties arise because of the wide range of normal values and the fact that the level of cholesterol in the circulating blood varies with age.

Cantarow and Trumper (1962) found that the serum cholesterol concentration increases with age, being somewhat higher in males and reaching a maximum in the sixth decade. After the menopause the values for females approach those for males. Carlson and Lindstedt (1968), in a prospective study of values for serum lipids, found that the level of serum cholesterol was the same in men and women between the ages of 25 and 49 years but that after the age of 50 there was a continuing increase in the level in women while there was a levelling off in men. Leren and Haabrekke (1971) also observed that blood lipid values rise in the healthy person with age, but they made the important point that as many as 20 per cent of 'normal' persons are shown to have an abnormal lipoprotein pattern which, of course, contributes to the difficulty of comparison between so-called normals and a series of patients.

Not only does the serum cholesterol rise with age but there is also apparently a seasonal variation. McDonough and Hames (1967) confirmed previous reports of a seasonal variation in serum cholesterol levels in an epidemiological study in Evans County, Georgia. They found a significant seasonal variation in both white and negro males but observed only borderline variations in females. To compound the difficulty in interpreting results they showed that the seasonal variation, which consisted of a fall in serum cholesterol in the late spring and summer, was confined to males in active occupation whereas it was not observed in males pursuing sedentary jobs.

However, despite the difficulties of assessing the significance of the levels of serum cholesterol it is generally believed that hyperlipidaemia is relevant to the development of coronary artery disease. The Framingham epidemiological study observed that an increased level of serum cholesterol was associated with an increased risk of developing arteriosclerotic heart disease and that although this was true at all ages it was more marked in the younger age groups (Dawber, Moore and Mann, 1957; Dawber et al, 1962; Kagan et al, 1962; Kannel et al, 1965). This point was also made in a prospective study of coronary heart disease of 1989 men by Paul et al (1963). They also showed that there was an association between an increased level of blood cholesterol and the development of coronary heart disease.

These prospective epidemiological studies provide strong support for the view that has held sway for many years that an increased incidence of hyperlipidaemia is important in relation to established coronary artery disease (Gertler, Garn and Lerman, 1950; Oliver and Boyd, 1953; Oliver and Stuart-Harris, 1965; Heinle et al, 1969).

Less attention has been given to a possible relationship between the level of the serum cholesterol and cerebral vascular disease and this applies to both transient cerebral ischaemia (TCI) and the established stroke. In the case of the latter there is little or no agreement in the literature as to the significance of the relation of the serum cholesterol.

Transient cerebral ischaemia and serum cholesterol

Relatively few observations have been made on the level of the serum cholesterol in patients presenting with TCI. Feldman and Albrink (1964) studied the serum lipids in 37 patients with completed strokes, 26 patients with TCI and 399 male controls. They found that there was not only no significant difference in the level of the serum cholesterol between the subgroups of patients with cerebral vascular disease but also that the incidence of raised serum cholesterol in patients with cerebral vascular disease was only slightly higher than in the group of normal male controls. Farid and Anderson (1972), in a pilot study of 13 men and 13 women whose ages ranged from 41 to 74 years, and who were suffering from either TCI or a stroke, found that in 6 females and 6 males the lipid patterns were normal and the abnormal lipid patterns appeared to be related to age.

In *the present series*, the level of the serum cholesterol was known in 96 per cent (55) of the 57 patients with a history of TCI only, and in 87 per cent (82) of the 94 patients who presented with TCI and later developed a stroke. The mean levels and also the distribution of patients according to the level of the serum cholesterol are shown (Table 10.1).

Table 10.1. The mean level of serum cholesterol in the clinical groups.

Clinical group	Total of cases in which recorded	Mean level of serum cholesterol (mg/100 ml)	Standard deviation
Males			
TCI only	43	248.30	46.23
TCI → stroke	64	244.71	46.53
Single stroke	95	245.78	51.88
Multiple stroke	107	238.65	46.77
All groups	309	243.44	48.11
	Not significant (Students' t-test)		
Females			
TCI only	12	272.08	44.75
TCI → stroke	18	281.66	41.73
Single stroke	39	276.00	74.59
Multiple stroke	39	274.61	46.52
All groups	108	276.00	56.91
	Not significant (Students' t-test)		

It will be seen that the mean level of the serum cholesterol for male patients with transient cerebral ischaemia only was 248.3 mg/100 ml and for female patients 272.1 mg/100 ml. The mean level of the serum cholesterol for male patients whose history was complicated later by a stroke was 244.7 mg/100 ml and for females 281.7 mg/100 ml. Although there were higher levels in females as compared with males of approximately the same age, it was noteworthy that there was no significant difference in the findings between the two groups of patients.

Stroke and serum cholesterol

There is no consistent agreement in the literature of an association between an elevation of serum lipids and the development of cerebral vascular disease. Broadly speaking, the information available can be divided into three areas. The first relates to studies where no association could be detected by observers between the level of serum cholesterol and other serum lipids, on the one hand, and cerebral vascular disease, on the other. The second group is of investigations where the observers believed that they did find a positive correlation. The third set of observations indicates that it may very well be that it is a combination of other risk factors with an elevated serum cholesterol level that is relevant, and that the most important of these is hypertension.

Several studies found no relationship between the level of the serum cholesterol in cases of established cerebral vascular disease. Marshall and Kaeser (1961), in a prospective study of 177 patients with cerebral infarction, observed that the level of the serum cholesterol had no influence on survival and that there was no significant difference in cholesterol levels between patients with a history of a single stroke or recurrent episodes. In elderly patients, Cutler (1967) studied 33 males and 29 females. No difference was observed in the serum cholesterol levels in male patients when compared with controls, and the female patients presenting with a stroke had a significantly lower mean level of serum cholesterol.

Liepelt, Skandsen and Julsrud (1972) carried out a detailed analysis using serum lipoprotein electrophoresis, cholesterol and triglyceride determinations in 54 patients with cerebral vascular disease and compared their findings with those in 94 patients with other neurological disorders. No significant difference in the two groups could be detected in lipoprotein patterns or in the mean values for cholesterol and triglyceride. A negative correlation has been reported in other control studies such as that of Meyer et al (1959) when 90 patients with cerebral vascular disease secondary to atheroma were compared with 79 control patients of comparable age. This was also true of the prospective study of Jacobson (1967) and that of Gertler et al (1968).

The observations of Kannel et al (1965) fell roughly into line with the series of negative observations since they, too, showed no significant difference in the number of brain infarctions in subjects with a serum cholesterol of 260 mg/100 ml or above when these were compared with patients showing levels below this figure. They did, however, observe an upward trend in the incidence of cerebral infarction in those patients who were below 50 years of age at the onset of their disease.

Observations which appeared to indicate an association between certain forms of cerebral vascular disease and significant elevations of the serum cholesterol have certainly been made. Heyman, Nefzger and Estes (1961) observed a significant difference in the results obtained in 68 male patients with cerebral infarction when compared with 83 male controls. Feldman and Albrink (1964) found a moderate elevation of the serum cholesterol level in patients with cerebral vascular disease compared with normal male controls. Pearce and Aziz (1970) examined the interrelationship between uric acid and serum lipids in 60 patients with cerebral vascular disease. They observed that although the level of the serum lipids was moderately higher in patients with cerebral vascular disease when compared with controls, ischaemia and infarction certainly occurred in patients with normal serum lipid values. Their view was that the elevated level of serum triglycerides was more closely associated with cerebral vascular disease than was elevation of the other lipid fractions.

The third group of observations relates to the association of risk factors of which the most important is considered to be hypertension. Cumings et al

(1967) thought that one reason for the variable findings of different observers could well be the fact that if patients are grouped clinically under the generic term of 'stroke' the process of cerebral infarction due to atheroma would obviously not be defined precisely. In an attempt to overcome this perennial difficulty they grouped together 29 patients with a diastolic blood pressure below 110 mm Hg, and 14 with a diastolic pressure of 110 mm Hg or more. They then compared the level of the serum lipids in both groups and the levels recorded in the 11 control patients. They could find no significant difference between the patients or between patients and controls. Kannel (1971), in an extension of the epidemiological studies of Framingham, felt that it was the combination of risk factors that caused an increased risk of brain infarction and that the most vulnerable groups of patients were subjects below the age of 50 with both hypertension and hyperlipidaemia. It was concluded by Kannel et al (1970) that there was no safe or critical level of either lipids or lipoprotein that could be identified in their study.

Finally, Cumings and Marshall (1968) grouped patients with clinical cerebral infarction according to the level of the diastolic blood pressure. They found that in patients with a diastolic blood pressure below 110 mm Hg the mean serum cholesterol was 228 mg/100 ml compared with 209 mg/100 ml in patients with a diastolic blood pressure greater than 110 mm Hg; the difference was not significant. They pointed out that since the difference between the serum lipid levels in patients with coronary artery disease and healthy controls vanishes with increasing age, and since patients with stroke are, on the whole, in an older age group than patients with coronary artery disease, a negative relationship could in fact be anticipated.

In the present series, the serum cholesterol was available in 81.7 per cent (134) of 164 patients with a history of single stroke only. As in TCI, the level for female patients was slightly higher than in the males, the male patients showing a figure of 245.8 mg/100 ml as compared with female patients, where the mean was 276.0 mg/100 ml. No significant difference was found between this group of patients with a history of single stroke when they were compared with the 500 patients with cerebral vascular disease (Table 10.1).

Similarly, in patients with a history of recurrent episodes, the levels were available in 78.9 per cent (146) of 185 patients with such a history (Table 10.1). Again, the female patients showed a moderate elevation as compared with the males, the figure for females being 274.6 mg/100 ml as compared with males with a mean level of 238.6 mg/100 ml. As with patients with a single stroke, no significant difference could be found in either male or female when they were compared with the total series.

If the ultimate outcome is examined in relationship to the level of the cholesterol, no significant relationship was observed (Table 10.2). Further, in examining a possible relationship between the level of serum cholesterol and the mode of dying, all deaths notified as cases of cerebrovascular disease were grouped together as were all cases of heart disease. Again, no significant association was found with the level of the serum cholesterol whether it was elevated or not.

These observations would seem to parallel the majority view expressed in the literature, that elevation of serum cholesterol does not appear to bear the

Table 10.2. Distribution of level of serum cholesterol and morbidity at end of study in 201 male and 85 female patients with cerebral vascular disease.

Final functional state	Total cases	Level of serum cholesterol—mg/100ml			
		< 200	200–249	250–299	300 or more
Males					
Complete functional recovery	134	20	47	53	14
Minimal residual disability	21	0	12	7	2
Marked disability	37	9	15	11	2
Confined to bed or chair	9	0	6	1	2
	201	29	80	72	20
	$\chi^2 = 3.28$; $v = 2$; $P > 0.05$				
Females					
Complete functional recovery	64	4	14	21	25
Minimal residual disability	0	0	0	0	0
Marked disability	10	3	2	3	2
Confined to bed or chair	11	1	1	5	4
	85	8	17	29	31
	$\chi^2 = 0.21$; $v = 1$; $P > 0.05$				

same close relationship to disease of the cerebral vasculature as it does in the case of coronary artery disease.

DIABETES MELLITUS

There is a widely held belief that the presence of overt or clinical diabetes mellitus is a significant factor in the development of atheromatous vascular disease and, by implication, ischaemic cerebral vascular disease.

The presence of overt diabetes mellitus in the community at large has been the subject of interest for some years. Pell and D'Alonzo (1960) found a prevalence in a selected population of 90 596 employees of 0.48 per cent for men and 0.27 per cent for women. A working party (Diabetes Survey Working Party, 1962) was set up by the Royal College of General Practitioners to investigate the incidence of diabetus mellitus, and it reported in 1962. In a population of 18 532 individuals, 0.64 per cent were known diabetics and in a further 0.69 per cent a diabetic abnormality was detected. The presence of glycosuria in this population was 2.6 per cent and if known diabetics were included this rose to 3.3 per cent.

From other evidence it is clear that the figures for incidence will vary with the degree of vigour with which the diagnosis of diabetes is pursued. Sharp, Butterfield and Keen (1964) conducted a survey of the incidence of diabetes mellitus in Bedford. The study was on a population of 25 701 people who were over the age of 21 years and the reported incidence of diabetes on clinical grounds only was 0.1 per cent. But, at the other extreme, where a combination of tests, culminating in the glucose tolerance test, were used to assess incidence, an incidence of up to 12 per cent was observed.

On whether the incidence of diabetes is related to the development of atheroma, opinion is divided. The variation in opinion is so wide on occasion that selection is clearly playing a major role. Grunnet (1963) studied 107 diabetic patients and was of the opinion that diabetes was definitely associated with an increase in the frequency and severity of atherosclerosis at all ages.

In contrast, however, Goldenberg, Alex and Blumenthal (1958) reported their findings in 3470 autopsies. They found an overall incidence of diabetes of 7.6 per cent but they could detect no significant difference between the diabetic and the non-diabetic with regard to the frequency of cerebral vascular disease. In sharp contrast, is a post-mortem study of 219 cases by Savre, Taveras and Stein (1964). They identified most of the cerebral vessels by post-mortem angiography. Their observations led them to conclude that, since the incidence of diabetes in their study was 23 per cent, diabetes mellitus was relevant to the development of stenotic vascular lesions.

In spite of these contrasting results the picture is clearer when clinical studies are examined. Baker, Ramseyer and Schwartz (1968), in 79 male patients presenting with TCI, found that 6.3 per cent had diabetes initially, and one further patient developed it during the period of follow-up study. Goldner, Whisnant and Taylor (1971), in 140 patients with TCI found that 8 per cent were diabetic. In the case of transient ischaemia, therefore, it would seem that the incidence of diabetes mellitus falls within the range observed by Sharp, Butterfield and Keen (1964) in the Bedford study.

In patients with an established stroke believed to be due to cerebral infarction, the observed incidence of diabetes mellitus is well above the anticipated range in the normal community with two exceptions (David and Heyman, 1960; Robinson, Demirel and LeBeau, 1968). These are shown in Table 10.3. However, it is clear that the factors of selection may very well account for the differences seen. For example, Silverstein and Doniger (1963), who found a 32 per cent incidence of diabetes mellitus in 100 patients, were studying patients with clear arteriographic evidence of occlusive vascular disease.

It is of some interest that Bental and Pillar (1972), in a study of 276 patients with an acute stroke, found the incidence of diabetes to be 27 per cent. Of this number, one-third were unaware of a diabetic state before the development of the cerebral vascular accident.

There is a suggestion, from the figures given, that the age at which the patient has the stroke may be relevant. Howard et al (1963) found that in six patients who developed 'cerebral thrombosis' below the age of 50 years, three were diabetics. Even more impressive was the study of stroke in young adults reported by Louis and McDowell (1967). In a series of 56 patients presenting with cerebral vascular disease below the age of 50, five were diabetic before the stroke occurred, six were found to have significant glycosuria in hospital, and a further ten developed diabetes during follow up, giving an incidence of diabetes for the whole group of 42 per cent.

Table 10.3. Percentage incidence of diabetes mellitus observed in patients with stroke.

	Per cent
Meyer, Waltz, Hess & Zak (1959)	12.2
David & Heyman (1960)	8.0
McDowell, Potes & Groch (1961)	15.0
Silverstein & Doniger (1963)	32.0
Baker, Schwartz & Ramseyer (1968)	13.3
Gertler, Rusk, Whiter, Leetma & Ehrenkranz (1968)	30.0
Robinson, Demirel & LeBeau (1968)	13.0
Moskowitz, Lightbody & Freitag (1972)	20.0
Bental & Pillar (1972)	27.0
Lavy, Melamed, Cahane & Carmon (1973)	20.0

The overall evidence in the established stroke would appear to indicate that the prevalence of diabetes mellitus is higher than might be expected in the general population. Several authors have taken the view that diabetes mellitus or an impaired glucose tolerance test play a role in causing cerebral infarction (Jacobson, 1967; Kannel, 1971; Kuller and Tonascia, 1971; Gertler, Rosenberger and Leetma, 1972; Gordon and Kannel, 1972). Not every report agrees on this and, for example, Root (1959) and Warren, Lecompte and Legg (1966), could find no evidence that the incidence of cerebral vascular disease was higher in the diabetics than the non-diabetics.

As far as the prognosis is concerned, Robinson et al (1959) analysed the records of 1018 hospital patients admitted in a 10-year period with a diagnosis of cerebral vascular disease, and could find no evidence that the presence of diabetes was in any way related to survival following the initial acute episode.

INTERMITTENT CLAUDICATION

Relatively little attention has been paid in the literature to the incidence of intermittent claudication and ischaemic cerebral vascular disease. Silverstein and Doniger (1963) found that in 100 patients with arteriographic evidence of occlusive cerebral vascular disease, 12 per cent also had peripheral vascular disease and six further patients showed a significant difference in the blood pressure recorded in the upper limbs. In elderly patients, Friedman, Loveland and Ehrlich (1968) found that in a control population of similar age the incidence of intermittent claudication was 2.1 per cent, whereas in patients who had sustained a stroke the incidence was 7.7 per cent.

The fact that the two diseases—which pathologically are closely related, if not identical, in all cases—should occur together occasions no surprise. In the Framingham Survey a history of intermittent claudication was associated with an increased incidence of stroke (Kannel et al, 1965; Kannel, 1966). They also made the interesting observation that although there was a predominance of males in coronary artery disease and intermittent claudication there was no male predominance in brain infarction. Gordon and Kannel (1972) came to the anticipated conclusion that atherosclerotic brain infarction, coronary heart disease and intermittent claudication appeared to have a common set of precursors, a statement that was true for both males and females.

It is of some interest to compare the natural history of intermittent claudication with cerebral vascular disease. Bloor (1961) studied 1476 patients who presented with intermittent claudication. Only 10.5 per cent of these were females, but it was clear in terms of survival rates that the presence of intermittent claudication significantly affected the outcome. In the 55 to 65 year age group the survival rate in his patients roughly paralleled that in the general population who were 10 years older. Although the incidence was much lower in females the disease pattern was very similar. Of the patients who died, the cause of death was cerebral vascular lesions in 16.6 per cent whereas in 59.5 per cent the cause of death was some form of cardiac lesion. In one-fifth of the patients who survived five years or more after the onset of symptoms a non-fatal coronary thrombosis or an intracranial vascular episode were observed.

Begg and Richards (1962) also examined the prognosis in 198 patients with intermittent claudication and in 20 per cent of these there was evidence of ischaemic heart disease when they first presented. They confirmed Bloor's finding that the commonest cause of death was ischaemic heart disease since 48.6 per cent of the patients who died did so as a result of coronary artery disease, whereas only 12 per cent of them died from an acute cerebral vascular accident.

In *the present series*, 34 patients gave a history of intermittent claudication, and specific enquiry was made in every case for the presence of the appropriate symptomatology.

In TCI without the history of a stroke there were only four male patients who gave a positive history of this disorder, whereas in 94 patients who subsequently developed a stroke there were seven patients with a history of intermittent claudication; this was not a particularly striking difference. In patients who presented with a stroke there were 22 males and 1 female patient with a history of intermittent claudication but there was no obvious difference in the incidence of intermittent claudication in the patients with a history of single stroke, on the one hand, or in those with recurrent episodes, on the other.

EPILEPSY

120 years ago, Copland (1850) commented that the association between apoplexy and epilepsy was closer than had previously been realised. He recognised that epilepsy could either precede apoplexy, occur at the onset of the stroke, or develop as a late complication of the episode. Hughlings Jackson (1881) agreed with him that the hemiplegic patient may develop convulsions but he felt that it was more likely when the hemiplegia was secondary to embolism or thrombosis. Gowers (1888) pointed out that in his experience convulsions that developed as a late complication following apoplexy were more likely to recur if the cortex of the brain was involved. He observed that epilepsy could continue indefinitely and 'such recurring convulsions are far more frequent after softening than after haemorrhage'.

Gowers's observation on involvement of the cortex has been confirmed by more modern neuropathological studies. Richardson and Dodge (1954) examined 561 autopsy records and in 427 cases the brain had been examined. In 27 per cent they found evidence of cerebral haemorrhage or cerebral infarction and on reviewing the clinical records found that a convulsion had occurred in 12.5 per cent of these as compared with 2.7 per cent of controls. They commented that the cortex of the brain was commonly involved in these cases.

Dodge, Richardson and Victor (1954) presented in detail the clinical and pathological findings in six cases of infarction and confirmed that involvement of the cortex was important in the pathogenesis of epilepsy following cerebral infarction but noted that the size of the lesion was not particularly relevant to the later development of epilepsy. They also felt that epilepsy during the acute episode should be considered as a clinical entity different from epilepsy resulting from an old vascular lesion. Louis and McDowell (1967) found an incidence of epilepsy of 7.7 per cent in 1000 patients with non-embolic cerebral infarction. The epilepsy was observed either in the acute phase or subsequently. Moskowitz, Lightbody and Freitag (1972), in 518 patients who had previously sustained a cerebral infarct, observed that epilepsy developed in 5 per cent of patients in a period of up to two years but this figure rose to 9.5 per cent five years later.

A direct relationship between epilepsy and a cerebral vascular lesion can, of course, only be inferred. Epilepsy arising *de novo* is not uncommon in the elderly. White, Bailey and Bickford (1953), in a series of 2700 patients with epilepsy, noted that 4 per cent of them had developed their first attack over the age of 50 years. Of these patients, 32 per cent had generalised cerebral vascular disease, and a further 8 per cent had a history of a focal vascular lesion. Schwade (1960) agreed that epilepsy was not uncommon in the elderly but, in his experience, carried a good prognosis in this age group. Fine (1966, 1967) agreed that epilepsy in the elderly was relatively common and it was his experience that the underlying cause was usually cerebral vascular disease.

In the present series, 11.6 per cent (58) patients in all had a history of epilepsy; the type of epilepsy was generalised convulsions in 45 patients and focal seizures in 13. The presence of epilepsy did not appear to affect the prognosis in any way and the attacks readily responded to routine anticonvulsant measures.

CONCLUSION

1. Abnormally high levels of serum cholesterol do not appear to have any relevance to the prognosis in TCI or stroke.
2. The combination of hypertension and a high serum cholesterol appear to have some significance in the development of cerebrovascular disease. In general, hypertension is the more important.
3. Opinion on the effect of diabetes mellitus in relation to the development of cerebrovascular disease is remarkably variable in the literature. Much of this confusion is due to varying methods of case selection for study. The weight of evidence is that, at the usual age of developing a stroke, the

incidence of diabetes is higher than in the general population. There is no evidence that diabetes is relevant in TCI.

4. There is suggestive evidence that diabetes in the relatively young may be important in relation to the development of cerebrovascular disease at an early age.

5. Intermittent claudication, not surprisingly, is found in 6 to 7 per cent of patients with TCI or stroke.

6. Cortical infarcts, as distinct from subcortical, are relevant to the development of epilepsy following a stroke. In general epilepsy following infarction, whether the lesion is large or small responds well to routine anticonvulsants. Cerebral infarction is probably the commonest cause of epilepsy developing in elderly subjects.

REFERENCES

Baker, R. N., Ramseyer, J. C. & Schwartz, W. S. (1968) Prognosis in patients with transient cerebral ischaemic attacks. *Neurology*, **18**, 1157–1165.

Baker, R. N. Schwartz, W. S. & Ramseyer, J. C. (1968) Prognosis among survivors of ischaemic stroke. *Neurology*, **18**, 933–941.

Begg, T. B. & Richards, R. L. (1962) The prognosis of intermittent claudication. *Scottish Medical Journal*, **7**, 341–352.

Bental, E. & Pillar, T. (1972) Symptoms and diseases accompanying arteriosclerotic cerebrovascular events. *Geriatrics*, **27**, 142–146.

Bloor, K. (1961) Natural history of arteriosclerosis of the lower extremities. *Annals of the Royal College of Surgeons of England*, **28**, 36–52.

Cantarow & Trumper (1962) *Clinical Biochemistry*. 6th edition. 99 ff. Philadelphia: W. B. Saunders.

Carlson, L. A. & Lindstedt, S. (1968) The Stockholm prospective study. I. The initial values for plasma lipids. *Acta Medica Scandinavica, Supplementum*, 493.

Copland, J. (1850) *Causes, Nature, and Treatment of Palsy and Apoplexy.* London: Longman, Brown, Green & Longmans.

Cumings, J. N., Grundt, I. K., Holland, J. T. & Marshall, J. (1967) Serum lipids and cerebrovascular disease. *Lancet*, **ii**, 194–195.

Cumings, J. N. & Marshall, J. (1968) Serum lipids in cerebrovascular disease. *American Heart Journal*, **76**, 584–585.

Cutler, J. L. (1967) Cerebrovascular disease in an elderly population. *Circulation*, **36**, 394–399.

David, N. A. & Heyman, A. (1960) Factors influencing the prognosis of cerebral thrombosis and infarction due to atherosclerosis. *Journal of Chronic Diseases*, **11**, 394–404.

Dawber, T. R., Moore, F. E. & Mann, G. V. (1957) Coronary heart disease in the Framingham study. *American Journal of Public Health*, **47**, 4–24.

Dawber, T. R., Kannel, W. B., Revotskie, N. & Kagan, A. (1962) The epidemiology of coronary heart disease, the Framingham study. *Proceedings of the Royal Society of Medicine*, **55**, 265–271.

Diabetes Survey Working Party (1962) Report of a Working party appointed by the College of General Practitioners. *British Medical Journal*, **i**, 1497–1503.

Dodge, P. R., Richardson, E. P. & Victor, M. (1954) Recurrent convulsive seizures as a sequel to cerebral infarction. A clinical and pathological study. *Brain*, **77**, 610–638.

Farid, N. R. & Anderson, J. (1972) Cerebrovascular disease and hyperlipoproteinaemia. *Lancet*, **i**, 1398–1399.

Feldman, R. G. & Albrink, M. J. (1964) Serum lipids and cerebrovascular disesae. *Archives of Neurology*, **10**, 91–100.

Friedman, G. D., Loveland, D. B. & Ehrlich, S. P. (1968) Relationship of stroke to other cardiovascular disease. *Circulation*, **38**, 533–541.

Fine, W. (1966) Epileptic syndromes in the elderly. *Gerontologia Clinica*, **8**, 121–133.

Fine, W. (1967) Post-hemiplegic epilepsy in the elderly. *British Medical Journal*, i, 199–201.

Gertler, M. M., Garn, S. M. & Lerman, J. (1950) The inter-relationships of serum cholesterol, cholesterol esters and phospholipids in health and in coronary artery disease. *Circulation*, **2**, 205–214.

Gertler, M. M., Rusk, H. A., Whiter, H. H., Leetma, H. E. & Ehrenkranz, M. (1968) Ischaemic cerebrovascular disease. The assessment of risk factors. *Geriatrics*, **23**, 135–141.

Gertler, M. M., Rosenberger, J. L. & Leetma, M. E. (1972) Identification of individuals with overt ischaemic thrombotic cerebrovascular disease. *Stroke*, **3**, 764–771.

Goldenberg, S., Alex, N. & Blumenthal, H. T. (1958) Sequelae of arteriosclerosis of the aorta and coronary arteries. A statistical study of diabetes mellitus. *Diabetes*, **7**, 98–108.

Goldner, J. C., Whisnant, J. P. & Taylor, W. F. (1971) Long term prognosis of transient cerebral ischaemic attacks. *Stroke*, **2**, 160–167.

Gordon, T. & Kannel, W. B. (1972) Predisposition to atherosclerosis from the head, heart and legs. The Framingham study. *Journal of the American Medical Association*, **221**, 661–666.

Gowers, W. R. (1888) *A Manual of Diseases of the Nervous System*, Vol. 2. London: Churchill.

Grunnet, L. M. L. (1963) Diabetes and cerebral atherosclerosis. *Neurology*, **13**, 486–491.

Heinle, R. A., Levy, R. I., Frederickson, D. S. & Gorling, R. (1969) Lipid and carbohydrate abnormalities in patients with angiographically documented coronary artery disease. *American Journal of Cardiology*, **24**, 178–186.

Heyman, A., Nefzger, M. D. & Estes, E. H. (1961) Serum cholesterol level in cerebral infarction. *Archives of Neurology*, **5**, 264–268.

Howard, F. A., Cohen, P., Hickler, R. B., Locke, S., Newcomb, T. & Tyler, H. R. (1963) Survival following stroke. *Journal of the American Medical Association*, **183**, 921–925.

Jackson J. Hughlings (1881) On temporary paralysis after epileptiform and epileptic seizure, a contribution to the study of dissolution of the nervous system. *Brain*, **3**, 433–451.

Jacobson, T. (1967) Glucose tolerance and serum lipid levels in patients with cerebrovascular disease. *Acta Medica Scandinavica*, **182**, 233–243.

Kagan, A., Dawber, T. R., Kannel, W. B. & Revotskie, N. (1962) A prospective study of coronary heart disease. The Framingham study. *Federation Proceedings*, **21**, 52–57.

Kannel, W. B., Dawber, T. R., Cohen, M. E. & McNamara, P. M. (1965) Vascular disease of the brain—epidemiological aspect. The Framingham study. *American Journal of Public Health*, **55**, 1355–1366.

Kannel, W. B. (1966) *Cerebral Vascular Diseases*. Transactions of the fifth conference of the American Neurological Association. (Eds.) Millikan, C. H.

Kannel, W. B., Wolf, P. A., Verter, J. & McNamara, P. M. (1970) Epidemiological assessment of the role of blood pressure in stroke. Framingham study. *Journal of the American Medical Association*, **214**, 301–310.

Kannel, W. B. (1971) Current status of the epidemiology of brain infarction associated with occlusive arterial disease. *Stroke*, **2**, 295–318.

Kuller, L. & Tonascia, S. (1971) Follow-up study of the commission on chronic illness, morbidity survey in Baltimore. *Journal of Chronic Diseases*, **24**, 111–124.

Lavy, S., Melamed, E., Cahane, E. & Carmon, A. (1973) Hypertension and diabetes as risk factors in stroke patients. *Stroke*, **4**, 751–759.

Leren, P. & Haabrekke, O. (1971) Blood lipids in normals. *Acta Medica Scandinavica*, **189**, 501–504.

Liepelt, F., Skandsen, S. & Julsrud, O. J. (1972) Lipoprotein patterns in cerebrovascular disorders. *Acta Neurologica Scandinavica*, **51**, 455–456.

Louis, S. & McDowell, F. (1967) Epileptic seizures in non-embolic cerebral infarction. *Archives of Neurology*, **17**, 414–418.

McDonough, J. R. & Hames, C. G. (1967) Influence of race, sex, and occupation on seasonal changes in serum cholesterol. *American Journal of Epidemiology*, **83**, 356–364.

McDowell, F. H., Potes, J. & Groch, S. (1961) The natural history of internal carotid and vertebro-basilar artery occlusion. *Neurology*, **11**, 153–157.

Marshall, J. & Kaeser, A. C. (1961) Survival after non-haemorrhagic cerebrovascular accidents—a prospective study. *British Medical Journal*, ii, 73–77.

218   STROKES

Meyer, J. S., Waltz, A. G., Hess, J. W. & Zak, B. (1959) Serum lipid and cholesterol levels in cerebrovascular disease. *Archives of Neurology*, **1**, 303–311.
Moskowitz, E., Lightbody, F. E. H. & Freitag, N. S. (1972) Long term follow up of the post-stroke patient. *Archives of Physical Medicine and Rehabilitation*, **53**, 167–172.
Oliver, M. F. & Boyd, G. S. (1953) Plasma lipids in coronary artery disease. *British Heart Journal*, **15**, 387–392.
Oliver, M. F. & Stuart-Harris, C. H. (1965) Present position concerning prevention of heart disease. *British Medical Journal*, **ii**, 1203–1208.
Paul, O., Lepper, M. H., Phelan, W. H., Dupertuis, G. W., Macmillan, A., McKean, H. & Park, M. S. (1963) A longitudinal study of coronary heart disease. *Circulation*, **28**, 20–31.
Pearce, E. & Aziz, H. (1970) Uric acid and serum lipids in cerebrovascular disease. *Journal of Neurology, Neurosurgery and Psychiatry*, **33**, 88–91.
Pell, S. & D'Alonzo, C. A. (1960) Diabetes mellitus in an employed population. *Journal of the American Medical Association*, **172**, 1000–1006.
Robinson, R. W., Cohen, W. D., Higano, N., Meyer, R., Lukowsky, G. H. & McLaughlin, R. B. (1959) Life table analysis of survival after cerebrothrombosis—10 year experience. *Journal of the American Medical Association*, **169**, 1149–1152.
Richardson, E. P. & Dodge, P. R. (1954) Epilepsy in cerebrovascular disease. *Epilepsia*, **3**, 1–26.
Robinson, R. W., Demirel, M. & Lebeau, R. J. (1968) Natural history of cerebral thrombosis 9–19 year follow up. *Journal of Chronic Diseases*, **21**, 221–230.
Root, H. F. (1959) The treatment of diabetes mellitus. In *The Nervous System and Diabetes*, **10**, 506. London: Henry Kimpton.
Schwade, E. D. (1960) Epilepsy in the ageing and the aged. *Geriatrics*, **15**, 11–18.
Sharp, C. L., Butterfield, W. J. H. & Keen, H. (1964) Diabetes survey in Bedford. *Proceedings of the Royal Society of Medicine*, **57**, 193–202.
Silverstein, A. & Doniger, D. E. (1963) Systemic and local conditions predisposing to ischaemic and occlusive cerebrovascular disease. *Journal of the Mount Sinai Hospital, New York*, **30**, 435–450.
Svare, G. T., Toveras, J. N. & Stein, B. M. (1964) Post mortem angiography of the cerebral vascular systems. *Neurology*, **14**, 1149–1151.
Warren, S., Lecompte, P. & Legg, M. A. (1966) *The Pathology of Diabetes Mellitus* 4th edition. London: Henry Kimpton.
White, P. T., Bailey, A. A. & Bickford, R. G. (1953) Epileptic disorders in the aged. *Neurology*, **3**, 674–678.

CHAPTER ELEVEN

Post-Mortem Findings

CAUSE OF DEATH IN SURVIVORS FROM 'STROKE'

In considering the cause of death in cerebral vascular disease we are not concerned with the large group of patients who die in the first acute episode. Clearly, in these circumstances the cause of death will be cerebral infarction or cerebral haemorrhage. More appropriate to the subject of the natural history is the ultimate cause of death in survivors and the knowledge this will contribute to the understanding of the problems of both pathogenesis and management

In this chapter it is proposed to examine first of all the overall picture as it can be interpreted from the published data, and thereafter, to attempt to define the role of hypertension in view of its undoubted association with a poor prognosis in patients with cerebral vascular disease, in terms of morbidity and mortality. Before doing so, a brief consideration of the problems of death certification is necessary.

The accuracy of death certificates in indicating the precise cause of death has been assailed so often that it is hardly necessary to consider it in detail. Within the problem of cerebral vascular disease, as it has been considered in this monograph, there are three main problems. The first, as Carroll (1962) pointed out, is that the immediate cause of death is often difficult to define since pneumonia may complicate a long-term disability following hemiplegia, and it is a matter of nice judgement as to which condition should be assigned the ultimate responsibility for the patient's death. Marquardsen (1969) also acknowledged this very real difficulty, and he used all the available hospital information to arrive at an opinion but accepted that allocating a single cause was often artificial.

The second is a differentiation between cerebral infarction and cerebral haemorrhage. There is no certain evidence that one can assume that the two conditions are directly related; indeed, much of the evidence available would indicate that the two processes are distinct nosological entities. There appears to be little doubt that cerebral haemorrhage is over-diagnosed and Whisnant et al (1971) provided convincing evidence that this is so.

The third is the tendency to ascribe sudden death to an acute intracerebral episode. While it is true that death in subarachnoid haemorrhage may be devastatingly sudden, it is equally true that in both cerebral haemorrhage and cerebral thrombosis death rarely, if ever, comes rapidly. A period of several hours usually elapses before death and this is true even in the majority of cases of spontaneous haemorrhage in the posterior fossa. The figures already given for the immediate mortality in cerebral infarction indicate that only a small percentage of deaths occur in the first 24 hours although, admittedly, the percentage rises rapidly over the next 14 days. Sudden deaths in patients known to be subject to vascular disease are commonly the result of coronary artery disease and it is probably this condition that is under-estimated in the certified causes of death, and hence, in studies based on death certificates.

CAUSES OF DEATH

The inaccuracies of death certificates, however, do not detract from the value of published figures if only because of the fact that the information obtained is so clear-cut.

To examine the overall causes of death in survivors from an acute stroke, the results of 10 series published over the past 17 years have been analysed. The total number of patients involved is over 2000. Many of the series contain details of initial deaths in the analysis as well as the fate of survivors, and the former have been removed from further consideration. Of necessity, the larger series dealing with general populations such as those reported by Whisnant et al (1971) and Matsumoto et al (1973), or large hospital population series such as that of Robinson, Demirel and LeBeau (1968), contain a significant number of patients with unknown causes of death where the final details could not be traced after a period of many years. Smaller series such as those of Marshall and Shaw (1959), David and Heyman (1960) and the present series, which are hospital-based, are able, because of close supervision, to present the cause of death in all. The unknown have therefore been removed leaving a total for consideration of 1631.

The details of the cause of death are shown in Table 11.1, which indicates whether or not the information provided was obtained from post-mortem examination or by death certificate. It should be noted that the publications of Whisnant et al (1971) and Matsumoto et al (1973) are all recorded as being based upon information obtained by death certificate but the diagnoses in these two series have been accurately monitored as a consequence of the high post-mortem rate, which is possible in a community relying mainly on one hospital service, namely, that based upon the Mayo clinic.

The designation in the table of a 'further cerebral episode' covers deaths from cerebral haemorrhage and cerebral infarction. It is not possible to refine the figures further than this except in the Mayo clinic series.

The differentiation in the table between myocardial infarction and other cardiac lesions is not as precise as it seems. Other cardiac lesions refer almost invariably to heart failure due to hypertension or to degenerative heart disease and no doubt include a significant percentage of cases of acute coronary

Table 11.1. Ultimate cause of death determined by autopsy or death certificate in 1631 patients surviving a stroke.

Author(s)	Total no. of cases	Autopsy (%)	Death certificate (%)	Further cerebral episode (%)	myocardial infarct (%)	Other cardiac lesion (%)	Other vascular disease (%)	Other causes (%)
Pincock, 1957	52	92	8	23	40			36.5
Marshall & Shaw, 1959	132	Not stated		52	21			26
David & Heyman, 1960	21	33	67	43	19			38
Marshall & Kaeser, 1961	28	53	47	46	18	22		14
Marquardsen, 1969	304	44.5	54.5	28	12	37.5		21.3
Robinson et al, 1968	474		100	45	33			22
Whisnant et al, 1971	218		100*	19	34		15	32
Matsumoto et al, 1973	269		100*	19	37			44
Present series	133	31	69	44	17	18		21

occlusion. 'Other causes' relate to the grouping together of diagnoses that have no immediate association, however tenuous, with cerebral vascular disease. Conditions such as carcinoma and chronic bronchitis are included under this heading.

From the results it can be seen that for practical purposes a recurrence of a cerebral vascular episode, recorded in 37 per cent of cases, was almost equalled by the incidence of cardiac deaths whether the latter were due to acute myocardial infarction or to the long-term effects of hypertension or coronary artery disease (Figure 11.1). Other vascular diseases, variously labelled as generalised atherosclerosis or peripheral vascular disease, have been noted in 2 per cent. Although no certain opinion can be offered about this finding, clinical experience would suggest that this is certainly an under-estimate of the importance of generalised vascular disease in the overall morbidity and mortality of this group of patients. The important fact that emerges is that survivors from an acute intracerebral episode do not commonly die from a recurrent episode. In fact, rather than a recurrence being inevitable, on the laws of chance it will occur in just over a third of the patients only. While this is clearly so, it should not obscure the important point that of all survivors from an acute stroke, 74 per cent will ultimately die from the consequences of degenerative vascular disease, however this is defined.

This last fact alone would indicate that in observing a group of patients, however large, with a common factor of cerebral vascular disease, we are still examining a pre-selected group. Although they are an important group they still represent only one clinical facet of the consequence of generalised vascular disease.

THE SIGNIFICANCE OF HYPERTENSION

Some definition that is by no means complete can be attempted of the precise significance of hypertension as it affects prognosis both in transient cerebral ischaemia (TCI) and in cerebral infarction on the basis of the information obtaining in the literature and in the present series.

Transient cerebral ischaemia

Neither Ziegler and Hassanein (1973) nor Baker, Ramseyer and Schwartz (1968) in their study of the natural history of cerebral vascular disease make any reference to the occurrence of cerebral haemorrhage as the cause of death in these patients. However, Goldner, Whisnant and Taylor (1971), using very precise criteria for the diagnosis of TCI, recorded five examples of cerebral haemorrhage in the 42 deaths reported.

It has often been noted in the past literature that short-lived episodes which would now possibly be accepted as TCI can precede cerebral haemorrhage. Aring and Merritt (1935), in their clinico pathological study of cerebral haemorrhage and cerebral infarction, discussed the question of premonitory symptoms which were recorded in 22 of the 116 cases of cerebral haemorrhage

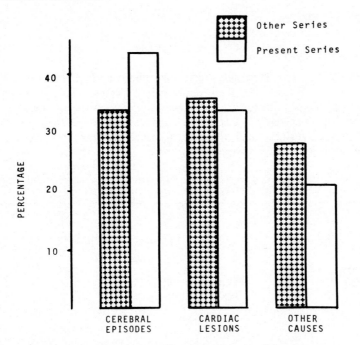

Figure 11.1. Histogram comparing incidence of causes of death in 1498 patients with stroke reported in literature with the findings in 133 patients in present series.

examined. Disregarding for the moment the symptom of headache, which was not infrequent, and mental disturbance and drowsiness, they record in one patient an episode of localised numbness and weakness of the left extremities for a period of a week before the cerebral haemorrhage occurred. In two others there were attacks of dizziness which were not, however, defined as vertigo. They made the point that many of the patients were admitted in coma so that any clear-cut history was difficult to obtain.

Marshall (1964) drew attention to the fact that transient ischaemic attacks (TIAs) within the modern definition of the syndrome could be a fore-runner of cerebral haemorrhage. He cited three personal cases. Two patients had an episode of transient hemi-paresis lasting, in one patient, for 24 hours but for a much shorter period in the other. The interval between the TIA and the fatal cerebral haemorrhage was three months in one patient and one year in the other. In a third patient the transitory episode lasted only one hour and was followed six hours later by a pontine haemorrhage which was proven at autopsy.

Although information on the subject is limited, it seems possible that Marshall's conjecture that TIAs may precede cerebral haemorrhage more frequently than is thought may ultimately prove to be correct.

PERSONAL SERIES

Transient cerebral ischaemia

The cause of death in 36 patients who presented with TCI and subsequently died is shown in Table 11.2. They require little comment as the number is small. Heart disease due either to myocardial infarction or degenerative vascular disease was the most frequent cause and was recorded in 14, and three of these certainly died of acute myocardial infarction, as this was confirmed by post-mortem examination.

Table 11.2. Cause of death determined by post-mortem examination or death certificate in 36 patients presenting with a history of transient cerebral ischaemic attacks.

Post-mortem examination				Death certificate		
TCI only	TCI → Stroke	Total		TCI only	TCI → Stroke	Total
0	1	1	Cerebral haemorrhage and	0	7	7
0	2	2	Cerebral infarction			
0	3	3	Cardiac infarct	2	5	7
1	0	1	Heart failure	1	2	3
3	4	7	Other causes	1	4	5
		14				22

One important point to which we will return when the individual clinical histories of patients are considered is that where patient presented with TCI and ultimately died from cerebral haemorrhage.

Stroke

Of patients who presented with a history of a stroke, 133 subsequently died and the cause of death was obtained from the death certificate or at post-mortem examination; the findings are detailed in Table 11.3. The general pattern is that already recorded and is depicted in Figure 11.1, and the distribution of causes of death follows that which had been observed in the general literature. The difference of 10 per cent between a further cerebral episode and a cardiac cause of death is hardly significant.

But the significant information, bearing in mind the role of hypertension, stems from the 54 patients who entered the study with a history of a stroke and then went on to recurrent episodes and who died subsequently in either the second episode or in episodes subsequent to this.

An autopsy examination was available in 16 of these, and in 7 of them, at autopsy, the cause of death was cerebral haemorrhage.

It is a somewhat trite saying to emphasise the difficulty on occasion of differentiating between cerebral infarction and cerebral haemorrhage. Presented with an unconscious patient with an illness of sudden onset and short duration, the physical signs and a bloodstained cerebrospinal fluid will

Table 11.3. Cause of death determined by post-mortem examination and death certificate in 42 patients with a history of a single stroke and in 91 patients with a history of multiple strokes.

| Post-mortem | | | Death certificate | | |
Single stroke (%)	Multiple stroke (%)		Single stroke (%)	Multiple stroke (%)
0 –	7 25.9	Cerebral haemorrhage and	1 3.3	38 59.4
3[a] 21.4	9 33.3	Cerebral infarction		
5 35.7	2 7.4	Myocardial infarction	7 25.0	9 14.1
2 14.3	4 14.8	Heart failure	10 35.7	8 12.5
0 –	1 3.7	Status epilepticus	0 –	0 –
4 28.6	4 14.8	Other causes	10 35.7	9 14.0
14	27		28	64

[a]Died in the acute stage of the stroke.

commonly settle the diagnosis. But in this study we are concerned with patients who presented with a history of the development of a focal neurological deficit, with or without recovery, without any loss of consciousness at the onset and where it seemed reasonable to accept a diagnosis of cerebral infarction.

To emphasise the difficulty some representative case histories are recorded.

Case 1. J. K., male, age at death 36 years. The patient, a Pole, was a poor linguist. He gave a history of dragging of the left leg for some six months. It was difficult to ascertain the precise mode of onset but there was no dramatic episode as far as could be ascertained, and certainly there had been no progression of symptoms. When first seen, the casual blood pressure reading was 230/130 mm Hg. In the central nervous system the positive physical signs were increased tone in the left arm and leg, increased reflexes in these limbs, and a left extensor plantar response. There was no sensory loss nor were there signs of cerebellar disorder.

In view of his relative youth the patient was put on the waiting list for urgent admission, but he suddenly became unconscious at home and was admitted in this state and died within three hours of admission.

Post mortem. General features. Left ventricular hypertrophy but no other remarkable features in the general post-mortem examination.

Brain: Gross atheroma of the Circle of Willis and of the intracranial portions of the carotid and vertebral arteries but no intravascular thrombi noted. There was an old vascular lesion in the right corpus striatum. There was recently clotted blood over the right lobe of the cerebellum and the underlying cerebellum was destroyed by an intracerebellar haemorrhage, and the blood had invaded the 4th ventricle and the pons.

Case 2. I.W., female, age at death 56 years. In June 1963 the patient noted a sudden onset of paraesthesiae of the right foot which, within a period of hours, was followed by paresis of the right arm and leg and transient loss of consciousness. On recovery of consciousness there was marked hemiparesis and dysphasia but these signs rapidly regressed and mobility was quickly restored.

In November 1963 she had a further episode of weakness in the right arm and leg which was followed by a typical thalamic syndrome involving the right arm and face, with troublesome contact dysaesthesiae.

Examination at this time revealed a hemiparesis with facial involvement together with contact dysaesthesiae of the right face and palm of the right hand with pin prick stimulation, which persisted until her death.

When reviewed in hospital in 1964 she complained of typical drop attacks. She described them as a sudden fall when the legs became useless and she fell to the ground. During the attack the power in her arms was perfectly normal. The duration of the drop attacks was for seconds only.

During her assessment the blood pressure was noted to be labile. A casual reading in the out-patients ranged from 220/160 to 220/140 but at rest this fell to 180/110 mm Hg.

She was admitted in deep coma of sudden onset on the 7th of April, 1965, and survived for 36 hours.

Post mortem. General findings: There was left ventricular hypertrophy and some terminal oedema of the lungs.

Brain: A massive cerebral haemorrhage had destroyed the left basal ganglia and erupted from this into the ventricular system, which was distended with blood.

Case 3. L. N., female, age at death 45 years. At the age of 43 she had an episode of sudden loss of use of the left arm and leg without loss of consciousness which completely recovered in four days. She gave a history of hypertension which extended back over the previous ten years. The blood pressure was 230/130 mm Hg.

Twelves months later she had a second episode of weakness in the left arm and leg but on this occasion she did not make a complete recovery and there was significant disability present.

Nine months later she was admitted to hospital with sudden loss of consciousness. When she was admitted she was in deep coma and the essential signs were of a left III nerve palsy and a dense left hemiplegia. She survived in hospital four days.

Post mortem. General findings: There was marked left ventricular hypertrophy. The carotid vessels in the neck showed only minimal atheroma.

Brain: There was an old cystic haemorrhage in the right corpus striatum and a recent massive cerebral haemorrhage into the left occipital pole. Gross atheroma of the intracranial vessels was present but no occlusion or significant stenosis were noted.

Case 4. J. W., male, age at death 60 years. Three years before his death the patient presented in the out-patient clinic with a history of recurring transient attacks of vertigo. In addition to these he complained of occasional attacks of sudden unsteadiness of the trunk. The majority of these attacks lasted for seconds only but in one attack the truncal ataxia persisted for 30 minutes. The attacks occurred at approximately monthly intervals and continued for a period of nine months. At this time the attacks ceased and he remained free of any neurological symptoms until his death nine months later. Eighteen months after the onset of symptoms he collapsed suddenly and died within an estimated period of three hours. The blood pressure was 230/160 mm Hg.

Post mortem. General findings: There was marked left ventricular hypertrophy but there were no other findings of note in the general post-mortem examination.

Brain: In the cerebellum there were three small cysts approximately 5 mm in diameter and two similar cysts were noted in the pons. There was marked atheroma of the intracranial blood supply but no significant stenosis of the vessels.

A massive haemorrhage into the left thalamic area had erupted into the ventricular system and, thence, into the third and fourth ventricles, where blood leaked into the subarachnoid space.

Case 5. W.E., male, age at death 50 years. Three years before death the patient presented with a three-week history of numbness of the left upper lip. This spread in a stepwise fashion over a period of four days to involve the whole of the sensory distribution of the left V cranial nerve. A week after the onset a similar sensation developed in the left hand and evolved in a similar manner, taking six days in all to reach its final distribution. The blood pressure at the initial examination was 250/125 mm Hg. There was sensory loss to all modalities over the area of numbness in the face but in spite of the symptoms in the· hand there were no objective abnormalities to be demonstrated there.

Detailed in-patient investigation proved non-contributory apart from the evidence of hypertension, and angiography was not carried out.

The second episode in 1960, which developed quite briskly, resulted in a disturbance of speech and a persisting dysarthria. He died, suddenly, three years after the onset of symptoms.

Post mortem. General findings: There was marked left ventricular hypertrophy but no other findings of note were observed in the general post-mortem examination.

Brain: There was a massive cerebral haemorrhage involving the right cerebral hemisphere. The ventricular system was filled with blood throughout and there were secondary brain stem haemorrhages. No comment was made in the post-mortem report as to previous vascular disturbance in the brain stem.

From these case histories it is evident that even had we fully appreciated the ability of hypertensive cerebral vascular disease to simulate not only restricted cerebral infarction but also TCI, there would have been no way at the moment in which we could have diagnosed between the nature of the lesions in these patients accurately on clinical grounds. The error rate is not small. In the post-mortem series (Table 11.3) it was 15 per cent and, since the diagnoses taken from the death certificate roughly paralleled those of the post-mortem study, this level of incorrect diagnosis almost certainly applies to the whole series. If patients with a history of recurrent episodes only are considered, then nearly half the patients (7 out of 16) died with a cerebral haemorrhage with evidence in some at post mortem that the initial episode was due to a localised intracerebral haematoma.

The blood pressure in all these patients was high, the diastolic blood pressure being over 120 mm Hg. The figures of Aring and Merritt (1935), however, offer no hope for the suggestion that the figures for the blood pressure during life would provide supporting clinical evidence for a diagnosis of cerebral haemorrhage. The blood pressure in cerebral infarction was frequently just as high in their patients. The experience in the present series would suggest that with a diastolic blood pressure of 120 mm Hg or more the chances of a given episode being directly due to hypertension lie between 40 and 50 per cent. It is important to recall, however, that in all the patients coming to post mortem, cerebral infarction exceeded cerebral haemorrhage as a cause of death (Table 11.3).

Marquardsen's (1969) results are very relevant here. In considering his results he observed that a considerable proportion of recurrent strokes were due to cerebral haemorrhage. In 23 out of 47 cases the fatal recurrence was a massive cerebral haemorrhage, most often found in the contralateral basal ganglia. Referring to the autopsy reports, an old haemorrhagic lesion could be demonstrated in one quarter of 24 patients with a verified cerebral haemorrhage, and of the remaining patients three-quarters showed either an old infarct or else the pathologist failed to demonstrate macroscopic signs of a previous vascular lesion.

Marquardsen (1969) concluded that it was 'tempting to assume that recurrent cerebrovascular accidents, whether infarcts or haemorrhage, had a common pathogenesis'. In the present series, as in many others, the post mortem examinations were part of the routine pathological service, and we believe that the final answer to this important point will come only from a prospective and combined clinical and neuropathological study.

CONCLUSION

1. Over 70 per cent of patients presenting with a stroke will ultimately succumb to the effects of either degenerative vascular disease or hypertension.
2. The cause of death will be either a recurrent stroke or a cardiac lesion; these two types of terminal illness occur in roughly equal numbers.
3. Localised intracerebral haematomas may mimic cerebral ischaemia exactly and may be responsible for recurrent episodes of stroke.
4. When the diastolic B.P. is 120 mm Hg or more the chances are about 50 per cent that a given episode, apparently ischaemic clinically, will be due to a localised intracerebral haematoma.
5. There is some clinical evidence that hypertension alone can cause TCI.

REFERENCES

Aring, C. D. & Merritt, H. H. (1935) Differential diagnosis between cerebral haemorrhage and cerebral thrombosis. *Archives of Internal Medicine*, **56**, 435–456.
Baker, R. N., Ramseyer, J. C. & Schwartz, W. S. (1968) Prognosis in patients with transient cerebral ischaemia. *Neurology*, **18**, 1157–1165.
Carroll, D. (1962) The disability in hemiplegia caused by cerebrovascular disease. A serial study of 98 cases. *Journal of Chronic Diseases*, **15**, 179–188.
David, J. N. & Heyman, A. (1960) Factors influencing the prognosis of cerebral thrombosis and infarction due to atherosclerosis. *Journal of Chronic Diseases*, **11**, 394–404.
Goldner, J. C., Whisnant, J. P. & Taylor, W. F. (1971) Long-term prognosis of transient cerebral ischaemic attacks. *Stroke*, **2**, 160–165.
Marquardsen, J. (1969) The natural history of acute cerebrovascular disease. A retrospective study of 769 patients. *Acta Neurologica Scandinavica*, **45**, 1–137.
Marshall, J. & Shaw, D. A. (1959) The natural history of cerebrovascular disease. *British Medical Journal*, **i**, 1614–1617.
Marshall, J. (1964) A trial of long-term hypotensive therapy in cerebrovascular disease. *Lancet*, **i**, 10–12.
Matsumoto, N., Whisnant, J. P., Kurland, L. T. & Okazaki, H. (1973) Natural history of stroke in Rochester, Minnesota, 1955 through 1969. An extension of a previous study, 1945 through 1954. *Stroke*, **4**, 20–29.
Robinson, R. W., Demirel, M. & LeBeau, R. J. (1968) Natural history of cerebral thrombosis nine to nineteen years follow-up. *Journal of Chronic Diseases*, **21**, 221–230.
Whisnant, J. P., Fitzgibbons, J. P., Kurland, L. T. & Sayre, G. P. (1971) Natural history of stroke in Rochester, Minnesota, 1945 through 1954. *Stroke*, **2**, 11–22.
Ziegler, D. K. & Hassenein, R. S. (1973) Prognosis in patients with transient ischaemic attacks. *Stroke*, **4**, 366–676.

CHAPTER TWELVE

Medical Management of Strokes

Although this monograph has been mainly concerned with the natural history of two varieties of cerebral ischaemia, namely, transient cerebral ischaemia (TCI) and stroke, consideration is now given to the problems of management. It is appropriate that our consideration of management should be confined to the problems of treating TCI and of attempting to modify the subsequent history in patients who present with a stroke. Thus, we do not propose to deal with the manifold problems that arise in the rehabilitation of stroke sufferers.

In the present state of knowledge there is no satisfactory evidence that the process of atheroma can be either prevented or even halted once it becomes clinically evident. In patients with TCI the development of a stroke is the generally accepted major complication. In the patients surviving an acute stroke it is the problem of recurrent episodes that is all-important.

The two concluding chapters will consider the medical and surgical treatment available to the two groups of patients. In this chapter three areas of medical management are examined. First, among these, is the value of treating hypertension in the presence of established stroke. Secondly, we shall consider the merits and results of reducing the levels of the blood cholesterol. Thirdly, we shall discuss the advisability of using anticoagulant drugs.

TREATMENT OF HYPERTENSION IN THE ESTABLISHED STROKE

The evidence that hypertension adversely affects the prognosis in established cerebral vascular disease has already been examined in this monograph. Most observers agree that this is an established clinical fact. The notable exceptions are Adams (1965) and Merrett and Adams (1966) but, as has been suggested previously, it may be that the age of their patients, since they were mainly drawn from geriatric practice, induced a different result from that obtained by most other observers.

Two studies have been published that seem to establish beyond reasonable clinical doubt that treatment of hypertension will improve the outcome. These studies have been reported by Carter (1970) and by Beevers et al (1973).

Carter (1970) began a prospective study in January 1964. He intended to treat hypertension in all patients with a presumed cerebral infarct who presented to him under 80 years of age. It was a randomised study but the results were so positively in favour of the effects of treating the hypertension that the trial was discontinued after four years.

Carter defined hypertension under the categories of diastolic and systolic hypertension. Diastolic hypertension was declared to be present with a diastolic reading of 110 mm Hg or more. Systolic hypertension was accepted when the systolic pressure exceeded 160 mm Hg but the diastolic pressure was below 110 mm Hg.

Out of a series of 244 patients, 99 patients entered the trial and were personally seen by Carter in the four-year period. Control of hypertension implied lowering the diastolic pressure to between 90 and 100 mm Hg in patients with diastolic hypertension and a reduction below 160 mm Hg in patients with systolic hypertension. Control was achieved in 82 per cent of the treated group.

Of the patients treated during the follow-up period, 26.5 per cent (13) died, which compared favourably with the corresponding figure of 46 per cent for the untreated group. The causes of death in the two groups were interesting. Causes unrelated to cerebral vascular disease were almost the same in both groups. Death from cardiac infarction or heart failure was observed in five of the treated and six of the untreated patients. The difference in mortality in the two groups was almost totally related to deaths from further intra-cerebral episodes. In the untreated group, seven patients had a recurrent cerebral infarct and three a cerebral haemorrhage. In the treated group, only one had a recurrent stroke but two sustained a cerebral haemorrhage. Carter (1970) did not give the precise number of post mortems carried out, but refers to a 'high proportion of necropsy confirmation'.

There were 18 non-fatal recurrences, of which 11 were in the non-treated group and 7 in the treated group. In the whole trial, 21 (44 per cent) of the recurrences occurred in the non-treated group as compared with 10 (20 per cent) in the treated group.

In the final analysis of his results Carter showed that the benefit of treating hypertension was to be found in patients who were aged 65 years or below.

Beevers et al (1973) reviewed 162 hypertensive patients, all of whom had survived an acute cerebral vascular episode, and were being treated for hypertension. They defined control as 'good' if the diastolic pressure fell below 100 mm Hg, 'fair' if the pressure fell to between 100 and 109 mm Hg, and 'poor' when the diastolic pressure was 110 mm Hg or more.

Twenty-nine per cent (47) of the 162 had recurrent episodes. When divided into groups according to the criteria laid down for control, 16 per cent of the 'good' control group had a further episode, as did 32 per cent of the 'fair' control group, and the number of recurrences in the 'poor' control group was 55 per cent.

It is of some interest that the time lapse between the first and second stroke also appeared to be related to the degree of control of hypertension. In the 'good' control group, only 5 per cent had a second stroke within two years, whereas in the 'poor' control group the second stroke was noted within two years in 28 per cent.

These two contributions alone seem to establish the merits of treating hypertension in patients with stroke under the age of 65 years. It is still curious, however, looking at Carter's results, that recurrent cerebral infarction was the hazard most significantly affected, whereas one might have expected that the major difference would relate to the incidence of cerebral haemorrhage. Future studies may clarify this particular point.

SERUM CHOLESTEROL

The published data on the interrelationship between serum cholesterol and stroke has already been reviewed. Unlike myocardial infarction, increased risk is not associated with a high cholesterol level according to most published work. A study in Los Angeles found the incidence rate of stroke to be more closely related to hypertension than a high serum cholesterol level (Chapman, 1970). In prospective studies, only one showed an association between the level of the serum cholesterol and the subsequent development of stroke, and this was in the 30 to 49-year-old age group (Dawber and Thomas, 1968).

Attempts to influence the course of ischaemic cerebral vascular disease by reducing the level of cholesterol have been reported rarely. Hirsch, Weschler and Tourtellotte (1972) described the use of clofibrate (Atromid-S) in a double-blind controlled trial conducted at a Veterans' Administration Hospital. Of 20 patients treated they refer to all as showing 'some improvement' in the initial symptoms and signs, and 8 returned to their previous occupation. In contrast, in the control group only 8 improved and only 3 returned to their previous occupation. Clearly, the number of patients treated were too small to establish with any certainty a beneficial effect and the authors did point out that in a comparative study of 541 patients no substantial benefit was observed by the use of Atromid-S.

Acheson and Hutchinson (1972) reported on a series of 95 patients (males 65; females 30) who were observed for a period of seven years. The patients were suffering from either TCI or had presented with a stroke. They entered the trial only if the blood cholesterol was 250 mg/100 ml or more. The patients were matched for age, sex and degree of functional recovery in cases where a stroke had occurred. The patients were also matched according to blood pressure. Forty-seven patients received clofibrate and 48 received the placebo. The mean duration of the disease at the close of the trial was $8\frac{1}{2}$ years (S.D. 3 years 3 months) in patients treated with Clofibrate, and 7 years 7 months (S.D. 3 years 4 months) in control patients.

The effect on the serum cholesterol is shown on Table 12.1. It can be seen that a significant lowering of the serum cholesterol was achieved in the treated patients in all the clinical groups. Although this can only be regarded as a pilot survey it was carried on for a lengthy time and there was certainly no encouragement from the results to extend it into a full-scale trial. Of the treated group, 66 per cent, and 60 per cent of the controls had further episodes

Table 12.1. Mean pre-treatment level of serum cholesterol and mean proportional change in level of serum cholesterol in treated and control patients.

Clinical category at time of entry into trial	Mean pre-treatment level of serum cholesterol		Mean proportional change in level of serum cholesterol	
	Treated patients	Control patients	Treated patients (%)	Control patients (%)
Single stroke	297.42 (S.D. 49.31)	291.33 (S.D. 41.48)	24.42[a]	14.5
Multiple strokes	290.33 (S.D. 28.31)	266.19 (S.D. 30.08)	19.47[a]	9.54
Onset with transient vascular ischaemia	284.78 (S.D. 34.82)	292.00 (S.D. 35.63)	20.34[a]	13.99

[a]Significant $P < 0.05$
By permission of *Atherosclerosis* (1972), **15**.

of ischaemia. Approximately the same number in both groups had further strokes, and of 15 patients who had further episodes of transient ischaemia 8 were receiving treatment.

The obvious conclusion, therefore, was that in this particular group of patients there was no discernible effect on the course of the disease as a result of administering clofibrate.

ANTICOAGULANTS

The value of anticoagulant drugs in the treatment of cerebral vascular disease has provoked controversy and disagreement since the introduction of these remedies. Shaw (1962), in a review of the subject up to that date, came to the conclusion that anticoagulants had not fulfilled their early promise. He examined the evidence available so far and felt that their use should be limited to TCI in both the vertebro-basilar and in the carotid territories and perhaps to a developing stroke in the vertebro-basilar territory.

Opinion about the use of anti-coagulants in cerebral vascular disease has diverged since that time. Clauss and Redisch (1971) state categorically that there is no evidence to suggest that anticoagulants are of any value in occlusive vascular disease. They wrote 'in cerebral as well as in peripheral manifestations of occlusive atherosclerosis their uselessness is well established'. To some, this would seem an extreme view, and certainly the evidence from clinical studies cannot be disposed of so easily. The weight of pathological evidence both at post mortem and from the results of histological studies of resected specimens at endarterectomy indicate that both platelet micro-emboli and solid fibrin and cholesterol emboli may arise from a common site of arterial disease. It has been assumed that anticoagulant drugs will prevent the further formation of platelet emboli but could hardly be expected to alter firm masses of fibrin or cholesterol. Since the syndrome of TCI differs so markedly in its clinical content from the developing or completed stroke it is usual to present the evidence in each of the three clinical categories, namely the established stroke and the ingravescent stroke and the syndrome of TCI.

Established stroke and ingravescent stroke

The wisdom and effectiveness of using anticoagulants in the established stroke was effectively questioned in a report by Hill, Marshall and Shaw (1960). They studied 142 patients randomly allocated to two groups. They could find no evidence that the incidence of recurrent episodes was affected in either group. Moreover, there were four deaths from cerebral haemorrhage in the high-dose anticoagulant group. The recent development in knowledge of hypertension and its effect on the cerebral blood vessels, particularly the development of miliary aneurysms, provide suggestive supporting evidence in the pathological field for the reason why cerebral haemorrhage should occur.

Millikan (1971) reviewed the evidence for the use of anticoagulants in all three categories of stroke. In the case of the established stroke he pointed out that Baker, Broward and Fang (1962) had shown that recurrence of a cerebral infarct occurred in 42 per cent in the treated group compared with 27 per cent of the controls. In addition to this there was an incidence of cerebral haemorrhage of 10 per cent in the treated group. In other series, the incidence of cerebral haemorrhage ranged from 4 per cent to 11 per cent (Hill, Marshall and Shaw, 1962; McDowell and McDevitt, 1965; Enger and Bøyesen, 1965; and Howell, Tatlow and Feldman, 1964). It would seem from the available evidence that the use of anti-coagulants in this variety of stroke is hardly justified.

In examining the evidence for the value of anticoagulants in the developing of ingravescent stroke Millikan (1971) is critical of the criteria for acceptance into this category in much published work. His criticism was mainly directed at the inclusion of patients where the neurological deficit was at its maximum 24 hours or more prior to admission to the trial. He argued that admitting these patients to a trial must prejudice the results against any form of treatment.

Millikan then examined five trials of anticoagulants where he felt the criteria for ingravescent stroke had been met (Millikan, 1965; Carter, 1961; Baker, Broward and Fang, 1962; Fisher, 1958; Fisher, 1961). There seemed to be clear evidence in favour of the treated group. Progression of signs occurred in numbers ranging from 14 per cent to 32 per cent whereas in the control group progression occurred in 40 per cent to 64 per cent. Somewhat surprisingly, only one patient in all the series examined died of cerebral haemorrhage. Many would feel that the difficulty in differentiating positively between an infarct and a localised intracerebral haematoma is such that the widespread use of anticoagulants in the ingravescent stroke is still a matter for discussion and further examination. The majority view seems to be hardening against their use in such cases.

Transient cerebral ischaemia

In TCI there is usually no serious diagnostic problem and it is simply a matter of deciding whether or not the acknowledged hazards of treatment with anticoagulants are outweighed by the benefits. This statement may have to be modified in the future if it does become possible to recognise a group of patients who present with TCI associated with the miliary aneurysms of hypertension rather than the micro-emboli of atheromatous ulceration. The largest series, that of Siekert, Whisnant and Millikan (1963) appeared to show undoubted benefit, in that 32 per cent of the control group developed a cerebral infarct compared with only 4 per cent of the treated group.

A further valuable contribution to the problem of treating TCI has been published recently from the Mayo Clinic by Whisnant, Matsumoto and Elveback (1973). Eighty patients received long-term anticoagulant, and 118 did not. There was no significant difference between the two groups in the distribution of diastolic blood pressure.

There was no overall difference in the survival rates in either group, but when the incidence of stroke was examined two important points emerged. They compared the treated and untreated groups with one another and with the expected probability of a stroke in the population by means of age-specific stroke rates for the population of Rochester based on the figures from 1955 to 1969 (Whisnant et al, 1973).

There was a significant difference between the 'net probabilities' at one, three, and five years respectively (Figure 12.1) in the treated and untreated groups. Whisnant, Matsumoto and Elveback (1973) then examined the behaviour of both the treated and untreated groups at two-monthly intervals throughout the first twelve months of the illness (Figure 12.2). They came to the important conclusion that most of the beneficial effect of anticoagulant therapy will occur in the first two months following the onset of TCI. Thereafter the two populations follow a similar course.

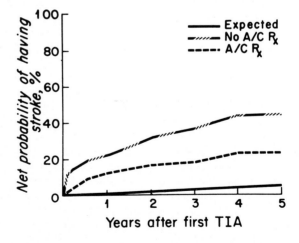

Figure 12.1. Conditional probability of occurrence of stroke after first TIA in patients treated and untreated with anticoagulants. Expected probability is for population of given age and sex and is based on stroke incidence rates of Rochester, Minnesota, 1955 through 1969 (From *Mayo Clinic Proceedings*, December, 1973, with permission of Dr Jack P. Whisnant).

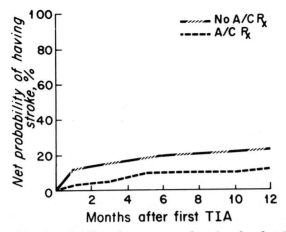

Figure 12.2. Conditional probability of occurrence of stroke after first TIA in patients treated and untreated with anticoagulants (From *Mayo Clinic Proceedings*, December, 1973, with permission of Dr Jack P. Whisnant).

CONCLUSION

1. The available evidence is beginning clearly to indicate that effective treatment of hypertension is both safe and valuable in patients with established cerebrovascular disease.
2. Successful treatment of the hypertension materially affects the incidence of recurrence of cerebrovascular episodes and, thus, the morbidity and ultimate mortality.
3. New evidence appears to substantiate the value of anticoagulants in TCI. The effect appears to take place in the first two to three months after the initial episode.

REFERENCES

Acheson, J. (1971) Factors affecting the natural history of focal cerebral vascular disease. *Quarterly Journal of Medicine*, **40**, 25–46.

Acheson, E. J. & Hutchinson, E. C. (1972) Control trial of Clofibrate in cerebral vascular disease. *Atherosclerosis*, **15**, 177–183.

Adams, F. G. (1965) Prospects for patients with strokes. With special reference to the hypertensive hemiplegic. *British Medical Journal*, **ii**, 253–259.

Baker, R. N., Broward, J. A. & Fang, H. C. (1962) Anticoagulant therapy in cerebral infarction. *Neurology*, **12**, 823–835.

Beevers, D. G., Hamilton, M., Fairman, M. J. & Harpur, J. E. (1973) Antihypertensive treatment and the course of established cerebral vascular disease. *Lancet*, **i**, 1407–1409.

Carter, A. B. (1961) Anticoagulant treatment in progressing stroke. *British Medical Journal*, **ii**, 70–73.

Carter, A. B. (1970) Hypotensive therapy in stroke survivors. *Lancet*, **i**, 485–489.

Chapman, J. M. (1970) Epidemiology of risk factors in ischaemic heart disease. *Annals of Internal Medicine*, **72**, 97–109.

Clauss, R. H., Redisch, W. (1971) *Remedial Arterial Disease*. p. 184. New York: Grune & Stratton.

Dawber, T. R. & Thomas, H. E. (1968) Prophylaxis of coronary heart disease, stroke and peripheral atherosclerosis. *Annals of the New York Academy of Science*, **149,** 1038–1057.

Enger, E. & Bøyesen, S. (1965) Long term anticoagulant therapy in patients with cerebral infarction, a controlled clinical study. *Acta Medica Scandinavica*, Supplementum **438,** 1–61.

Fisher, C. M. (1958) The use of anticoagulants in cerebral thrombosis. *Neurology*, **8,** 311–322.

Fisher, C. M. (1961) Anticoagulant therapy in cerebral thrombosis and cerebral embolism. A national cooperative study, interim report. *Neurology*, **11** (Part 2), 119–131.

Hill, A. B., Marshall, J. & Shaw, D. A. (1962) Cerebrovascular disease: Trial of long-term anticoagulant therapy. *British Medical Journal*, **ii,** 1003–1006.

Hirsch, S. B., Wechsler, A. F. & Tourtellotte, W. W. (1972) Clofibrate for the treatment of occlusive cerebrovascular disease. *New England Journal of Medicine*, **287,** 671.

Howell, D. A., Tatlow, W. F. T. & Feldman, S. (1964) Observations on anticoagulant therapy in thromboembolic disease of the brain. *Journal of Canadian Medical Association*, **90,** 611–614.

McDowell, F. & McDevitt, E. (1965) Treatment of the completed stroke with long-term anticoagulants. *Transactions of the Fourth Princeton Conference on Cerebrovascular Disease*, 185–199.

Marshall, J. & Shaw, D. A. (1960) Anticoagulant therapy in acute cerebrovascular accidents, a controlled trial. *Lancet*, **i,** 995–998.

Merrett, J. D. & Adams, G. F. (1966) Comparison of mortality rates in hypertensive and normotensive hemiplegic patients. *British Medical Journal*, **ii,** 802–805.

Millikan, C. H. (1971) Reassessment of anticoagulant therapy in various types of occlusive cerebrovascular disease. *Stroke*, **2,** 201–208.

Millikan, C. H. (1965) Therapeutic agents—current status: anticoagulant therapy in cerebrovascular disease. *Transactions of the Fourth Princetown Conference on Cerebrovascular Disease*, ed. Millikan, C. H., Seikert, R. G. & Whisnant, J. P. New York: Grune & Stratton. pp. 181–184.

Shaw, D. A. (1962) The use of anticoagulants in neurology. In *Modern Trends io Neurology*, ed Williams, D. London: Butterworth.

Sierkert, R. G., Whisnant, J. P. & Millikan, C. H. (1963) Surgical and anticoagulant therapy of occlusive cerebrovascular disease. *Annals of Internal Medicine*, **58,** 637–641.

Whisnant, J. P., Matsumoto, N. & Elveback, L. R. (1973) The effect of anticoagulant therapy on the prognosis of patients with transient cerebral ischaemic attacks in a community, Rochester, Minnesota, 1955 through 1969. *Mayo Clinic Proceedings*, **48,** 844–848.

CHAPTER THIRTEEN

The Surgical Treatment of Extracranial Cerebrovascular Disease

L. J. LAWSON

This chapter deals with the surgical treatment of cerebral ischaemia. The rationale for attempting such intervention is discussed together with the relative importance of structural change in vessel size and embolic complications secondary to mural damage. The methods of radiographic investigation and techniques for protection of the cerebral cells are reviewed. Reconstruction of the diseased carotid arteries and modern procedures for relief of subclavian and vertebral artery disease are considered in detail. The results of seven years experience with such methods are then analysed.

The interest shown by surgeons in disease of the extracranial carotid artery has increased progressively since Eastcott, Pickering and Rob (1954) first demonstrated that surgical treatment was possible. The association of cerebrovascular accidents with stenosis of the extracranial carotid artery has been known for many years. It was recorded by Virchov (1856) and Gowers (1875) in the nineteenth century, Chiari (1905) referred to the problem, and Hunt (1914) discussed stenosis of the carotid vessels in relation to stroke. Yates and Hutchinson (1961) reported their findings in 100 cases in whom death was thought to be due to cerebral ischaemia. They demonstrated that nearly all infarcts of the brain were associated with stenosis or occlusion of the extracranial cerebral arteries. Severe obstructive disease was present in the carotid arteries in 51 patients as well as in 40 vertebral arteries. Schwartz and Mitchell (1961) in the same year published details of a comparable autopsy study with similar results. Both studies underlined the accessibility of common sites of extracranial arterial stenosis to surgical exploration. Such intervention when appropriate might prevent a major stroke or a cerebral infarct. Equally disturbing, but less dramatic in impact, is the effect of obstruction of the vertebral or subclavian vessels. Hind-brain ischaemia causes unpleasant symptoms, and the effects of reverse flow in the vertebral arteries have been recognised since 1960, when the features were first described by Contorni. The possibility of direct relationship between narrowing of the extracranial cerebral vessels and neurological syndromes focuses the need for investigation and diagnosis of such cases at an early stage, and for surgical intervention if appropriate.

MECHANISMS OF CEREBRAL ISCHAEMIA

The classic concept of aetiology of stroke syndromes is concerned with the reduction of blood flow to the cerebral arteries via the circle of Willis. The circulatory effects of an atheromatous plaque in an extracranial feeding artery or reverse flow in a vertebral artery may reduce total cerebral perfusion pressure. This might cause acute thrombosis of the internal carotid artery or of the vertebral artery. Alterations in body posture may temporarily reduce flow through narrow segments, but the relationship of transient symptoms to persistent anatomical defect is more obscure. The demonstration of a surgically correctable and accessible lesion is not uncommon but the selection of those cases suitable for surgery is more of a problem. The precise relationship between atherosclerosis of the major cervical vessels and cerebral infarction is uncertain. Schwartz and Mitchell (1961) in their pathological study of an unselected group of patients demonstrated that the incidence of atheroma of the major cerebral vessels increased with age and stenosis did not necessarily produce cerebral infarction. Millikan (1965) suggested that the importance of stenosis due to atheroma of the cervical vessels in the pathogenesis of cerebral ischaemia was overemphasised. Several further studies demonstrate that significant stenosis can be present in the cervical vessels without histological or pathological evidence of ischaemia during life (Hutchinson and Yates, 1957; Martin, Whisnant and Sayer, 1960; and McGee, McPhedran and Hoffman, 1962).

The association between atheroma and the development of cerebral infarction may be merely a matter of degree. Batacharji, Hutchinson and McCall (1967) demonstrated that atheromatous ulceration of the cervical vessels is significantly more frequent and severe in cases with cerebral infarction than in a controlled series of patients without the evidence of such infarction. The presence of a stenosis in the cervical vessels in itself, therefore, is of dubious importance but the complications of such stenosis may be critical. The high incidence of stenosis of the carotid artery in persons with infarct-free brains has been noted. It has been suggested that episodic hypotension could complicate such lesions and produce thrombosis, but Vost, Wolochow and Howell (1964) found no evidence to support this hypothesis. The significance of arterial narrowing *per se* has also been questioned by the observation of Brice, Dowsett and Lowe (1964), that a 95 per cent reduction in lumen is required to produce demonstrable pressure change. Moreover, total occlusion of a carotid artery that is the subject of stenosis often leads to the complete cessation of all symptoms, and ligation of the vertebral artery has been advocated and practised for the relief of hind-brain ischaemia.

In recent years there has been an increased awareness of the importance of emboli arising from ulcerated atheromatous plaques in the cervical portion of the cerebral blood supply. Fisher (1954) published a clinical and pathological study of carotid artery disease emphasising the importance of emboli arising from such changes at the origin of the internal carotid artery that could cause cerebral infarction . Millikan and Siekert (1955) suggested that an embolus may fragment and pass through the cerebral circulation, causing only transient ischaemia. Examination of the fundus oculi by ophthalmoscope has revealed within the retinal vessels small emboli that have later disappeared (Russell, 1961; Ashby et al, 1963). Gunning et al (1964) have reviewed the concept of the cerebral vascular insufficiency and, from their evidence and other observations, concluded that friable micro-emboli detached from mural · thrombi are the commonest cause of transient blindness and contralateral hemiparesis. McBrien, Bradley and Ashton (1963) demonstrated that such emboli may consist of aggregation of platelets. Permanent arterial occlusion may be produced by larger embolic fragments. Many patients with small vessel occlusion within the brain also have ulcerating lesions in the internal carotid artery or aortic arch vessels (Soloway and Aronson, 1964).

There is good evidence, therefore, for regarding atheromatous ulceration of the cervical blood supply as a common cause of both cerebrovascular insufficiency and cerebral infarction by providing a source for micro-emboli. The fact that post-mortem examination may demonstrate that those vessels immediately supplying an area of infarction are patent does not run counter to this thesis, since Bladin (1964) has shown by serial carotid angiography that emboli may disappear from the circulation within a period of several weeks; this is in accord with known clot removal by fibrinolysis. A constant feature of the clinical history given by patients presenting with transient ischaemic episodes, is the repetitive similarity on each occasion. The explanation probably lies in the 'stream' effect of blood flow so that detached particles of mural thrombi follow laminar flow patterns to identical areas of distribution in each occasion (Luessenhop and Spense (1960)

The appreciation of the role of embolisation and the possibility of surgical intervention renders assessment of cases presenting with transient stroke particularly important. The separation of other causes of focal cerebral pathology and the selection of cases for surgery is essential. The association of hypertension and focal cerebrovascular disease is known to be adverse. The relationship has been clarified by Cole and Yates (1967); they showed that there are changes in the brain associated with systemic hypertension which are specific to that process and are distinct from those found with cerebral infarction. They consist of cystic lesions related to the micro-aneurysms of hypertension; they are found when the diastolic blood pressure is 100 mm Hg or more. The coexistence of ischaemic and hypertensive lesions is extremely rare. The separation of these two groups is clinically, therefore, very important. There is some evidence from Acheson and Hutchinson (1971) that repeated episodes of cerebrovascular insufficiency in normotensive patients affect one anatomical territory, whereas in the hypertensive group the involvement of the three major territories occurs in random fashion. This may be of help in differentiating patients in whom surgery will be indicated. It is unlikely that surgical correction of anatomical deformity in the cervical arteries would affect the outcome in cases with diffuse arterial disease.

The survival rates of patients with transient ischaemic attacks, simple stroke, or multiple strokes, show progressive worsening with the passage of time. It is known (Lyons, 1965; Gurdjian et al, 1965; and Acheson and Hutchinson, 1971) that up to 60 per cent of patients who experience a completed stroke give a history of previous episodes. The prevention of repeated strokes is, therefore, of great importance, and the surgical correction of anatomical abnormality in those cases with appropriate symptoms should be associated with an improved morbidity or significant increase in survival. The essential concept of such surgical treatment is *prophylactic* and in this respect differs fundamentally from more usual surgical practice.

CLINICAL FEATURES

The features of occlusive cerebrovascular disease are determined by the location, severity and extent of cerebral ischaemia. The clinical diagnosis during episodes of short duration rests upon the patient's symptom description. With persistent defects analysis of the residual signs is of value. Three categories of symptom complex may be identified—

1. Transient neurological abnormality (TIA).
2. Stroke in evolution—a picture of pathological instability and fluctuation in symptoms.
3. A completed stroke with fixed neurological deficit.

Patients in categories 1 and 2 commonly present with the following symptoms:

1. Transient paresis affecting the upper or lower limb or both.
2. Transient monocular blindness.
3. Paraesthesiae.

They are frequently repetitive and have been encountered as often as 12 times during a 24-hour period. Table 13.1 shows their relative incidence. Less constant features were dizziness, dysarthria and, occasionally, bilateral episodes of visual blurring. Most of the patients with these symptoms had evidence of vertebro-basilar insufficiency in addition.

Table 13.1. Frequency of presenting symptoms in 70 cases.

Contralateral hemiparesis	52
Contralateral paraesthesiae	46
Monocular blindness (ipsilateral)	18

INVESTIGATION

The initial assessment of the patient's condition should be made by a neurologist. The separation of neurological syndromes due to other forms of pathology requires specialist diagnostic and investigatory techniques. These will usually have included clinical assessment of cardiovascular function for abnormal bruits, hypertension, heart block, or cardiac arrhythmia. EEG, ECG and biochemical/haematological profiles should also have been routinely performed.

The surgeon may also help, by virtue of his experience, in delineating unusual bruits in the neck vessels or upper limbs. Bruits localised to the area of the carotid bifurcation are of significance but on the right side may be transmitted from innominate lesions, and, occasionally, on the left from the subclavian artery. Stenosis of the external carotid artery may also be responsible. Palpation of neck arteries is of little value. A pulse may be felt from the more superficial external carotid artery even when the internal carotid artery is occluded. Superficial temporal pulsation may be a help, however, in the assessment of postoperative patency, since acute occlusion of vessel after operation usually involves the external carotid origin as well as the internal.

Compression of either carotid artery in an attempt to assess the cerebral blood flow or the response to clamp occlusion during prospective surgery is of little value. It may, indeed, be dangerous and may produce dislodgement of an embolus or a syncopal attack resulting from stimulation of the carotid sinus. The blood pressure should be measured routinely in both arms, and significant pressure differences from unsuspected subclavian stenoses are not uncommon. It should be remembered that vertebral artery lesions, total carotid occlusion, or ulcerating atheroma of the carotid artery may be impossible to detect by physical means and the absence of a bruit does not exclude the presence of significant intravascular lesions.

Radiographic examination

The purpose of angiography is to confirm the diagnosis and to provide detailed information for subsequent surgical exploration. The investigation may include arch angiography, four-vessel selective angiography, or bilateral selective carotid angiography. The techniques have been well described by Sutton and Davies (1966). Whatever method is employed it should be simple and safe, and provide anatomical clarity and full demonstration of all the components of the intra- and extra-cranial circulation. It is important to examine the cerebral vessels for evidence of space-occupying lesions and for evidence of atherosclerotic narrowing of the major branches of the internal carotid artery or of the siphon of this artery. Demonstrable lesions here are associated with an adverse prognosis.

The limitations of arch angiography are well recognised. Detail of atheromatous lesions within the arch is often obscured by the density of opacification, and two oblique projections are essential. Stenosis in the major aortic branches can be identified in this way (Figure 13.1) but detail of internal carotid abnormalities are often poorly demonstrated by this method. Micro-emboli may not infrequently arise from ulcerating atheroma within the arch and the demonstration of such defects is extremely difficult, if not impossible. The routine use of subtraction techniques has proved of some help in this area and in the detection of reverse flow, as found in subclavian steal syndromes. Selective low puncture radiography of both carotid arteries is perhaps the most useful method of detailing treatable lesions at the bifurcation of the carotid artery. Two-plane radiography and, in particular, the horizontal beam techniques have proved to be of great help (Figure 13.2). The trickle method described by Hugh (1970) in this context is of great assistance in localising marginal stenosis as well as in highlighting focal stasis (Figure 13.3), or adherent thrombi (Figure 13.4), attached to what can be quite superficial areas of ulceration (Figure 13.5). The details that have been

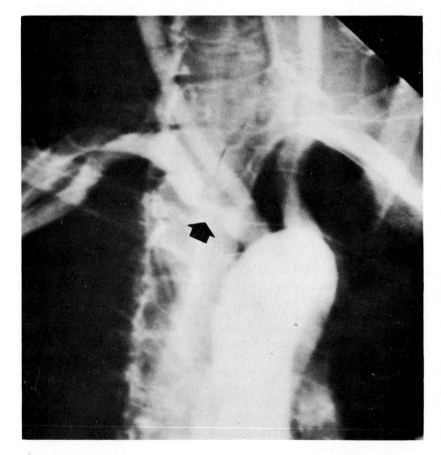

Figure 13.1. Arch angiogram showing severe stenosis of the right subclavian artery.

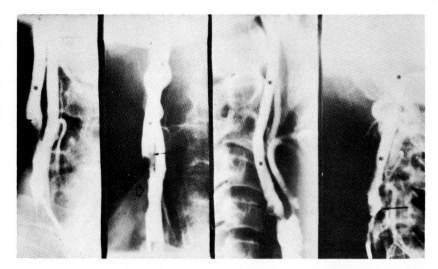

Figure 13.2. Selective carotid angiograms demonstrating the appearance seen in antero-posterior and lateral projections. The two films on the left and the two films on the right of the illustration are from similar carotid arterial systems. The degree of stenosis and the presence of mural thrombus is highlighted by alteration of projection.

shown by these techniques have correlated well with the macroscopic pathological appearance revealed by surgery (Figure 13.6). Equally as important is the demonstration of inoperable lesions such as are found when total occlusion of the internal carotid artery is present (Figure 13.7).

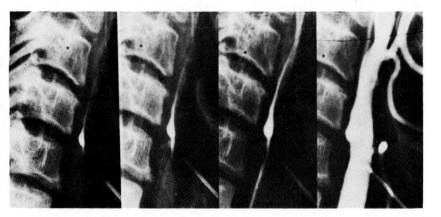

Figure 13.3. Trickle angiography (Hugh, 1970) demonstrating a small mural ulcer with contrast stasis. The exposures were made at 0, 2, 4 and 6 seconds after injection and are to be viewed from right to left.

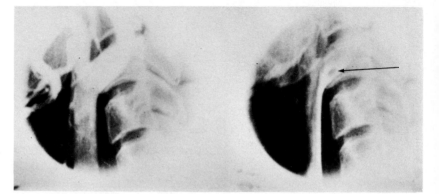

Figure 13.4. Comparison of conventional (left) with trickle carotid angiogram. A small thrombus is clearly seen in the right-hand picture, taken during trickle angiography, which was not apparent during conventional radiology of the same vessel.

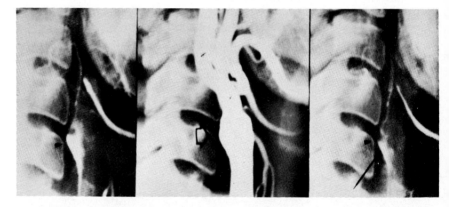

Figure 13.5. Trickle angiogram of carotid artery. Note the presence of contrast stasis and mural thrombus seen during the 4 and 6 second angiograms. These are on the extreme left and extreme right of the illustration.

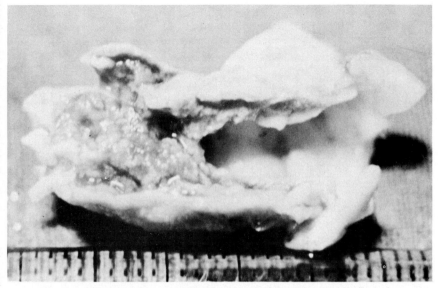

Figure 13.6. Operative specimen showing adherent mural thrombus and shallow ulcer crater.

SURGICAL TECHNICAL CONSIDERATIONS

It must be remembered that the surgical treatment of carotid artery disease has been developed only during the past 20 years. The first successful record of surgical relief of carotid artery stenosis was by Eastcott, Pickering and Rob in 1954 and the first successful endarterectomy for this condition was performed by Cooley, Al-Naaman and Carton (1956). An earlier attempt at reconstruction by endarterectomy by Strully, Hurwitt and Blankenberg (1953) was unsuccessful. Other reports of successful surgical intervention appeared in the literature at about the same time (Gurdjian and Webster, 1958; Rob and Wheeler, 1957). Since then, debate has waxed and waned about the techniques available for the procedure. Most debate has probably centred about the technique that should be employed to protect the cerebral circulation and oxygenation during operation, and this is considered next.

ANAESTHESIA FOR CAROTID RECONSTRUCTION

Local anaesthesia was employed in the early stages of surgery, using either a field block or a cervical plexus block. One theoretical advantage was that the method allowed the surgeon to evaluate the effects of his procedure while it was taking place. The effects of trial occlusion of the internal carotid or common carotid arteries upon responses to questions or upon volitional movement were assessed and if any neurological deficit occurred the clamp was removed. Patients prefer to be asleep, however, and trial clamping is no guarantee of safety during prolonged occlusion at operation.

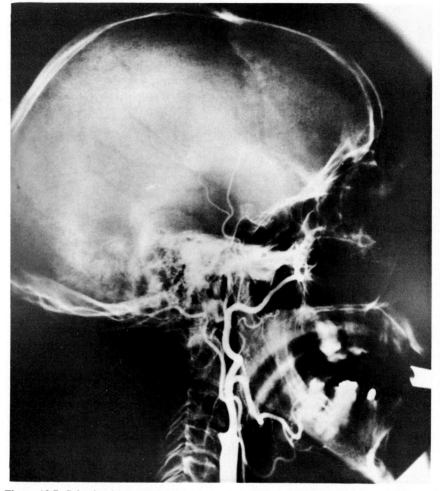

Figure 13.7. Selective low puncture right carotid angiogram. Note the total occlusion of the internal carotid artery.

General anaesthesia with hypothermia induced by surface cooling had a vogue for some time. Body temperature was reduced to 30 to 32°C, as at these temperatures the cerebral consumption of oxygen is reduced to about 50 per cent of normal. The total period of anaesthesia for operation is prolonged by this method and may induce the added risks of hypotension, cardiac arrhythmia, and abnormal blood clotting. It is a surgically cumbersome method.

General anaesthesia with the use of an intracarotid shunt has many advocates, and will maintain flow during operation. The Javid, Ostermiller and Henish (1970) shunt is probably the best available at present. The insertion of the shunt is not always easy, however, and the author has certainly produced microembolisation by dislodgement of fragments during the insertion of shunts. Magowan, Lynch and Staunton (1971) report similar difficulties.

Adequate protection is afforded to the cerebral cortex by modern anaesthetic methods. Wells, Keates and Cooley (1963) originally suggested hypercarbic anaesthesia, using cyclopropane and a high oxygen content. Hypercarbia is a potent means of increasing cerebral blood flow and elevation of pCO_2 to 60 mm Hg is associated with doubling of the cerebral blood flow (Larsen, 1970; Hutchinson, personal communication). For this to hold true it is important to maintain systemic blood pressure at or slightly above normal values. In the conscious patient fluctuation in blood pressure has little effect on cerebral blood flow due to autoregulation. There is evidence, however, that under anaesthesia this regulation is absent (Wylie and Ehrenfeld, 1970) and that the pressure in the occluded carotid artery is influenced by a fall in the systemic blood pressure. Debakey et al (1965) and Wylie and Ehrenfeld (1970), have published the results of operations upon large series of cases, using these methods without complication.

We have used a modification of this technique for the past seven years. The method has been developed by my colleague Dr W. K. Merifield, and is as follows—

Premedication, using pethidine 50 mg and promethazine 50 mg is given one hour preoperatively. Anaesthesia is induced with sodium methohexital and atropine 0.6 mg, followed by 50 mg suxemethonium chloride. The vocal cords are then sprayed with 4 per cent lignocaine, an oral endotracheal tube is inserted, and the cuff is inflated. Inhalational anaesthesia is started, using a gas/oxygen mixture with 1 to 1.5 per cent halothane. An intravenous infusion of dextrose/saline is started and the patient is placed on the operating theatre table. Anaesthesia is continued, using the Magill semi-open circuit. Nitrous oxide is then discontinued and the patient is given a mixture of 1 per cent halothane and 99 per cent oxygen, supplied at a rate of 4 litres/min. Respiration is reduced to about 12 breaths per min with incremental doses of phenoperidine and droperidol. These drugs depress the patient's respiratory rate and help to maintain a satisfactory level of anaesthesia. This technique is used continuously for the remainder of the operation until final extubation in theatre. It was our original practice to increase the pCO_2 to a level above 60 mm Hg by the addition of extra CO_2 from the anaesthetic machine, in order to achieve maximal increase in cerebral blood flow. Experience has led us to modify this procedure and to allow spontaneous increase of the patient's alveolar CO_2, by diminished respiratory rate resulting in less elevation of the carbon dioxide tension in the blood. The advantages are seen in a markedly reduced incidence of cardiac arrhythmias.

Blood pressure maintenance is essential. Larsen (1970) points out that autoregulation of the cerebral blood flow is affected by carotid occlusion. As a result of this, if variations occur in systemic blood pressure, the stump pressure in the occluded artery will be affected and cerebral perfusion will drop. Should systemic pressure fall, therefore, it is artificially raised. Simple augmentation of intravenous fluid therapy is usually sufficient but if this is not the case then incremental 10 mg doses of methyl amphetamine are given as necessary.

Measurement of venous oxygen tension in jugular blood has been suggested as an index of cerebral blood flow (Viancos et al, 1966). Measurements we have taken show an increased pVO_2 of up to 110 mm Hg (range 60 to 110 mm Hg). This is taken to indicate an increase in mean cerebral blood flow and reflects an arteriovenous difference of 400 to 500 mm Hg. Failure adequately to maintain blood pressure is demonstrably harmful. Stump pressure falls and back bleeding is virtually non-existent. In one case in which this was experienced through a technical error, there was a markedly delayed recovery following anaesthesia and temporary paresis of an arm was present for 24 hours. Complete recovery, however, ensued after this period. This was the only case in our experience in which the cerebral perfusion pressure has been inadequate and the only one in which the features of impaired perfusion have been encountered. This was also the only patient in whom there was not immediate recovery from anaesthesia and in whom full consciousness was not restored within 30 minutes. Following extubation at the conclusion of surgery, all remaining patients would respond to simple commands and were fully conscious and responsive two hours later.

TECHNIQUE OF CAROTID ENDARTERECTOMY

After induction of anaesthesia the operative area is prepared and draped and a 5 to 10° head-up tilt established, with the appropriate side of the neck rotated away from the surgeon. The relevant carotid artery is then exposed through an oblique incision centred on the anterior border of sterno-mastoid at the level of the angle of the jaw and angled a little towards the horizontal. This incision heals well and does not form the unpleasant scar which might be anticipated by those surgeons unfamiliar with this route. The incision is deepened, the platysma muscle divided, and superficial nerves avoided where possible. The carotid sheath is identified and opened, the internal jugular vein and common facial vein being dissected carefully. The latter is separated for a length of 1 to 2 cm and then divided between ligatures. As long a piece as possible is preserved in normal saline in readiness for use later as patch angioplasty.

The common carotid artery is cleaned by sharp dissection of its adventitial attachment about 3 to 4 cm below the bifurcation; this can usually be identified as a widening in the course of the artery and the external division may be identified by the presence of its first branch, the superior thyroid artery. Nylon tapes are passed around the common carotid artery and the external carotid artery as far distant as possible from the carotid sinus. The superior thyroid artery and, occasionally, the ascending pharyngeal vessels are temporarily occluded by silk ligature. Traction is then exerted to the external carotid artery, which permits dissection into the adventitial plane of the internal carotid artery. Care is taken to pass the instruments and subsequent nylon tapes around this vessel as far distant from the bifurcation itself as the limit of dissection will permit. By these means it is possible to avoid alterations in pulse rate or rhythm which can occur due to stimulation of the carotid sinus. It also obviates the need to infiltrate local anaesthetic to this area as advocated by Eastcott (1969).

When all three vessels have been isolated and taped, provided the systemic blood pressure is at least equal to the pre-operative value, occlusion clamps are applied. A vertical arteriotomy is then made in the common carotid artery proximal to the bifurcation and is extended into the internal carotid vessel. The ulcerated or stenotic areas of diseased intima are then gently separated from the outer arterial coats. Particular attention is taken at the distal attachment to produce a clean separation and the first centimetre or so of the external carotid artery is also cleared of intima. The distal line of separation is divided smoothly and then all adherent fragments are carefully removed. The divided distal layer of intima is fixed into position to prevent flap lifting with several sutures of 6 × 0 Ethiflex. Careful irrigation of this zone with saline will usually demonstrate any non-adherent portions.

The arteriotomy is then closed with the insertion of a diamond-shaped piece of vein, so as to widen its termination. The piece of common facial vein, which has been preserved from the start of the operation, is used for this purpose; it is attached with two running 6 × 0 Ethiflex sutures starting at the distal end of the arteriotomy and sutured evenly to ensure a smooth entrance to the internal carotid vessel itself. The angioplasty extends proximally to the bifurcation of the common carotid artery. It was former practice to extend the angioplasty to include the entire arteriotomy, but experience has shown this to be unnecessary and even undesirable, since abnormal dilatation may be produced with excessive turbulence of blood. It may be argued that angioplasty closure is unnecessary, and in many cases this may well be correct, but if the internal carotid artery is of small calibre any build-up of fibrin or blood particles at the distal suture line may cause progressive narrowing of the lumen. In critical cases this may go on to thrombosis or may accentuate otherwise minimal degrees of distal intimal separation. The effects of postoperative occlusion of the operated artery are extremely serious and usually cause an acute hemiparesis. Prevention of this complication is highly desirable and, since we have established that the length of time during which the internal carotid artery is occluded does not influence the outcome of surgery, there is no reason to hasten closure by avoiding the extra time required to insert a small vein patch.

The suture line is continued until 3 or 4 sutures only are required for completion and then the clamps occluding external, internal and common carotid vessels are released in order that any debris or blood clot that may have formed adjacent to them can be expelled. The vessel is washed out with heparinised saline and the final few sutures are then inserted. When the clamps are finally removed, the flow into the external carotid artery from the common carotid artery is always restored before that to the internal carotid vessel. If the pressure is measured in the internal carotid artery at clamp release, it is found to be about 70 per cent of the systemic blood pressure, and the jet released by back bleeding is an excellent guide to this value. Use has been made of this so-called stump pressure by Wylie and Ehrenfeld (1970) as a prognostic guide to cerebral perfusion pressure during clamp occlusion. After the completion of anastomosis, it is our practice to delay wound closure for 20 to 30 min so that any detectable fault of technique that may lead to thrombosis can be recognised. If the anastomosis remains satisfactory for this period the wound is then closed in layers, using a subcuticular skin closure and suction drainage.

During the surgical exploration of the carotid system, using this technique, the blood pressure is monitored continuously. The pressure is maintained at or above the preoperative level; this can usually be done with intravenous saline solution or Dextran but, occasionally, sympathomimetic amines, such as Methedrine, are required. Spontaneous respiration also contributes to this, as there is a slight elevation of pCO_2, usually to the upper 50 or lower 60 mm Hg range. This may add to cerebral vasodilatation but is probably far more important for its hypertensive effect. Samples were taken from a percentage of cases during the series, to measure arterial and venous pO_2. Systemic pO_2 is usually in excess of 600 mm Hg (450 to 710 range). Venous pO_2 is usually above 100 mm Hg (60 to 110 mm Hg). Arterial samples were taken from the common carotid artery and venous samples from the upper jugular vein. The measurements were made by radiometer Clark electrode.

It is not our practice to use anticoagulants during surgery, other than a small amount of heparin in the irrigating solutions. These are prepared using a dose of 10 000 i.u./litre of saline. Systemic heparin is not given and no heparin solutions are injected into the distal carotid arteries. Kenyon, Thomas and Goodwin (1972) have reported 34 explorations of the carotid artery using systemic heparin for brain protection. Minor complications occurred postoperatively but no significant neurological sequelae occurred. The possibility of haemorrhage from infarcted areas does exist, however, and we prefer to avoid the risk presented by the use of this drug since from our experience there is no evidence of intracerebral coagulation during temporary occlusion of carotid flow. When surgery is performed for transient ischaemic attack alone, as in the Kenyon et al series, this risk is certainly very small.

On completion of the operative manoeuvre the patient is extubated in Theatre and at this stage will usually respond to simple stimuli. Full consciousness is resumed in the Recovery Ward, and all limb movements are checked prior to the return to the main ward. Blood pressure is monitored during this period and intravenous therapy continued. It is usually necessary to allow for bladder emptying at this time, since the maintenance of blood pressure during surgery by intravenous routes gives a high rate of urinary secretion.

EXAMPLES OF SURGICAL TREATMENT

Case 1
A 57-year-old housewife was admitted to hospital as an emergency, with a left hemiparesis involving predominantly the left upper limb. There was a previous history of two similar but transient episodes three and five months earlier, consisting of loss of use of the left hand and forearm for half an hour on one occasion, and one hour on the second occasion. She was normotensive on admission to hospital, and no other features of note were found. After 48 hours, the movement of the upper and lower limbs had virtually returned to normal. Bilateral carotid angiography was performed at this stage, and demonstrated a severe lesion at the origin of the right internal carotid artery (Figure 13.8). One week later the right carotid artery was explored surgically. At that time, no neurological abnormality was found on clinical examination. The operation was uneventful and an ulcerated, thickened area of intima with adherent thrombus was excised (Figure 13.9). The carotid artery blood flow was interupted for 44 minutes and a full length angioplasty was performed in this case (Figure 13.10). The post-operative course was uncomplicated and she was discharged home on the 9th post-operative day. The appearances of the operated vessels are shown in Figure 13.11. Follow-up has been for five years and no further neurological features have occurred during this time.

Comment
The cerebral ischaemic episodes in this case were typical of microembolisation. The persistence of the neurological signs suggested that it fitted into the category of 'stroke in evolution'. Many of these cases improve quite rapidly and are well worth investigating and treating by surgery. The ulcerated area of atheroma with fibrin, red and white blood cells, platelets and cholesterol elements adherent to its surface provided a ready source of emboli, and subsequent symptoms could well have proved serious with permanent features. The likelihood in this case of an eventual stroke was high, and five post-operative years follow-up without further problem confirmed that surgical treatment was beneficial.

Case 2
F.R. A 48-year-old man was referred to the neurologists after multiple episodes of loss of vision in the left eye. Physical examination revealed a harsh bruit over the left carotid artery. No other physical signs were found, apart from the remains of a small cholesterol embolus detected on ophthalmological examination of the left fundus oculi. The patient was normotensive and had no other evidence of arterial pathology on clinical examination. Bilateral selective carotid angiography was performed and the appearances of the left carotid system are shown in Figure 13.12. Surgery was advised and performed one week later, and an area of ulcerated atheroma was removed from the carotid bifurcation (Figure 13.13). The carotid artery was occluded for a period of 38 min and patch angioplasty was performed. Recovery was uneventful and follow-up for $3\frac{1}{2}$ years postoperatively has shown no recurrence of symptoms.

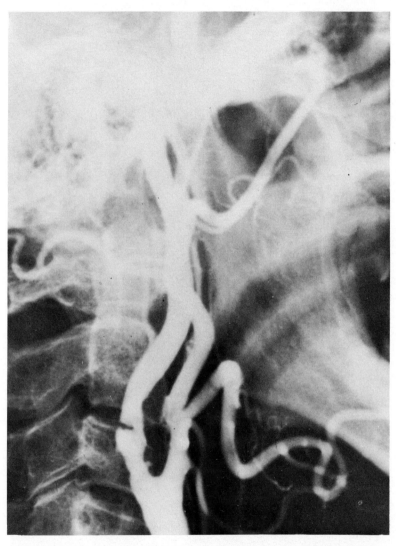

Figure 13.8. Selective low puncture right carotid angiogram. Note the degree of stenosis and double ulcer craters which are visible just distal to the carotid bifurcation.

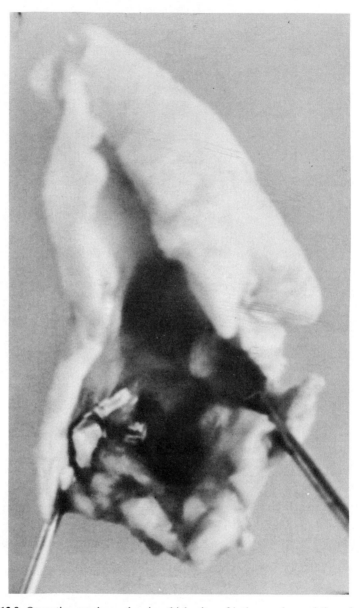

Figure 13.9. Operative specimen showing thickening of intima and mural thrombus.

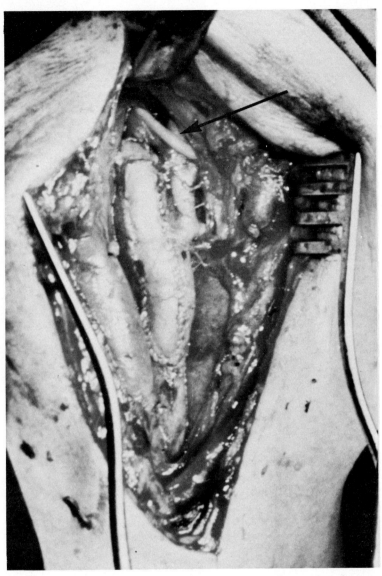

Figure 13.10. The appearance of carotid vessels after endarterectomy. Note the appearance of full length angioplasty and the close proximity of the hypoglossal nerve to the upper limit of the arteriotomy.

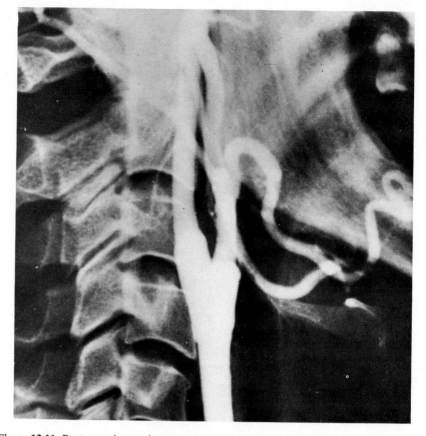

Figure 13.11. Postoperative angiogram taken 1 week after surgical exploration.

Comment

The visual features in this case were typical of recurrent peripheral micro-embolisation of the retinal vessels. The glistening appearance shown in the pathological specimen removed from the carotid vessels was typical and is produced by adherent red cells and thrombus upon an ulcerated area of atheroma. A comparatively large area was involved in this instance, but cases have been seen in which the ulcerated intima was quite superficial but with obvious adherent thrombus.

Case 3

F.D. A retired professional man of 73 years was first seen after recurrent episodes of transient blindness and three episodes of paraesthesia and difficulty in moving the left upper limb. There were no abnormal neurological features on first clinical examination, and the blood pressure was normal. Bruits were present over both carotid bifurcations. He had a history of myocardial infarction but an ECG showed minimal change. Bilateral selective low puncture carotid angiography was performed and showed that a severe stenosis was present on the inappropriate side, and ulcerating atheroma was demonstrated in the right internal carotid artery. In view of the previous history and the patient's age, together with the

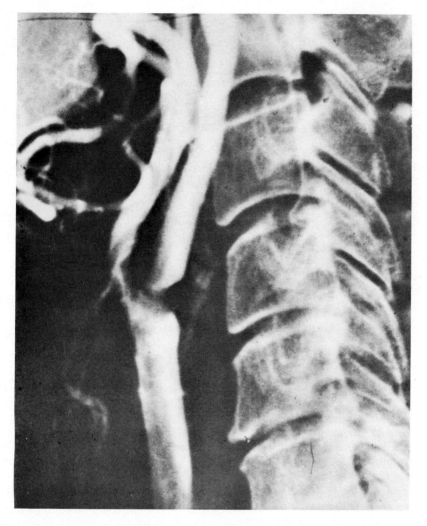

Figure 13.12. Left carotid angiogram. Note the severe degree of stenosis present at both internal and external carotid artery origins.

possibility of occlusion of the stenotic vessel during reconstruction of the ulcerated internal carotid artery, it was decided to operate upon both vessels. The symptomless left carotid system was explored first as a precaution. A 2 cm stenosis was excised, and reconstruction included a vein patch angioplasty. The carotid flow was occluded for a total of 58 min on this side. No neurological features were encountered in the postoperative period and one month later the opposite side was explored. The appearances of the excised intimal segment from this side are shown in Figure 13.14. The carotid artery flow on this side was occluded for 49 min. Recovery, as in the first operation, was uneventful. The post-operative follow-up has been for two years to date and no recurrent symptoms have been encountered during this period.

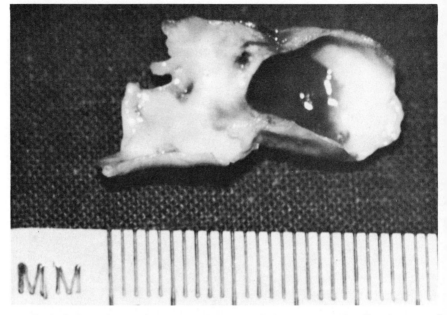

Figure 13.13. Operative specimen. Note the degree of narrowing and the glistening area of mural thrombus.

Comment

The appearances of the carotid system on the symptomless side are shown in Figure 13.15. It will be noted that a severe degree of stenosis was present and it was feared that in a man of this age, with a previous history of myocardial infarction, the control of blood pressure might be difficult. Any attendant drop in systemic arterial pressure during the operation could have precipitated total occlusion of this segment if the side producing symptoms were dealt with in the first instance. At operation, however, although the blood pressure tended to be labile, there was no undue difficulty in maintaining an adequate perfusion pressure and no complications ensued. The postoperative angiographic appearances of the reconstructed vessel on this side are shown in Figure 13.16. The reconstruction of the side with relevant symptoms was carred out a month later, and proceeded uneventfully even though the source for cerebral microembolisation, which is shown in Figure 13.14, was quite severely ulcerated. It is of interest, also, that no problems have occurred to date with regard to maintenance of blood pressure during changes of posture.

Case 4
S.D. A somewhat overweight man of 57 years was referred for a neurological assessment after a transient loss of use of his left arm. There was also a history of episodic blindness affecting the right eye on several occasions during the previous four weeks. A bruit was present over the right internal carotid artery but no other relevant physical signs were present. Bilateral carotid angiography was performed and showed a narrowing of the origin of the right internal carotid vessel (Figure 13.17) and an unexpected total occlusion

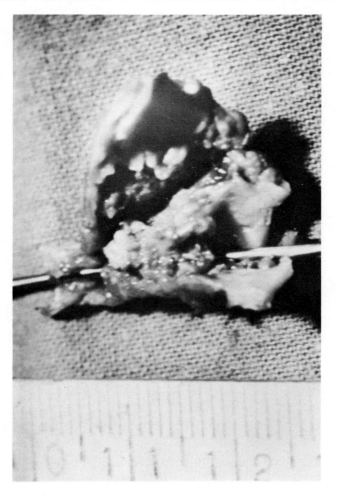

Figure 13.14. Operative specimen. The probe passes through the small residual channel and is surrounded by thrombus.

of the left internal carotid artery. In view of these findings, arch angiography was performed to determine the adequacy of vertebral blood flow. Operation was subsequently advised and exploration of the right internal carotid artery was performed in the usual way. The total occlusion time was 48 min and a very good back bleed was obtained from the stump of the internal carotid artery during clamp release. Recovery from anaesthetic was rapid, following extubation and, by return to the ward, the patient was conversing. The appearances of the internal carotid artery and its origin during exploration are shown in Figure 13.18 in which it will be noted that there is a ball thrombus visible. The close-up details of this are shown in Figure 13.19. At the conclusion of the surgical procedure, closure included the small diamond angioplasty which is our current standard practise, and a close-up detail of which is shown in Figure 13.20.

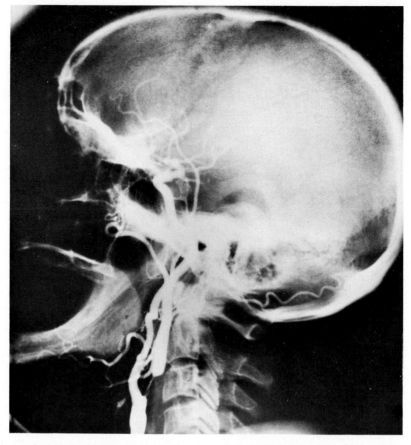

Figure 13.15. Left carotid angiogram showing severe stenosis of the internal carotid artery.

Comment

This case is interesting in that it is one of several that demonstrate that cerebral blood flow can be maintained during reconstructive surgery by vertebral flow alone. The arch angiogram performed pre-operatively demonstrated that both vertebral arteries were patent with evidence of good flow rate. The patent carotid artery was occluded for a total of 48 min and extensive atheromatous disease with thrombus formation was excised during this period. Blood pressure was maintained at 10 mm above the patient's normal resting arterial pressure for the whole of this period, and stump pressure appeared to be adequate during trial clamp release. pO_2 was measured in the arterial and venous blood during this case and the pAO_2 was 610 mm Hg and pVO_2 110 mm Hg. Recovery following surgery was rapid and uneventful. It was considered essential in this case to perform patch angioplasty since it is highly probable that a postoperative thrombotic complication at the site of operation could have produced disastrous effects.

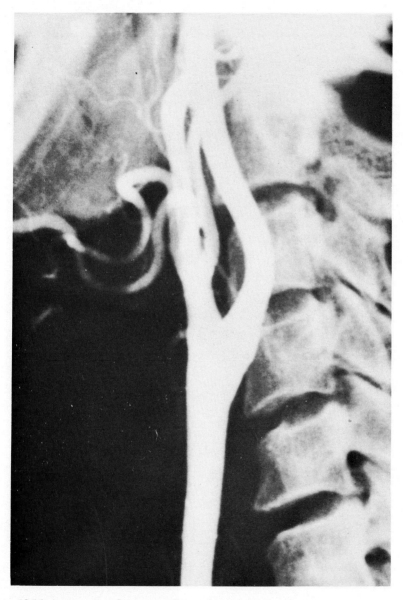

Figure 13.16. Appearance of postoperative angiogram.

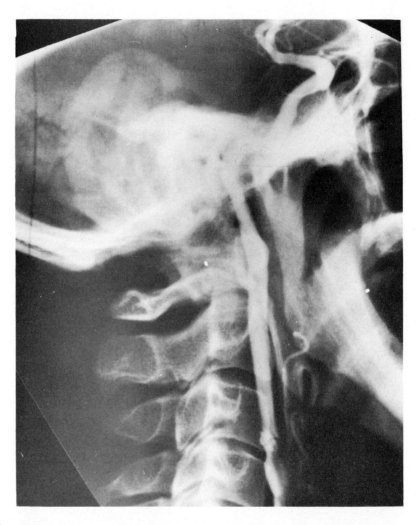

Figure 13.17. Lateral carotid angiogram with stenosis of the internal carotid artery origin.

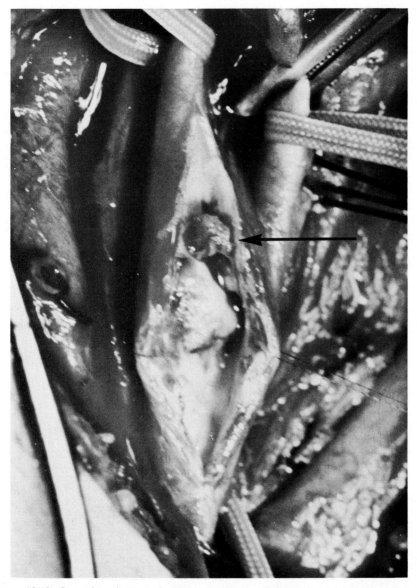

Figure 13.18. Operative photograph. Note the degree of thickening of intima with ball thrombus attached to the wall.

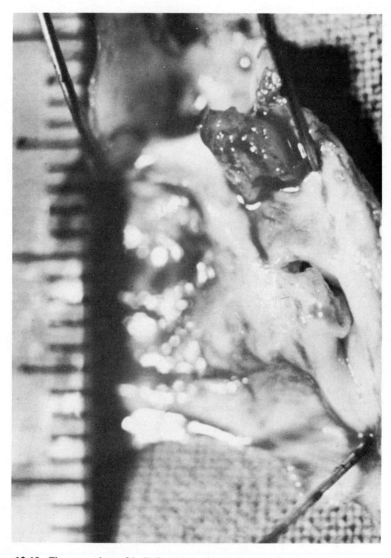

Figure 13.19. Close-up view of ball thrombus shown in Fig. 13.18.

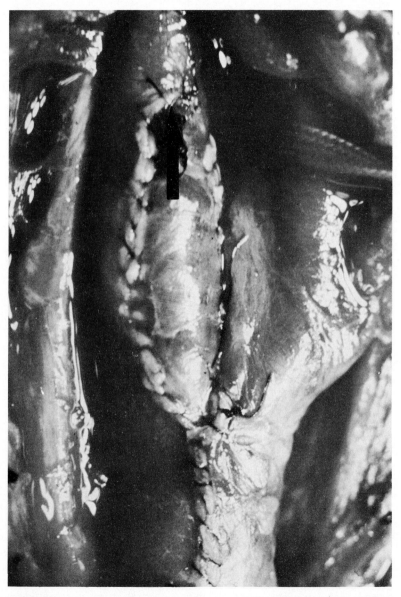

Figure 13.20. The appearance of carotid vessels on completion of operation. Small diamond-shaped angioplasty to the upper half of the arteriotomy is visible, terminating at the carotid bifurcation.

Case 5

J.D. A young man of 23 was referred from another hospital after admission with a left hemiparesis. This was beginning to recover by the time of transfer and was the third such episode of hemiparesis the patient had experienced within nine months. The left lower limb had regained coarse movements, but the left upper limb had only a minimal degree of movement when he was first seen. The previous two episodes had been very similar, but complete recovery had ensued in each case. Examination of the patient showed the presence of a small swelling in the right side of the neck, over which a bruit was clearly audible. He was normotensive and no other physical signs of note, other than those relevant to the hemiparesis, were apparent. The presumptive diagnosis was of an aneurysm of the common or internal carotid arteries with microembolisation of the cerebrum. Surgical exploration was advised and performed ten days after admission. It was confirmed that an aneurysm was present arising from the internal carotid artery 5 mm after its origin from the common carotid artery and extending distally to within 1.5 cm of the base of skull. The aneurysm was mobilised with care and was then resected after interruption of carotid blood flow with occlusion clamps. The usual anaesthetic procedure was followed and blood pressure was carefully maintained at the pre-operative level. The length of aneurysm measured some 5.5 cm in length and it was decided to restore the deficit in the internal carotid artery by means of autogenous saphenous vein. The appropriate length of saphenous vein was then removed from the upper part of the right thigh and cleaned of its adentitial layer. It was then sutured end to end between the stump of the internal carotid artery and the transected upper portion about 1.5 cm below the base of the skull (Figure 13.21). The carotid flow was interrupted for a total of 78 min while this procedure was performed. This patient awoke within half an hour of the completion of the anaesthetic and was fully conversational. There were no additional neurological deficits to those which had been present at the beginning of the operation. The appearances of the excised aneurysm are shown in Figure 13.22.

Comment

Aneurysms of the internal carotid artery are comparatively rare but are seen from time to time. They may give rise to microembolisation of cerebral tissue in a similar manner to that associated with ulcerated atheroma. The important difference in their surgical management is the method of reconstruction. Autogenous saphenous vein is a very satisfactory substitute for the normal carotid artery in this situation, and is used as a total replacement for the excised segment of diseased artery.

RESULTS OF SURGERY FOR CAROTID ARTERY DISEASE

Since 1968 we have operated on 70 patients with carotid artery disease; 54 were male and the remainder female. The right side was involved primarily in 37 and the left in 33. There was evidence of bilateral disease in 24 cases. There were no immediate operative deaths. Two patients developed neurological deficits at 16 and 18 hours postoperatively and were re-submitted to surgery. Occlusion of the operated vessel occurred in both cases due to a dissection of the distal intimal flap. In both cases clots were evacuated and vein patch angioplasty was performed. In neither case had angioplasty been performed at the original operation and in no case in whom an angioplasty had been part of the operative procedure had similar thrombosis of the operated segment occurred. The remaining patients were all satisfactory postoperatively. One had a secondary haemorrhage at 5 days, requiring re-exploration and suture. One death occurred 3 weeks after operation from cardiac arrest. The majority of the patients had been explored because of

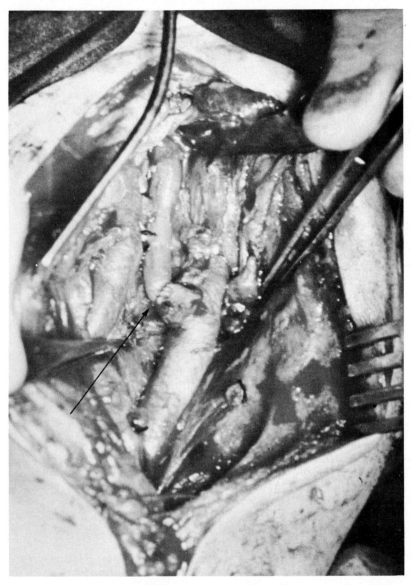

Figure 13.21. Operative photograph of reconstructed internal carotid artery using autogenous saphenous vein. The proximal suture line is clearly visible.

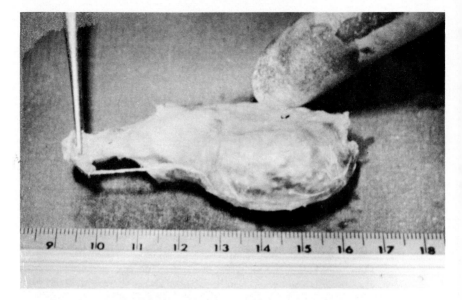

Figure 13.22. Aneurysm of the internal carotid artery (postoperative specimen).

episodes of TIA. The remainder were submitted to surgery after completed strokes. Of 70 patients, 5 have died subsequently, 3 from progressive neurological lesions, and 2 from coronary artery occlusion. All had presented with episodes of frank stroke. In those patients presenting with transient ischaemic episodes, further symptoms have occurred during the follow-up period in 4 of 40. Thus, approximately 90 per cent have remained symptom free. By comparison, 8 patients presenting with completed strokes have had further symptoms or subsequent strokes. No patients were made actively worse by surgery and no additional neurological deficits were produced. Prior to this series an attempt had been made to operate on acute thrombosis of the internal carotid artery and the occasional case of total occlusion. No improvement was produced in either of these types of patient and in the latter group it is not possible to achieve a flow through the diseased and occluded artery. The results are in general agreement with other published series.

The operative mortality is 1 case in 70 operations, representing a mortality rate of 1.4 per cent. This compares with a range of 1.5 per cent in a series by Thomson, Austin and Patman (1970) to 5.6 per cent for Bloodwell et al's series (1968). Eastcott refers to 4 deaths in his first 80 cases but like our single death all these occurred in patients submitted to surgery for completed stroke. Wylie and Ehrenfeld (1970) report a mortality of 0.5 per cent in their last 219 operations. Our technique of surgical treatment is similar to that of Wylie and Ehrenfeld (1970) and Debakey et al (1965). Routine use of patch angioplasty increases the time of carotid occlusion. A mean figure of 43 min with a range of 20 to 78 min has been recorded. No neurological deficits have been associated with this length of occlusion, and all patients, save 1 who was hypotensive during clamp occlusion, have awoken instantly at the end of the operation. The 2 cases who suffered occlusion of the endarterectomised segment of carotid artery in the postoperative period both woke instantly after surgery and became hemiparetic after 12 to 18 hours. Neither case had been treated with angioplasty and minimal intimal dissection produced their post-operative thrombosis. It is thought that patch angioplasty in these cases would have prevented the complication. Both were treated by this method at a second procedure. They eventually recovered completely, although recovery of speech defects in both cases was slow.

SELECTION OF CASES FOR SURGERY AND COMPARISONS OF SURGICAL AND CONSERVATIVE TREATMENT

The best results following surgery are seen when operation is performed for transient ischaemic attack. Wylie and Ehrenfeld (1970), Eastcott (1969) and Deweese et al (1973) have all published results which support this conclusion. Surgical intervention in patients with acute stroke or completed stroke failed to show improvement and indeed in a combined study of surgical and non-surgical cases (Bauer et al, 1969) there was a definitely less favourable outcome after surgery, and in bilateral carotid disease with occlusion of one artery a mortality rate of 45 per cent was experienced in the operative group. In patients with signs of improvement after an initial hemiparesis there may be a place for prophylactic surgery but they must be chosen directly on individual merit. Surgery in the case of complete occlusion of the appropriate artery is definitely contraindicated.

Support for operative treatment is obtained from the low morbidity and mortality of the operative procedure and statistical evidence of an improved prognosis when compared with non-operative methods. Bauer (Figure 13.23)

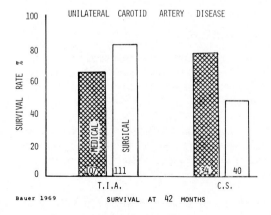

Figure 13.23. Comparative survival rates in unilateral carotid artery disease. On the left, data from cases presenting with transient ischaemic episode. On the right, similar data from cases presenting with completed stroke. Taken from Bauer et al, 1969.

has reported that of 218 patients presenting with transient ischaemic attacks and having unilateral carotid artery disease, random medical or surgical treatment showed a 17 per cent difference in favour of surgery. The cumulative survival rate at 42 months was 83 per cent in the group having surgery compared with a 50 per cent survival in those treated medically. This is significant at the 5 per cent confidence level in favour of surgery. Long-term results again show a bias in favour of the surgical group in patients presenting with transient ischaemic attacks. None of our cases who presented with these features have had further strokes or neurological episodes. A much smaller percentage of those treated who had persistent deficits remained symptom-free and further episodes of stroke occurred. Three of our patients died from this cause. Deweese et al (1973) have recently given evidence of an 84 per cent 5-year symptom-free rate for those patients presenting with transient ischaemic episodes and having classical symptoms. The mortality rate in this series was 34 per cent, mainly from myocardial infarction. This probably reflected the age structure of the series, since 70 per cent of their group and about 90 per cent of the deaths occurred in the 60 to 80 age group. The mean age of our series was 56 years, and 70 per cent of patients were in fact under 60 years of age. Eastcott and Kenyon (Eastcott, 1974) report a 60 per cent neurologically 'intact' rate at 5 years and Wylie and Ehrenfeld published a 90 per cent success rate at 4 years.

The figures from all centres, therefore, favour surgical intervention, particularly in those patients with transient ischaemic attacks. It is to be expected that patients in this category who are untreated will show at least a 35 per cent stroke rate over a 5-year period and a 60 per cent incidence has been reported in this country. The reduction in incidence in all reported groups treated by surgery appears, therefore, to be well worth while. Even when diffuse arterial disease is present in the elderly patient, it is worth remembering that in cerebrovascular insufficiency morbidity is almost as important as mortality and the quality of survival without stroke is worth pursuing.

HIND-BRAIN ISCHAEMIA

The prognosis and symptoms of hind-brain ischaemia are in general less serious than those of carotid insufficiency. Considerable discomfort and disability may be experienced by the patient, however. Two mechanisms are probably responsible—

1. Embolisation of the basilar territory from vertebral origin disease.
2. Haemodynamic change in the same territory produced by reverse flow in the vertebral artery when this vessel itself is normal and in the presence of occlusion or near occlusion of the proximal subclavian artery.

The former condition may be resolved spontaneously by occlusion of the vertebral artery or by ligation of this vessel in some cases, or endarterectomy in others. The latter state of affairs is remediable by subclavian endarterectomy or, better, by carotid subclavian by-pass.

VERTEBRAL ARTERY DISEASE

The place of surgery in the treatment of this condition is by no means established. Exploration is indicated when symptoms are definite and angiography confirms localised disease at the vertebral origin. The surgical approach to the vessel is identical to that to be described subsequently for exploration of the subclavian artery during by-pass. Two procedures are available to deal with the atheromatous area—

1.Trans-subclavian endarterectomy, in which the affected portion of intima is excised across the lumen of the subclavian artery. This is a technically difficult procedure, due to the characteristic softness of the subclavian arterial wall rendering lateral tearing a definite hazard. Moreover, the intimal separation line tends to be uncertain and occlusion of the vessel itself is not uncommonly the outcome after surgery.

2. Flush ligation of the vertebral origin from the subclavian artery, and transplantation of the distal portion of the vessel into the side of the adjacent common carotid artery. By careful dissection, 3 to 4 cm of the vertebral artery can be mobilised. It will then swing freely and can be anastomosed by interrupted sutures to the side of the carotid artery. As Wylie (1970) reports, this is a more satisfactory procedure than endarterectomy, since a clean anastomosis can be effected and overcomes the uncertainty of the intimal separation zone during vertebral endarterectomy. Two cases have been treated by this method. Both have been relieved of symptoms, and the vertebral arteries are patent at twelve months. Wylie and Ehrenfeld (1970) report successful use of this method on three occasions.

SUBCLAVIAN ARTERY OBSTRUCTION

Atheromatous lesions develop within the subclavian artery at any point from its origin, from the arch of the aorta on the left side or from the innominate bifurcation on the right. When symptoms develop they may involve the upper limb alone, giving rise to pain on use of the arm, or may be associated with dizziness or visual disturbance. When the latter symptoms of hind brain ischaemia are present the term 'subclavian steal syndrome' is frequently applied. The condition was first reported by Contorni (1960). Surgical correction of ipsilateral reversed flow caused by occlusive disease of the subclavian artery was first suggested by Reivich et al (1961). The intermittent neurological changes that occur can quite definitely be related to haemodynamic shifts within the arterial system. When the pressure falls in one subclavian artery, the flow is reversed in its vertebral branch, and this vessel acts as a large collateral to the deprived upper limb. When the atheromatous process has spread more distally along the subclavian artery to involve the origin of the vertebral artery itself, the only symptoms complained of by the patient may be those of claudication of the upper limb. In either situation the symptoms produced can be quite debilitating and demand relief if practicable. The condition is more common on the left side than the right. A bruit is invariably present over the subclavian artery behind the sterno-mastoid and a pressure difference of 40 mm Hg or more should be present between the two arms. The diagnosis may be confirmed by aortography (Figure 13.24) and this requires two oblique projections of the arch and subtraction techniques (Figures 13.25 and 26) to give additional clarity. Selective angiography may be necessary on occasion to clarify the extent of the disease (Figure 13.27).

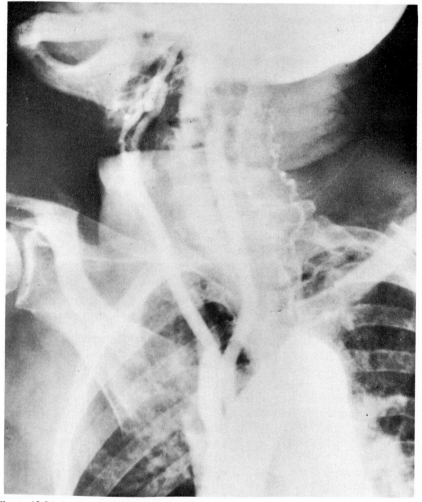

Figure 13.24. Right oblique arch angiogram. Note good filling of both common carotid arteries and no opacification of the subclavian arteries.

Surgical treatment

The classical surgical approach involves a direct reconstruction of the origin of the subclavian artery. On the right side this may not be too difficult from the supraclavicular route, but upper sternotomy may be required. The

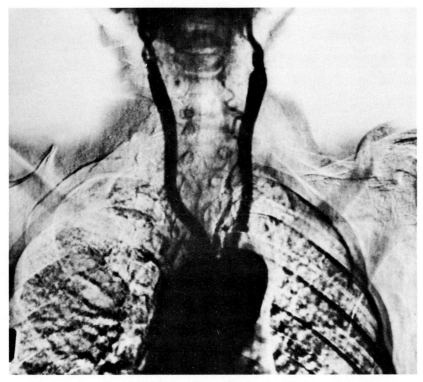

Figure 13.25. Subtraction techniques applied following reverse projection during arch angiogram. Note the lack of opacification of subclavian vessels.

patients, on the whole, tolerate this exposure well and certainly better than the transthoracic route, which is required for similar operations on the left subclavian artery. Adequate control and exposure may be achieved only on the left side by use of a posterior, third space thoracotomy. The morbidity of this procedure can be as high as 50 per cent (Fields, 1972) with a reported mortality of 8 per cent and is to be regarded now as of historical interest only. The surgical treatment of choice is a by-pass graft, carried out through a supraclavicular incision (Figure 13.28). Direct carotid subclavian by-pass is preferred, but if proximal disease is present in carotid arteries, subclavian to subclavian by-pass across the neck is an adequate alternative.

The technique of the procedure is identical whether performed on left or right, and the incision is similar to that used for cervical sympathectomy or direct approach to the vertebral artery. A skin-crease incision in the neck centred medially at a point about 2 cm above and medial to the clavicular attachment of the sterno-mastoid to the clavicle is extended laterally for a distance of some 20 cm. The platysma is divided and subcutaneous fat is separated and superficial veins are occluded with diathermy. The scalenus anterior muscle is then divided, care being taken to preserve the phrenic nerve, and the subclavian artery is exposed as it arches above the clavicle. In order to facilitate this exposure, it is helpful to place a narrow sandbag between the shoulder blades and to hyperextend the neck slightly. The clavicular fibres of the sterno-mastoid are divided, the sternal head being retracted medially.

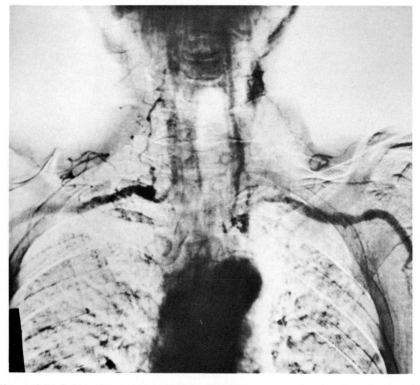

Figure 13.26. Subtraction technique of later film in the same series of arch angiogram as in Figure 13.25. Note the filling of both vertebral vessels and subclavian vessels by the retrograde route. This is a good example of the subclavian steal syndrome.

The carotid sheath is then dissected and opened with care. The common carotid artery is separated from the nerves and internal jugular vein and a tape is passed around it to facilitate subsequent manoeuvre. A 10 to 12 cm length of saphenous vein, which has been removed at the beginning of the operation by an incision in the upper part of the thigh, is then cleaned of attached fat particles and adventitia and its patency is tested by distending the graft with saline. The subclavian artery and vertebral artery are then occluded between clamps, and a longitudinal arteriotomy equal in size to the diameter of the autogenous saphenous vein is made in the former vessel. The reversed end of this vein is then sutured to the artery, using continuous 6×0 suture material. On completion of the suture line, the arterial occlusion clamps are released, first distally, and then proximally, and the efficacy of the anastomosis is tested. When the suture line is leak-proof and satisfactory flow has been demonstrated along the subclavian artery, a temporary occlusion clamp is placed adjacent to the anastomosis and the graft is distended tensely with saline. The common carotid artery is then clamped at an appropriate level in relation to the proposed site of anastomosis to the saphenous vein. The autogenous saphenous vein is placed in a temporary position against the artery, passing in front of the jugular vein and bowing around it in a gentle curve. It is important that the vein be distended at this point so that the correct length of graft may be accurately ascertained. Once this has been done the redundant vein tissue is excised and the carotid artery is opened by a vertical incision, again coincident in length with the diameter of the saphenous vein. The end-to-side anastomosis is then effected between the two structures. The posterior anastomosis is completed first from within the vessel, and anchored to two equatorial stitches placed in the 12 and 6 o'clock positions in

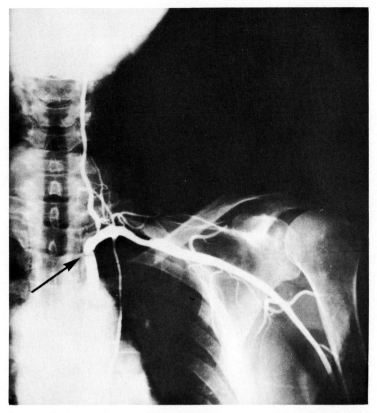

Figure 13.27. Selective angiogram of left subclavian artery. A severe stenosis is present in the proximal portion of this artery and a lesser degree of narrowing is demonstrated at the origin of the vertebral artery.

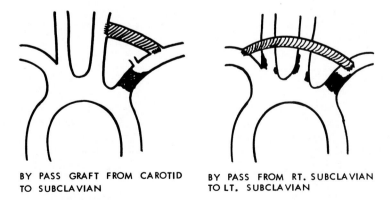

BY PASS GRAFT FROM CAROTID
TO SUBCLAVIAN

BY PASS FROM RT. SUBCLAVIAN
TO LT. SUBCLAVIAN

Figure 13.28. Supraclavicular by-pass routes for relief of disease of the proximal subclavian arteries.

relation to the anastomosis. The anterior suture line is completed and a precaution is taken to flush the artery both proximally and distally before the final sutures are placed in position. When the clamps are removed, a satisfactory pulsatile flow should be obtained from the carotid into the subclavian artery along the autogenous graft passing anterior to the jugular vein (Figure 13.29).

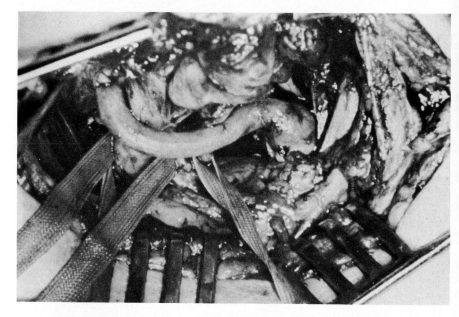

Figure 13.29. Operative appearance of completed left carotid subclavian by-pass graft. The curve taken by the vein graft passes in front of the internal jugular vein which is clearly seen on the left of this photograph.

The anaesthetic technique for the procedure is identical to that employed by us for the relief of carotid artery insufficiency.

The saphenous vein is particularly suitable for the operation, although the literature contains reports of Dacron prosthetic by-pass. Knitted Dacron velour grafts have been advocated in this respect, owing to the softness of texture and the ease of suture (McMullan and Hardy, 1973).

Results

Fourteen patients have been submitted to surgery for this condition. They appeared to compare favourably with those reported in other series. Santschi et al (1966) reported 74 cases, pointing out that the left side was more commonly affected than the right, and this is the distribution in our group. The essential features for diagnosis, namely that of pressure difference between the two arms or absence of pulse at the wrist, were present in all cases. When the subclavian steal syndrome was present, the history as regards the hind-brain ischaemia was quite long and extended back as far as 18 months. All such cases were considerably debilitated by the dizziness and were anxious

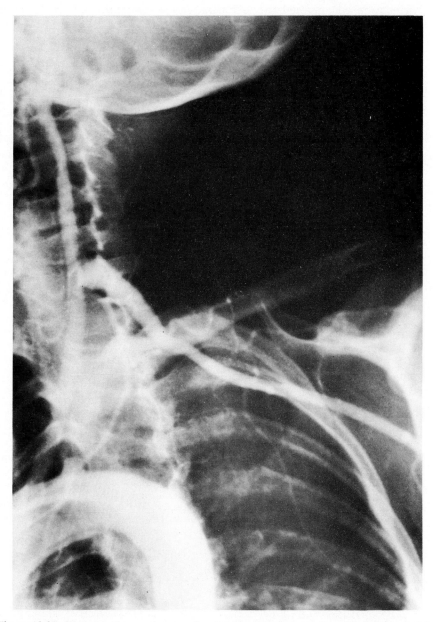

Figure 13.30. Postoperative angiogram showing the appearance of a patent left carotid subclavian by-pass graft. The stump of the occluded subclavian artery is seen as well as the retrograde filling of the internal mammary and vertebral arteries. This film was taken 4 months after completion of surgery.

for effective therapy. The symptoms were relieved in all cases. No neurological deficits were encountered or postoperative complications. All grafts have remained patent from 12 months to five years. One late death has occurred due to a contra-lateral cerebral haemorrhage, and autopsy showed that the graft was patent.

The fear that a carotid steal situation might be produced has not been realised, and there appears to be an increased flow in the proximal carotid artery when the graft is established. Studies of flow rate, through these vessels and through the graft, have been reported by Barner, Kaiser and Willmer (1971). They demonstrate quite clearly that reverse flow through the vertebral artery is corrected and that the increase takes place in the mean proximal carotid flow. In no case were pressure decreases observed in the distal carotid artery. The results have been confirmed by Cordell (1971). The radiological appearances of the functioning shunt are shown in (Figure 13.30), taken some four months postoperatively.

The advantage of supraclavicular reconstruction of vertebral or vertebral/ subclavian disease are thus to be seen in the simplicity of approach and the relative absence of morbidity. The discomfort to the patient and a 50 per cent morbidity rate after transpleural approach to the subclavian origin must militate against this method. The absence of significant morbidity in our series, supported by similar favourable results in the literature (McMullan and Hardy, 1973; Fields, 1972; Cordell, Hudspeth and Johnston, 1971) suggests that this is a superior surgical procedure. Experience may well give similar support for vertebral transplantation instead of endarterectomy for the relief of localised disease of this vessel.

REFERENCES

Acheson, J. & Hutchinson, E. C. (1971) Natural history of focal cerebro-vascular disease. *Quarterly Journal of Medicine*, (40), **157**, 15–23.
Ashby, M., Oakley, N., Lorentz, I. & Scott, D. (1963) Recurrent transient monocular blindness. *British Medical Journal*, **ii**, 894.
Barner, H. B., Kaiser, G. C. & Willman, V. L. (1971) Haemodynamics of carotid-sub-clavian by-pass. *Archives of Surgery*, **103**, 248–251.
Batacharji, S. K., Hutchinson, E. C. & McCall, A. J. (1967) Stenosis and occlusion of vessels in cerebral infarction. *British Medical Journal*, **iii**, 270.
Bauer, R. B., Meyer, J. S., Fields, W. S., Remington, R., McDonald, M. C. & Callen, P. (1969) Joint study of extracranial arterial occlusion. Progress Report of controlled study of long-term survival with or without operation. *Journal of the American Medical Association*, **208**, 509.
Bladin, P. F. (1964) Radiological and pathological study of embolism of the internal carotid-middle cerebral artery axis. *Radiology*, **82**, 615–625.
Bloodwell, R. D., Haleman, G. D., Keats, A. S. & Cooley, D. A. (1968) Carotid endarterec-tomy without a shunt. Results using hypercarbic general anaesthesia to prevent cerebral ischaemia. *Archives of Surgery*, **96**, 344.
Brice, J. G., Dowsett, D. J., Lowe, R. D. (1964) Haemodynamic effects of carotid artery stenosis. *British Medical Journal*, **ii**, 1363.
Chiari, H. (1905) Über das Verhalten des Teilungswinkels der Carotid communis bei der Endarteritis chronica deformans. *Verhandlungen Deutschen Gesellschaft fur Pathologie*, **9**, 326–330.
Cole, F. M. & Yates, P. O. (1967) Intracerebral micro-aneurysms and small cerebrovascular lesions. *Brain*, **90**, 759.

Contorni, L. (1960) The vertebro-basilar circulation in obliteration of the subclavian artery at its origin. *Minerva Chirurgica*, **15**, 268–271.

Cooley, D. A., Al-Naaman, Y. D. & Carton, C. A. (1956) Surgical treatment of arteriosclerotic occlusion of the common carotid artery. *Journal of Neurosurgery*, **13**, 500–506.

Cordell, A. R., Hudspeth, A. S. & Johnston, F. R. (1971) Current status of surgery for subclavian steal syndrome. *Surgical Clinics of North America*, **51**, 1415.

Debakey, M. E., Crawford, E. S., Cooley, D. A., Morris, G. C., Garrett, H. E. & Fields, W. S. (1965) Cerebral arterial insufficiency; one to eleven year results following arterial reconstructive operations. *Annals of Surgery*, **611**, 921.

Deweese, J. A., Rob, C. G., Satran, R., Marsh, D. O., Joynt, R. J., Summers, D. & Nichols, C. (1973) Results of carotid endarterectomies for transient ischaemic attacks.—Five years later. *Annals of Surgery*, **178**, 258–264.

Eastcott, H. H. G., Pickering, G. W. & Rob, C. G. (1954) Reconstruction of internal carotid artery in a patient with intermittent attacks of hemiplegia. *Lancet*, **ii**, 994–996.

Eastcott, H. H. G. (1969) *Arterial Surgery*. London: Pitman.

Eastcott, H. H. G. (1974) *Arterial Surgery*, 2nd edition. London: Pitman.

Fields, W. S. (1972) Joint study of extracranial arterial occlusion. *Journal of the American Medical Association*, **222**, 1139–1142.

Fisher, M. (1954) Occlusion of the carotid artery. Further experiences. *Archives of Neurology and Psychiatry*, **72**, 187.

Gowers, W. R. (1875) On a case of simultaneous embolism of central retinal and middle cerebral arteries. *Lancet*, **ii**, 794–796.

Gunning, A. J., Pickering, G. W., Robb-Smith, A. H. T. & Russell, R. W. R. (1964) Mural thrombosis of the internal carotid artery and subsequent embolisation. *Quarterly Journal of Medicine*, **33**, 155–195.

Gurdjian, E. S. & Webster, J. E. (1958) Thrombo-endarterectomy of the carotid bifurcation, and the internal carotid artery. *Surgery, Gynecology and Obstetrics*, **106**, 421–426.

Gurdjian, E. S., Darmody, W. R., Linder, D. W. & Thomas, L. M. (1965) The fate of patients with carotid and vertebral artery surgery for stenosis or occlusion. *Surgery, Gynecology and Obstetrics*, **121**, 326.

Hugh, A. E. (1970) Trickle arteriography; demonstration of thrombi in the origin of the internal carotid artery. *British Medical Journal*, **ii**, 574.

Hunt, J. R. (1914) The role of the carotid arteries in the causation of vascular lesions of the brain. *American Journal of the Medical Sciences*, **147**, 704.

Hutchinson, E. C. & Yates, P. O. (1957) Caroticovertebral stenosis. *Lancet*, **i**, 2.

Javid, H., Ostermiller, W. G. & Hensish, J. W. (1970) Natural history of carotid bifurcation atheroma. *Surgery*, **67**, 80–86.

Kenyon, J. R., Thomas, A. B. W. & Goodwin, D. P. (1972) Heparin protection for the brain during carotid artery reconstruction. *Lancet*, **ii**, 153.

Larson, C. P. (1970) Anaesthesia and control of cerebral circulation. Chapter 8. In *Extracranial occlusive Cerebrovascular Disease*. (Eds.) Wylie, E. J. & Ehrenfeld, W. K. Philadelphia: W. B. Saunders.

Luessenhop, A. J. & Spense, W. T. (1960) Artificial embolisation of cerebral arteries. *Journal of American Medical Association*, **172**, 1153–1155.

Lyons, C. (1965) Some surgical aspects of the stroke problems. *Alabama Journal of Medical Science*, **2**, 119–26.

Magowan, W. ,Lynch, G. & Staunton, H. (1971) Review of 36 cases with extra-cranial arterial occlusion. *Journal of the Irish Medical Association*, **54**, 487.

Martin, M. J., Whisnant, J. P. & Sayre, G. P. (1960) Occlusive vascular disease in the extracranial cerebral circulation. *Archives of Neurology*, **3**, 530.

McBrien, D. J., Bradley, R. D. & Ashton, N. (1963) The nature of retinal emboli in stenosis of the internal carotid artery. *Lancet*, **i**, 697.

McGee, D. A., McPhedran, R. S. & Hoffman, H. J. (1962) Carotid and vertebral artery disease. A clinico-pathological survey of 70 cases. *Neurology, Minneapolis*, **12**, 848.

McMullan, M. H. & Hardy, J. D. (1973) Lesions of the subclavian artery—Survey of 131 cases. *Annals of Surgery*, **178**, 80–86.

Millikan, C. H. (1965) The pathogenesis of transient focal cerebral ischaemia. *Circulation*, **32**, 438.

Millikan, C. H. & Siekert, R. G. (1955) Studies in cerebro-vascular disease IV. The syndrome of intermittent insufficiency of the carotid arterial system. *Proceedings of the Mayo Clinic*, **30**, 186–191.

Reivich, M., Holling, H. E., Roberts, B. & Toole, J. F. (1961) Reversal of blood flow through the vertebral artery and its effect on cerebral circulation. *New England Journal of Medicine*, **265**, 878.

Rob, C. & Wheeler, E. B. (1957) Thrombosis of the internal carotid artery treated by arterial surgery. *British Medical Journal*, **ii**, 264–266.

Russell, R. W. R. (1961) Observations on the retinal blood vessels in monocular blindness. *Lancet*, **ii**, 1422.

Santschi, D. R., Frahm, C J , Pascale, L. R. & Dumanian, A. V. (1966) The subclavian steal syndrome; clinical and angiographic considerations in 24 cases in adults. *Journal of Thoracic and Cardiovascular Surgery*, **51**, 103.

Schwartz, C. J. & Mitchell, J. R. A. (1961) Atheroma of the carotid and vertebral arterial systems. *British Medical Journal*, **ii**, 1057.

Soloway, H. B. & Aronson, S. M. (1964) Atheromatous emboli to central nervous system. Report of 16 cases. *Archives of Neurology*, **11**, 657–667.

Strully, K. J., Hurwitt, E. S. & Blankenberg, H. W. (1953) Thromboendarterectomy for thrombosis of the internal carotid artery in the neck. *Journal of Neurosurgery*, **10**, 474–482.

Sutton, D. & Davies, E. R. (1966) Arch aortography and cerebrovascular insufficiency. *Clinical Radiology*, **17**, 330.

Thomson, J. E., Austin, D. J. & Ratman, P. D. (1970) Carotid endarterectomy for cerebrovascular insufficiency. Long-term results in 592 patients followed-up to 13 years. *Annals of Surgery*, **172**, 663.

Viancos, J. G., Sechzer, P. H., Keats, A. S. & DeBakey, M. (1966) Internal jugular venous oxygen tension as an index of cerebral blood flow during carotid endarterectomy. *Circulation*, **34**, 875–882.

Virchov, R. (1856) (Cited by Haser, H.) Die Diagnose der Karotisthrombose durch den Ausenarzt. *Alin. Mbl. Ausenheilk*, **141**, 801–840 (1962).

Vost, A., Wolochow, A. & Howell, D. A. (1964) Incidence of infarcts of the brain in heart disease. *Journal of Pathology and Bacteriology*, **88**, 463.

Wells, B. A., Keates, A. S. & Cooley, D. A. (1963) Increased tolerance to cerebral ischaemia produced by general anesthesia during temporary carotid occlusion. *Surgery*, **54**, 216.

Wylie, E. J., Ehrenfeld, W. K. (1970) *Extracranial Occlusive Cerebrovascular Disease: Diagnosis and Management*. Philadelphia: W. B. Saunders.

Yates, P. O. & Hutchinson, E. C. (1961) *Cerebral Infarction. The Role of Stenosis of the Extracranial Cerebral arteries*. Medical Research Council Special Report Series No. 300. London: H.M.S.O.

Index